Year Book of Psychiatry and Applied Mental Health®: Drs Talbott, Ballenger, Buckley, Frances, Krupnick, and Mack

Year Book of Pulmonary Disease®: Drs Barker, Jones, Maurer, Raza, Tanoue, and Willsie

Year Book of Sports Medicine®: Drs Shephard, Cantu, Feldman, Jankowski, Khan, Lebrun, Nieman, Pierrynowski, and Rowland

Year Book of Surgery®: Drs Copeland, Behrns, Daly, Eberlein, Fahey, Huber, Jones, Mozingo, and Pruett

Year Book of Urology®: Drs Andriole and Coplen

Year Book of Vascular Surgery®: Drs Moneta, Gillespie, Starnes, and Watkins

2011

The Year Book of
CRITICAL CARE
MEDICINE®

Editors-in-Chief

R. Phillip Dellinger, MD

Professor of Medicine, Robert Wood Johnson Medical School, University of Medicine and Dentistry of New Jersey; Professor of Medicine, Cooper Medical School of Rowan University; Head, Division of Critical Care Medicine, and Director, Medical/Surgical Intensive Care Unit, Cooper University Hospital, Camden, New Jersey

Joseph E. Parrillo, MD

Professor of Medicine, Robert Wood Johnson Medical School, University of Medicine and Dentistry of New Jersey; Professor of Medicine and Chairman, Department of Medicine, Cooper Medical School of Rowan University; Chief, Department of Medicine, Edward D. Viner MD Chair, Department of Medicine, and Director, Cooper Heart Institute, Cooper University Hospital, Camden, New Jersey

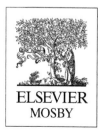

ELSEVIER
MOSBY

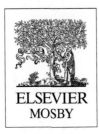

ELSEVIER
MOSBY

Vice President, Continuity: Kimberly Murphy
Developmental Editor: Patrick Manley
Production Supervisor, Electronic Year Books: Donna M. Skelton
Electronic Article Manager: Jennifer C. Pitts
Illustrations and Permissions Coordinator: Dawn Vohsen

Composition by TNQ Books and Journals Pvt Ltd, India

Printed and bound by CPI Group (UK) Ltd, Croydon, CR0 4YY

Transferred to Digital Print 2011

Editorial Office:
Elsevier
Suite 1800
1600 John F. Kennedy Blvd.
Philadelphia, PA 19103-2899

International Standard Serial Number: 0734-3299
International Standard Book Number: 978-0-323-08409-3

Associate Editors

Robert A. Balk, MD

J. Bailey Carter, MD, Professor of Medicine, Rush Medical College; Director, Division of Pulmonary and Critical Care Medicine, Rush University Medical Center, Chicago, Illinois

Todd Dorman, MD

Associate Dean and Director of Continuing Medical Education; Professor and Vice-Chair for Critical Care Services; Departments of Anesthesiology/Critical Care Medicine, Internal Medicine, Surgery, and the School of Nursing, Johns Hopkins University, Baltimore, Maryland

David J. Dries, MSE, MD

John F. Perry, Jr. Professor, Department of Surgery, University of Minnesota; Assistant Medical Director for Surgical Care, HealthPartners Medical Group, Minneapolis, Minnesota; Director of Critical Care Services and Director of Academic Programs, Department of Surgery, Regions Hospital, St Paul, Minnesota

Sergio L. Zanotti-Cavazzoni, MD

Assistant Professor of Medicine, Robert Wood Johnson Medical School, University of Medicine and Dentistry of New Jersey; Assistant Professor of Medicine, Cooper Medical School of Rowan University; Program Director, Critical Care Medicine Fellowship, Division of Critical Care Medicine, Cooper University Hospital, Camden, New Jersey

Guest Editors

Guest Editor for Gastroenterology
Christopher W. Deitch, MD
Assistant Professor of Medicine, Robert Wood Johnson Medical School, University of Medicine and Dentistry of New Jersey; Assistant Professor of Medicine, Cooper Medical School of Rowan University; Division of Gastroenterology, Cooper University Hospital, Camden, New Jersey

Guest Editor for Transfusion in the Critically Ill
David R. Gerber, DO
Associate Professor of Medicine, Robert Wood Johnson Medical School, University of Medicine and Dentistry of New Jersey; Associate Professor of Medicine, Cooper Medical School of Rowan University; Associate Director, Medical/Surgical Intensive Care Unit, Cooper University Hospital, Camden, New Jersey

Guest Editor for Infection
Anand Kumar, MD
Associate Professor of Medicine, Robert Wood Johnson Medical College, University of Medicine and Dentistry of New Jersey; Associate Professor of Medicine, Cooper Medical School of Rowan University; Division of Critical Care Medicine and Division of Infectious Diseases, Cooper University Hospital, Camden, New Jersey; Associate Professor of Medicine, Sections of Critical Care Medicine and Infectious Disease, University of Manitoba, Winnipeg, Canada

Guest Editor for Burns
Barbara A. Latenser, MD
Clara L. Smith Professor of Burn Treatment, Department of Surgery, University of Iowa; Director, Burn Treatment Center, University of Iowa Healthcare, Iowa City, Iowa

Guest Editor for Neurologic Care
Kiwon Lee, MD, FACP, FAHA
Assistant Professor, Neurology and Neurological Surgery, Columbia University College of Physicians and Surgeons; Faculty Attending Staff, Neurological Intensive Care Unit, New York Presbyterian Hospital, Columbia University Medical Center, New York, New York

Guest Editor for Postoperative Critical Care
Elizabeth A. Martinez, MD, MHS
Associate Professor of Anesthesia, Critical Care and Pain Medicine, Massachusetts General Hospital, Harvard University, Boston, Massachusetts

Guest Editor for Ethics
Vijay K. Rajput, MD
Associate Professor of Medicine, Robert Wood Johnson Medical School, University of Medicine and Dentistry of New Jersey; Associate Professor of Medicine and Assistant Dean for Curriculum, Cooper Medical School of Rowan University; Program Director, Internal Medicine Residency, Cooper University Hospital, Camden, New Jersey; Associate Fellow, Center for Bioethics, University of Pennsylvania, Philadelphia, Pennsylvania

Guest Editor for Critical Care Performance Improvement and ICU Administration
Christa A. Schorr, RN, MSN
Assistant Professor of Medicine, University of Medicine and Dentistry of New Jersey; Assistant Professor of Medicine, Cooper Medical School of Rowan University; Director of Databases for Quality Improvement and Research, Program Director of Clinical Industry Trials in Critical Care, Cooper University Hospital, Camden, New Jersey

Guest Editor for Emergency Medicine
Stephen Trzeciak, MD, MPH
Assistant Professor of Medicine and Emergency Medicine, Robert Wood Johnson Medical School, University of Medicine and Dentistry of New Jersey; Assistant Professor of Medicine and Emergency Medicine, Cooper Medical School of Rowan University; Department of Emergency Medicine and Division of Critical Care Medicine, Cooper University Hospital, Camden, New Jersey

Guest Editor for Nephrology and Poisoning/Overdose
Lawrence S. Weisberg, MD
Professor of Medicine, Robert Wood Johnson Medical School, University of Medicine and Dentistry of New Jersey; Professor of Medicine and Assistant Dean for Curriculum, Cooper Medical School of Rowan University; Head, Division of Nephrology, Cooper University Hospital, Camden, New Jersey

Guest Editor for Cardiology
Steven W. Werns, MD
Professor of Medicine, Robert Wood Johnson Medical School, University of Medicine and Dentistry of New Jersey; Professor of Medicine, Cooper Medical School of Rowan University; Director, Invasive Cardiovascular Services, Cooper University Hospital, Camden, New Jersey

Contributing Editors

Zoulficar A. Kobeissi, MD

Assistant Professor of Clinical Medicine, Weill-Cornell School of Medicine, New York, New York; Intensivist, Division of Critical Care Medicine, The Methodist Hospital, Houston, Texas

Sundip N. Patel, MD

Assistant Professor of Emergency Medicine, Robert Wood Johnson Medical School, University of Medicine and Dentistry of New Jersey; Assistant Professor, Cooper Medical School of Rowan University; Director, Medical Student Programs, Department of Emergency Medicine, Cooper University Hospital, Camden, New Jersey

Collaborative Reviewers

Marguerite Balasta, BA
Medical Student, Robert Wood Johnson Medical School, University of Medicine and Dentistry of New Jersey, Piscataway, New Jersey

Travante Cartwright, MD
Resident, Department of Medicine, Division of Internal Medicine, Cooper University Hospital, Camden, New Jersey

Mariane Charron, MD
Postdoctoral Fellow, Department of Medicine, Division of Critical Care Medicine, Cooper University Hospital, Camden, New Jersey

Maher Dahdel, MD
Postdoctoral Fellow, Department of Medicine, Division of Pulmonary/Critical Care Medicine, Cooper University Hospital, Camden, New Jersey

Seraj M. El-Oshar, MD
Postdoctoral Fellow, Department of Medicine, Division of Critical Care Medicine, Cooper University Hospital, Camden, New Jersey

Andrew D. Fesnak, BA
Medical Student, Robert Wood Johnson Medical School, University of Medicine and Dentistry of New Jersey, Camden, New Jersey

Travis C. Foster, PhD
Medical Student, Robert Wood Johnson Medical School, University of Medicine and Dentistry of New Jersey, Piscataway, New Jersey

Kerri Keselowsky, BS
Medical Student, Robert Wood Johnson Medical School, University of Medicine and Dentistry of New Jersey, Piscataway, New Jersey

Michael E. Kwiatt, MD
Resident, Department of Surgery, Cooper University Hospital, Camden, New Jersey

John E. McGinniss, BS
Medical Student, Robert Wood Johnson Medical School, University of Medicine and Dentistry of New Jersey, Camden, New Jersey

Nitin Puri, MD
Postdoctoral Fellow, Department of Medicine, Division of Pulmonary/Critical Care Medicine, Cooper University Hospital, Camden, New Jersey

Ricardo R. Sanga, MD
Postdoctoral Fellow, Department of Medicine, Division of Critical Care Medicine, Cooper University Hospital, Camden, New Jersey

Arun Sharma, MD
Postdoctoral Fellow, Department of Medicine, Division of Critical Care Medicine, Cooper University Hospital, Camden, New Jersey

Brett J. Smith, BA

Medical Student, Robert Wood Johnson Medical School, University of Medicine and Dentistry of New Jersey, New Brunswick, New Jersey; Graduate Student, Center for Bioethics, University of Pennsylvania, Philadelphia, Pennsylvania

Moussa F. Yazbeck, MD

Postdoctoral Fellow, Department of Medicine, Division of Critical Care Medicine, Cooper University Hospital, Camden, New Jersey

Table of Contents

Journals Represented

Journals represented in this YEAR BOOK are listed below.

Acta Anaesthesiologica Scandinavica
AJR American Journal of Roentgenology
American Heart Journal
American Journal of Cardiology
American Journal of Emergency Medicine
American Journal of Obstetrics and Gynecology
American Journal of Respiratory and Critical Care Medicine
American Journal of Surgery
American Journal of Transplantation
American Surgeon
Anaesthesia and Intensive Care
Anesthesia & Analgesia
Anesthesiology
Annals of Emergency Medicine
Annals of Internal Medicine
Annals of Neurology
Annals of Surgery
Annals of Thoracic Surgery
Archives of Neurology
Archives of Surgery
British Journal of Anaesthesia
Burns
Canadian Journal of Surgery
Canadian Medical Association Journal
Chest
Circulation
Clinical Endocrinology
Clinical Infectious Diseases
Clinical Therapeutics
Critical Care Medicine
Digestive Diseases and Sciences
European Journal of Internal Medicine
European Heart Journal
European Respiratory Journal
Heart
Injury
Intensive Care Medicine
International Journal of Cardiology
Journal of Burn Care & Research
Journal of Cardiothoracic and Vascular Anesthesia
Journal of Clinical Anesthesia
Journal of Clinical Microbiology
Journal of Emergency Medicine
Journal of Medical Ethics
Journal of Neurosurgery
Journal of Surgical Research
Journal of the American College of Cardiology

Journal of the American College of Surgeons
Journal of the American Medical Association
Journal of Thoracic and Cardiovascular Surgery
Journal of Trauma
Journal of Urology
Journal of Vascular Surgery
Kidney International
Lancet
Neurology
New England Journal of Medicine
Pediatrics
Radiology
Spine
Stroke
Thrombosis Research
Transfusion
Transplantation
Transplantation Proceedings
World Journal of Surgery

STANDARD ABBREVIATIONS

The following terms are abbreviated in this edition: acquired immunodeficiency syndrome (AIDS), cardiopulmonary resuscitation (CPR), central nervous system (CNS), cerebrospinal fluid (CSF), computed tomography (CT), deoxyribonucleic acid (DNA), electrocardiography (ECG), health maintenance organization (HMO), human immunodeficiency virus (HIV), intensive care unit (ICU), intramuscular (IM), intravenous (IV), magnetic resonance (MR) imaging (MRI), and ribonucleic acid (RNA).

NOTE

The YEAR BOOK OF CRITICAL CARE MEDICINE® is a literature survey service providing abstracts of articles published in the professional literature. Every effort is made to assure the accuracy of the information presented in these pages. Neither the editors nor the publisher of the YEAR BOOK OF CRITICAL CARE MEDICINE® can be responsible for errors in the original materials. The editors' comments are their own opinions. Mention of specific products within this publication does not constitute endorsement.

To facilitate the use of the YEAR BOOK OF CRITICAL CARE MEDICINE® as a reference tool, all illustrations and tables included in this publication are now identified as they appear in the original article. This change is meant to help the reader recognize that any illustration or table appearing in the YEAR BOOK OF CRITICAL CARE MEDICINE® may be only one of many in the original article. For this reason, figure and table numbers will often appear to be out of sequence within the YEAR BOOK OF CRITICAL CARE MEDICINE®.

1 Airways/Lungs

Acute Lung Injury/Acute Respiratory Distress Syndrome

A systematic review to inform institutional decisions about the use of extracorporeal membrane oxygenation during the H1N1 influenza pandemic

Mitchell MD, Mikkelsen ME, Umscheid CA, et al (Univ of Pennsylvania Health System, Philadelphia; Hosp of the Univ of Pennsylvania, Philadelphia)
Crit Care Med 38:1398-1404, 2010

Objectives.—To systematically evaluate the effect of extracorporeal membrane oxygenation on survival in adults with acute respiratory failure and to help inform institutional decisions about implementing an extracorporeal membrane oxygenation program or transferring patients to experienced extracorporeal membrane oxygenation centers during the H1N1 influenza pandemic.

Data Sources.—National Guideline Clearinghouse, MEDLINE, EMBASE, Agency for Healthcare Research and Quality Evidence-based Practice reports, National Institute for Health and Clinical Excellence, Cochrane Library, International Network of Agencies for Health Technology Assessment, and citation review.

Study Selection.—Studies of extracorporeal membrane oxygenation in adult acute respiratory failure, reporting mortality rates for at least 10 patients in extracorporeal membrane oxygenation and nonextracorporeal membrane oxygenation groups.

Data Extraction.—Mortality rates were abstracted for all patients and for patients with influenza. Risk ratios were meta-analyzed using random-effects methods and assessed for heterogeneity.

Data Synthesis.—There are no evidence-based clinical guidelines on the use of extracorporeal membrane oxygenation in patients with influenza. Three randomized controlled trials and three cohort studies evaluated extracorporeal membrane oxygenation in patients with acute respiratory failure; none reported specifically on patients with influenza. Meta-analysis of the randomized controlled trials revealed significant heterogeneity in risk of mortality. The summary risk ratio found by the meta-analysis was 0.93 (95% confidence interval, 0.71 to 1.22). The most recent trial found a reduction in mortality and severe disability at 6 months among patients in whom extracorporeal membrane oxygenation was considered. Observational studies suggest that extracorporeal membrane oxygenation for acute respiratory failure resulting from viral pneumonia is associated with improved mortality compared with other etiologies of acute respiratory failure.

Conclusions.—The best evidence to guide decisions regarding the use of extracorporeal membrane oxygenation for patients with influenza stems from trials of extracorporeal membrane oxygenation for acute respiratory failure of all etiologies, among which significant heterogeneity exists, and from case series describing outcomes of extracorporeal membrane oxygenation in patients with influenza. Thus, there is insufficient evidence to provide a recommendation for extracorporeal membrane oxygenation use among patients with respiratory failure resulting from influenza. However, clinicians should consider extracorporeal membrane oxygenation within the context of other salvage therapies for acute respiratory failure.

▶ The recent pandemic of influenza A (H1N1) infection in the United States and other parts of the world stressed the health care system and its ability to provide sufficient ventilatory support.[1,2] Unfortunately, we found that large numbers of H1N1-infected patients required significant ventilatory support and not infrequently required the use of salvage measures to improve oxygenation.[3] One of the salvage remedies is the use of extracorporeal membrane oxygenation (ECMO). While this technique may have been put on a back burner after the National Institutes of Health (NIH)-sponsored ECMO trial in the 1970s, a recent report by English investigators suggests a benefit associated with ECMO use in severe acute respiratory distress syndrome.[3,4] This article reviews the current evidence for and against the use of ECMO in managing patients with severe lung injury associated with H1N1 infection. Hopefully, the reader will not have to consult this reference as we move into the next flu season.

R. A. Balk, MD

References

1. Australia New Zealand Extracorporeal Membrane Oxygenation (ANZ ECMO) Influenza Investigators, Davies A, Jones D, Baily M, et al. Extracorporeal membrane oxygenation for 2009 influenza A (H1N1) acute respiratory distress syndrome. *JAMA.* 2009;302:1888-1895.
2. Kumar A, Zarychanski R, Pinto R, et al. Critically ill patients with 2009 influenza A(H1N1) infection in Canada. *JAMA.* 2009;302:1872-1879.
3. Peck CJ, Mugford M, Tiruvoipati R, et al. Efficacy and economic assessment of conventional ventilatory support versus extracorporeal membrane oxygenation for severe adult respiratory failure (CESAR): a multicentre randomised controlled trial. *Lancet.* 2009;374:1351-1363.
4. Zapol WM, Snider MT, Hill JD, et al. Extracorporeal membrane oxygenation in severe acute respiratory failure: a randomized prospective study. *JAMA.* 1979; 242:2193-2196.

Central Extracorporeal Membrane Oxygenation for Septic Shock in an Adult With H1N1 Influenza

MacLaren G, Cove M, Kofidis T (Natl Univ Health System, Singapore)
Ann Thorac Surg 90:e34-e35, 2010

Extracorporeal membrane oxygenation has been used as rescue therapy for respiratory failure caused by pandemic hemagglutanin-1 and neuroaminadase-1 (H1N1) influenza, but it is unclear as to whether it can be also used for refractory circulatory failure. A previously healthy 29-year-old woman presented with pneumonitis and septic shock. She deteriorated, despite multiple pharmacologic and ventilatory strategies, so she was placed on central (atrio-aortic) extracorporeal membrane oxygenation for 4 days. After a protracted intensive care stay, she recovered and is undergoing rehabilitation. In particularly severe cases of H1N1 influenza, central extracorporeal membrane oxygenation can completely supplant both cardiac and pulmonary function until the patient recovers from the infection.

▶ During the influenza H1N1 pandemic of 2009, many reports indicated that critically ill patients with severe respiratory failure often received salvage therapy modalities such as extracorporeal membrane oxygenation (ECMO).[1] Multiple ECMO modalities exist, but venovenous is the predominant mode used in patients with severe pulmonary failure but preserved cardiovascular function (hemodynamically stable). Patients with circulatory shock can be treated with venoarterial ECMO to help support them hemodynamically. In this article, the authors report the use of central ECMO (atrio-aortic cannulation) for a patient with H1N1 influenza with both respiratory and circulatory failure. The authors used this modality because of the patient's biventricular failure and their concern that the patient may receive deoxygenated coronary perfusion with the standard venoarterial approach. This case report highlights our need to better understand the indications of different modalities of ECMO and points out the potential use of central venoarterial ECMO in patients with both circulatory and respiratory failure such as the one reported in this case.

S. L. Zanotti-Cavazzoni, MD

Reference

1. Australia and New Zealand Extracorporeal Membrane Oxygenation (ANZ ECMO) Influenza Investigators. Extracorporeal membrane oxygenation for 2009 influenza A(H1N1) acute respiratory distress syndrome. *JAMA*. 2009;302: 1888-1895.

Pandemic 2009 Influenza A in Argentina: A Study of 337 Patients on Mechanical Ventilation

Estenssoro E, for the Registry of the Argentinian Society of Intensive Care (SATI) (Hosp Interzonal San Martin de La Plata, Buenos Aires, Argentina; et al)
Am J Respir Crit Care Med 182:41-48, 2010

Rationale.—The rapid spread of the 2009 Influenza A (H1N1) around the world underscores the need for a better knowledge of epidemiology, clinical features, outcomes, and mortality predictors, especially in the most severe presentations.

Objectives.—To describe these characteristics in patients with confirmed, probable, and suspected viral pneumonia caused by 2009 influenza A (H1N1) admitted to 35 intensive care units with acute respiratory failure requiring mechanical ventilation in Argentina, between June 3 and September 7.

Methods.—Inception-cohort study including 337 consecutive adult patients. Data were collected in a form posted on the Argentinian Society of Intensive Care website.

Measurements and Main Results.—Proportions of confirmed, probable, or suspected cases were 39%, 8%, and 53% and had similar outcomes. APACHE II was 18 ± 7; age 47 ± 17 years; 56% were male; and 64% had underlying conditions, with obesity (24%), chronic obstructive respiratory disease (18%), and immunosupression (15%) being the most common. Seven percent were pregnant. On admission, patients had severe hypoxemia (Pa_{O_2}/Fi_{O_2} 140 [87–200]), extensive lung radiologic infiltrates (2.87 ± 1.03 quadrants) and bacterial coinfection, (25%; mostly with *Streptococcus pneumoniae*). Use of adjuvants such as recruitment maneuvers (40%) and prone positioning (13%), and shock (72%) and acute kidney injury requiring hemodialysis (17%), were frequent. Mortality was 46%, and was similar across all ages. APACHE II, lowest Pa_{O_2}/Fi_{O_2}, shock, hemodialysis, prone positioning, and *S. pneumoniae* coinfection independently predicted death.

Conclusions.—Patients with 2009 influenza A (H1N1) requiring mechanical ventilation were mostly middle-aged adults, often with

TABLE 2.— Different Time Periods Elapsing Between Hospital Admission, ICU Admission, and Onset of Mechanical Ventilation

	All ($n = 337$)	Survivors ($n = 181$)	Nonsurvivors ($n = 156$)	P Value
Days from symptom start to hospital admission	6 [3–8]	6 [3–7]	6 [4–10]	0.13
Days from hospital admission to start of MV	1 [0–2]	0.5 [0–12]	1 [0–2]	0.33
Days from hospital to ICU admission	0 [0–2]	0 [0–1.5]	1 [0–2]	0.05

Definition of abbreviations: ICU = intensive care unit; MV = mechanical ventilation.
Data are expressed as median and interquartile ranges [IQR].

TABLE 6.— Independent Predictors of Hospital Mortality

	Odds Ratio	*P* Value	95% Confidence Interval
APACHE II	1.08*	<0.001	1.03–1.12
Lowest Pa_{O_2} FI_{O_2}	0.98[†]	<0.001	0.98–0.99
Use of inotropic drugs	2.32	0.01	1.23–4.38
Hemodialysis	2.85	<0.01	1.30–6.25
Prone positioning	4.07	<0.01	1.55–10.68
Coinfection with *S. pneumoniae* at admission	2.72	0.04	1.05–7.06

Definition of abbreviation: APACHE = Acute Physiology and Chronic Health Evaluation.
*Per point APACHE II.
[†]Per point Pa_{O_2} FI_{O_2}.

comorbidities, and frequently developed severe acute respiratory distress syndrome and multiorgan failure requiring advanced organ support. Case fatality rate was accordingly high (Tables 2 and 6).

▶ The Argentinean, Canadian, and Australian experiences with a large number of patients with life-threatening H1N1 acute respiratory distress syndrome have once again allowed the health care community to appreciate the devastating consequences of pandemic influenza. Although what we learn from the straightforward demographics (incidence of shock or renal failure, laboratory abnormalities, etc) is clearest, what we learn from application of sophisticated ventilation support techniques is less clear as it could not only potentially save lives but also would be expected to be applied to patients with a greater risk of death.

R. P. Dellinger, MD

Critically Ill Patients With 2009 Influenza A(H1N1) Infection in Canada

Kumar A, for the Canadian Critical Care Trials Group H1N1 Collaborative (Health Sciences Centre and St Boniface Hosp, Winnipeg, Manitoba, Canada; et al)
JAMA 302:1872-1879, 2009

Context.—Between March and July 2009, the largest number of confirmed cases of 2009 influenza A(H1N1) infection occurred in North America.

Objective.—To describe characteristics, treatment, and outcomes of critically ill patients in Canada with 2009 influenza A(H1N1) infection.

Design, Setting, and Patients.—A prospective observational study of 168 critically ill patients with 2009 influenza A(H1N1) infection in 38 adult and pediatric intensive care units (ICUs) in Canada between April 16 and August 12, 2009.

Main Outcome Measures.—The primary outcome measures were 28-day and 90-day mortality. Secondary outcomes included frequency and duration of mechanical ventilation and duration of ICU stay.

Results.—Critical illness occurred in 215 patients with confirmed (n=162), probable (n=6), or suspected (n=47) community-acquired 2009 influenza A(H1N1) infection. Among the 168 patients with confirmed or probable 2009 influenza A(H1N1), the mean (SD) age was 32.3 (21.4) years; 113 were female (67.3%) and 50 were children (29.8%). Overall mortality among critically ill patients at 28 days was 14.3% (95% confidence interval, 9.5%-20.7%). There were 43 patients who were aboriginal Canadians (25.6%). The median time from symptom onset to hospital admission was 4 days (interquartile range [IQR], 2-7 days) and from hospitalization to ICU admission was 1 day (IQR, 0-2 days). Shock and nonpulmonary acute organ dysfunction was common (Sequential Organ Failure Assessment mean [SD] score of 6.8 [3.6] on day 1). Neuraminidase inhibitors were administered to 152 patients (90.5%). All patients were severely hypoxemic (mean [SD] ratio of Pao_2 to fraction of inspired oxygen [Fio_2] of 147 [128] mm Hg) at ICU admission. Mechanical ventilation was received by 136 patients (81.0%). The median duration of ventilation was 12 days (IQR, 6-20 days) and ICU stay was 12 days (IQR, 5-20 days). Lung rescue therapies included neuromuscular blockade (28% of patients), inhaled nitric oxide (13.7%), high-frequency oscillatory ventilation (11.9%), extracorporeal membrane oxygenation (4.2%), and prone positioning ventilation (3.0%). Overall mortality among critically ill patients at 90 days was 17.3% (95% confidence interval, 12.0%-24.0%; n=29).

Conclusion.—Critical illness due to 2009 influenza A(H1N1) in Canada occurred rapidly after hospital admission, often in young adults, and was associated with severe hypoxemia, multisystem organ failure, a requirement for prolonged mechanical ventilation, and the frequent use of rescue therapies.

▶ One of the biggest health care–related stories of 2009 was the emergence of the influenza (H1N1) global pandemic. The largest numbers of confirmed cases were initially documented in the United States, Mexico, Canada, and Australia. This study reported the epidemiological characteristics, clinical features, treatments, and outcomes of a multicentered cohort of critically ill (adults and pediatrics) Canadian patients. Although ultimately many of the fears relating to the potential impact of this pandemic were not fulfilled, the influenza (H1N1) did have a significant impact on critical care resources in various regions in the world. This is the largest reported cohort of critically ill patients with H1N1, and important lessons can be learned from the results of this observational study. As in other reports, in the Canadian cohort, influenza (H1N1) occurred more commonly in younger patients (median age of 32 years), more frequently in women, and in those requiring critical care, it was associated with severe respiratory failure. Although the great majority of patients infected with H1N1 did not develop critical illness, those who did, required very aggressive critical care support.

In addition to the very important epidemiological data reported from this study, important information for the critical care practitioner that was identified in the study include the course of illness and the treatment for the affected patients. In this study, the patients showed a short median time from symptom onset to hospital admission (4 days). Furthermore, the time from hospitalization to intensive care unit (ICU) admission was only 1 day. This suggests that in those patients who developed the more severe form of influenza (H1N1), the progression to severe respiratory failure requiring critical care level of care can be very quick. The level of care that these patients require was extremely high, over 80% of them were mechanically ventilated on the first day of ICU admission. Even more striking was the fact that over a third of the patients with respiratory failure from influenza (H1N1) required some form of salvage therapy, such as neuromuscular blockade, inhaled nitric oxide, high-frequency oscillatory ventilation, extracorporeal membrane oxygenation, or prone positioning ventilation. Of these salvage therapies, the most frequently used were neuromuscular blockade and inhaled nitric oxide. The study does not provide any further data on which salvage therapies were most effective or how these were selected. However, the study does support the notion that these young patients with few comorbidities can survive if supported aggressively during their acute illness. The overall mortality for the critical care cohort was 14.3%. Finally, this study also identified a greater proportion of pregnant women requiring admission to the hospital who died compared with the proportion among all of those infected.

This study is a seminal report that outlined some of the salient clinical features of critically ill patients during the 2009 influenza (H1N1) pandemic. Perhaps the most important take-home message from this report is that a pandemic such as this has a high potential of overloading the capacity of a regional ICU. Careful planning must be implemented by critical care physicians and hospitals so that we have the ability to meet future threats.

S. L. Zanotti-Cavazzoni, MD

Cardiopulmonary Effects of Matching Positive End-Expiratory Pressure to Abdominal Pressure in Concomitant Abdominal Hypertension and Acute Lung Injury
da Silva Almeida JR, Machado FS, Schettino GPP, et al (Hosp Sirio-Libanes, Bela Vista, São Paulo, Brazil)
J Trauma 69:375-383, 2010

Background.—To evaluate the cardiopulmonary effects of positive end-expiratory pressure (PEEP) equalization to intra-abdominal pressure (IAP) in an experimental model of intra-abdominal hypertension (IAH) and acute lung injury (ALI).

Methods.—Eight anesthetized pigs were submitted to IAH of 20 mm Hg with a carbon dioxide insufflator for 30 minutes and then submitted to lung lavage with saline and Tween (2.5%). Pressure × volume curves of the respiratory system were performed by a low flow method during

IAH and ALI, and PEEP was subsequently adjusted to 27 cm · H_2O for 30 minutes.

Results.—IAH decreases pulmonary and respiratory system static compliances and increases airway resistance, alveolar-arterial oxygen gradient, and respiratory dead space. The presence of concomitant ALI exacerbates these findings. PEEP identical to AP moderately improved oxygenation and respiratory mechanics; however, an important decline in stroke index and right ventricle ejection fraction was observed.

Conclusions.—Simultaneous IAH and ALI produce important impairments in the respiratory physiology. PEEP equalization to AP may improve the respiratory performance, nevertheless with a secondary hemodynamic derangement.

▶ Physiologic data supporting the importance of compartment pressures and their interrelatedness in the progression of cardiopulmonary collapse are provided. Intra-abdominal hypertension is a major factor determining pulmonary response to mechanical ventilation with positive end-expiratory pressure (PEEP) manipulation in lung injury. Cardiovascular limitations of administration of high PEEP are effectively demonstrated. PEEP will help address compliance and gas exchange changes associated with abdominal compartment pressure elevation. Unfortunately, this comes at the cost of cardiovascular compromise and collapse.[1,2]

In this model of multicompartment dysfunction, the clinician should note the value and limitations of PEEP and abdominal pressure control in the management of thoracoabdominal inflammatory insults.

D. J. Dries, MSE, MD

References

1. Dries DJ, Mathru M. The right ventricle: selected issues. In: Dries DJ, Mathru M, eds. *Right Ventricle: The Neglected Neighbor of the Left*. Austin: RG Landes Company; 1994:1-14.
2. Mutoh T, Lamm WJ, Embree LJ, Hildebrandt J, Albert RK. Abdominal distension alters regional pleural pressures and chest wall mechanics in pigs in vivo. *J Appl Physiol*. 1991;70:2611-2618.

Clinical Characteristics and Outcomes of Sepsis-Related vs Non-Sepsis-Related ARDS

Sheu C-C, Gong MN, Zhai R, et al (Harvard School of Public Health, Boston, MA; Montefiore Med Ctr, Bronx, NY; et al)
Chest 138:559-567, 2010

Background.—ARDS may occur after either septic or nonseptic injuries. Sepsis is the major cause of ARDS, but little is known about the differences between sepsis-related and non-sepsis-related ARDS.

Methods.—A total of 2,786 patients with ARDS-predisposing conditions were enrolled consecutively into a prospective cohort, of which

736 patients developed ARDS. We defined sepsis-related ARDS as ARDS developing in patients with sepsis and non-sepsis-related ARDS as ARDS developing after nonseptic injuries, such as trauma, aspiration, and multiple transfusions. Patients with both septic and nonseptic risks were excluded from analysis.

Results.—Compared with patients with non-sepsis-related ARDS (n = 62), patients with sepsis-related ARDS (n = 524) were more likely to be women and to have diabetes, less likely to have preceding surgery, and had longer pre-ICU hospital stays and higher APACHE III (Acute Physiology and Chronic Health Evaluation III) scores (median, 78 vs 65, $P < .0001$). There were no differences in lung injury score, blood pH, PaO_2/FIO_2 ratio, and $PaCO_2$ on ARDS diagnosis. However, patients with sepsis-related ARDS had significantly lower PaO_2/FIO_2 ratios than patients with non-sepsis-related ARDS patients on ARDS day 3 ($P = .018$), day 7 ($P = .004$), and day 14 ($P = .004$) (repeated-measures analysis, $P = .011$). Compared with patients with non-sepsis-related ARDS, those with sepsis-related had a higher 60-day mortality (38.2% vs 22.6%; $P = .016$), a lower successful extubation rate (53.6% vs 72.6%; $P = .005$), and fewer ICU-free days ($P = .0001$) and ventilator-free days ($P = .003$). In multivariate analysis, age, APACHE III score, liver cirrhosis, metastatic cancer, admission serum bilirubin and glucose levels, and treatment with activated protein C were independently associated with 60-day ARDS mortality. After adjustment, sepsis-related ARDS was no longer associated with higher 60-day mortality (hazard ratio, 1.26; 95% CI, 0.71-2.22).

Conclusion.—Sepsis-related ARDS has a higher overall disease severity, poorer recovery from lung injury, lower successful extubation rate, and higher mortality than non-sepsis-related ARDS. Worse clinical outcomes in sepsis-related ARDS appear to be driven by disease severity and comorbidities.

▶ Despite important advances in treatment, the mortality for acute respiratory distress syndrome (ARDS) remains high, varying based on different reports from 35% to 45%.[1] Perhaps an important contributor to the lack of more drastic effects on mortality is related to the heterogeneity of patients with ARDS and the multiple different causes of this syndrome.[2] Teasing out the impact that different causes of ARDS have on patient outcomes seems an important step toward a better understanding of this complex disease.

Sheu et al, in this 10-year prospective cohort study, attempted to characterize the differences between patients with sepsis and nonsepsis-based causes of ARDS. They enrolled 2876 patients of whom 736 developed ARDS. One hundred and eight patients were excluded secondary to having both sepsis and nonsepsis-related risk factors for development of ARDS. Significantly, more patients had sepsis-related causes of ARDS ($P = 524$) than nonsepsis-related causes ($P = 62$). The authors compared multiple variables between survivors ($P = 372$) and nonsurvivors ($P = 214$).

They found multiple statistically significant differences between survivors and nonsurvivors with ARDS, including higher body mass index and Acute Physiology and Chronic Health Evaluation III in nonsurvivors. A statistically significant number of patients in the survivor group had trauma as their cause of ARDS. More patients in the nonsurvivor group had sepsis-related ARDS, but statistical significance was not achieved. No difference existed in the Pao_2/Fio_2 ratio upon diagnosis between the sepsis and nonsepsis ARDS groups. Yet, by day 7 and persisting through day 14, the sepsis group had statistically significantly lower Pao_2/Fio_2 ratios. A Kaplan-Meier estimate showed that patients with sepsis ARDS had a statistically significant higher mortality at 60 days. However, a multivariate analysis did not show that sepsis was an independent predictor of mortality in patients with ARDS.

The importance of this study is that it provides epidemiological data about patients with ARDS in a prospective study. The authors noted that both activated protein C therapy and an elevated serum glucose level upon admission were independently associated with higher mortalities in patients with ARDS. These hypothesis-generating findings are important for future studies involving ARDS. The authors noted multiple limitations with their study, the most important being the small number of nonsepsis patients in this study. Limited conclusions can only be drawn from the analysis of the 62 patients with nonsepsis-related ARDS. This study does not definitively prove that sepsis and nonsepsis-related ARDS are different syndromes, but it highlights the need for further studies to understand the causes of ARDS.

S. L. Zanotti-Cavazzoni, MD

References

1. Phua J, Badia JR, Adhikari NK, et al. Has mortality from acute respiratory distress syndrome decreased over time? A systematic review. *Am J Respir Crit Care Med.* 2009;179:220-227.
2. Phua J, Stewart TE, Ferguson ND. Acute respiratory distress syndrome 40 years later: time to revisit its definition. *Crit Care Med.* 2008;36:2912-2921.

Clinical Characteristics and Outcomes of Sepsis-Related vs Non-Sepsis-Related ARDS
Sheu C-C, Gong MN, Zhai R, et al (Harvard School of Public Health, Boston, MA; Montefiore Med Ctr, Bronx, NY; et al)
Chest 138:559-567, 2010

Background.—ARDS may occur after either septic or nonseptic injuries. Sepsis is the major cause of ARDS, but little is known about the differences between sepsis-related and non-sepsis-related ARDS.

Methods.—A total of 2,786 patients with ARDS-predisposing conditions were enrolled consecutively into a prospective cohort, of which 736 patients developed ARDS. We defined sepsis-related ARDS as ARDS developing in patients with sepsis and non-sepsis-related ARDS as ARDS developing after nonseptic injuries, such as trauma, aspiration, and multiple transfusions. Patients with both septic and nonseptic risks were excluded from analysis.

Results.—Compared with patients with non-sepsis-related ARDS (n = 62), patients with sepsis-related ARDS (n = 524) were more likely to be women and to have diabetes, less likely to have preceding surgery, and had longer pre-ICU hospital stays and higher APACHE III (Acute Physiology and Chronic Health Evaluation III) scores (median, 78 vs 65, $P < .0001$). There were no differences in lung injury score, blood pH, PaO_2/FIO_2 ratio, and $PaCO_2$ on ARDS diagnosis. However, patients with sepsis-related ARDS had significantly lower PaO_2/FIO_2 ratios than patients with non-sepsis-related ARDS patients on ARDS day 3 ($P = .018$), day 7 ($P = .004$), and day 14 ($P = .004$) (repeated-measures analysis, $P = .011$). Compared with patients with non-sepsis-related ARDS, those with sepsis-related had a higher 60-day mortality (38.2% vs 22.6%; $P = .016$), a lower successful extubation rate (53.6% vs 72.6%; $P = .005$), and fewer ICU-free days ($P = .0001$) and ventilator-free days ($P = .003$). In multivariate analysis, age, APACHE III score, liver cirrhosis, metastatic cancer, admission serum bilirubin and glucose levels, and treatment with activated protein C were independently associated with 60-day ARDS mortality. After adjustment, sepsis-related ARDS was no longer associated with higher 60-day mortality (hazard ratio, 1.26; 95% CI, 0.71-2.22).

Conclusion.—Sepsis-related ARDS has a higher overall disease severity, poorer recovery from lung injury, lower successful extubation rate, and higher mortality than non-sepsis-related ARDS. Worse clinical outcomes in sepsis-related ARDS appear to be driven by disease severity and comorbidities.

▶ Previous studies have shown that the underlying cause of the acute respiratory distress syndrome (ARDS) is the most common cause of death among patients who die early in the course of ARDS. In contrast, nosocomial pneumonia and sepsis are the most common causes of death among patients who die later in the clinical course of ARDS. Respiratory failure is an uncommon cause of mortality.[1] It is not surprising to find a higher mortality in sepsis-induced ARDS, as mortality due to severe sepsis is greater than mortality due to most other causes of ARDS.

The results of this study are consistent with the observations above. However, this is the first study that gives a comprehensive, direct, comparative assessment of mortality in sepsis-related versus nonsepsis-related ARDS.

R. P. Dellinger, MD

Reference

1. Bersten AD, Edibam C, Hunt T, Moran J. Incidence and mortality of acute lung injury and the acute respiratory distress syndrome in three Australian States. *Am J Respir Crit Care Med.* 2002;165:443-448.

Do hypooncotic fluids for shock increase the risk of late-onset acute respiratory distress syndrome?
Schortgen F, For the CRYCO Study Group (Groupe Hospitalier Albert Chenevier-Henri Mondor, Créteil, France; et al)
Intensive Care Med 36:1724-1734, 2010

Objective.—In patients with shock, late-onset acute respiratory distress syndrome (ARDS) carries poor prognosis. Hypooncotic fluids may improve kidney function preservation, whereas hyperoncotic fluids may in theory decrease the risk of late-onset ARDS. Our objective was to determine whether predominant or exclusive use of crystalloids and/or hypooncotic colloids for shock resuscitation influenced the risk of late-onset ARDS.

Participant and Settings.—International prospective cohort of consecutive adults who were free of ARDS on admission and who received fluid resuscitation for shock in 115 intensive care units (ICUs) during a 4-week period.

Measurements and Results.—Severity scores, hemodynamic status, indication for fluids, risk factors for ARDS, plasma expander use, transfusions, and late-onset ARDS were recorded prospectively. Logistic regression models were tested to determine whether predominant or exclusive use of hypooncotic fluids was associated with higher incidence of late-onset ARDS. Of 905 patients, 81 [8.9%; 95% confidence interval (CI) 7.2–11.0] developed ARDS, with no difference between patients given only hypooncotic fluids (10.4%; 95% CI 7.6–13.7) and the other patients (7.7%; 95% CI 5.5–10.5; $p = 0.16$). Late-onset ARDS was significantly associated with sepsis [odds ratio (OR) 1.90; 95% CI 1.06–3.40], worse chest X-ray score at fluid initiation (1.55; 95% CI 1.27–1.91), positive fluid balance (1.06 per l; 95% CI 1.02–1.09), and greater transfusion volume (1.14 per l; 95% CI 1.01–1.29). The proportion of hypooncotic fluids in the plasma expander regimen was not associated with late-onset ARDS (1.01 per %; 95% CI 0.99–1.01).

Conclusions.—Based on this observational study, there is no evidence that in patients with shock the use of hypooncotic fluids increases the risk of late-onset ARDS. This finding needs to be confirmed.

▶ The choice of fluid resuscitation between crystalloids and colloids in patients with shock has been the subject of controversy over many decades. To date, there is no evidence to support one more than the other in terms of effect on morbidity or mortality.[1] Though, there is enough evidence to suggest that net fluid balance after fluid resuscitation is the most significant risk factor for late-onset acute respiratory distress syndrome (ARDS).

Despite this, some still hypothesize that colloids and hyperoncotic fluids, such as starches, dextrans, and 20% as well as 25% albumin could decrease the risk of edema (including in the lungs) by increasing oncotic pressure gradient and perhaps preserving the integrity of the alveolocapillary membrane.[2]

In this international, prospective, observational study, there was no increase in development of late-onset ARDS with the use of hypooncotic fluids (crystalloids and 4% albumin) when compared with hyperoncotic fluids during shock resuscitation. Despite some limitations of this study, mostly the low incidence of late-onset ARDS development, which may limit the statistical power and the inclusion of 4% albumin, a colloid, in the hypooncotic group, the results are not surprising and are in tandem with previous studies as described above.[1]

This will not change our current clinical practice of aggressive fluid resuscitation with crystalloids or colloids in early shock with use of vasopressors and/or inotropes as clinically indicated. Hemodynamic stability should take priority, and once this is achieved, a dryer approach should be followed with less liberal fluid administration, use of diuretics, and mostly increasing blood transfusion threshold.

Finally, it is important to be reminded that mortality in ARDS is usually secondary to the underlying cause rather than the lung injury itself.[3] Therefore, treatment should be directed to the underlying cause even if this entails aggressive fluid resuscitation.

R. P. Dellinger, MD

References

1. Finfer S, Bellomo R, Boyce N, French J, Myburgh J, Norton R. The SAFE Study Investigators. A comparison of albumin and saline for fluid resuscitation in the intensive care unit. *N Engl J Med.* 2004;350:2247-2256.
2. Jia X, Malhotra A, Saeed M, Mark RG, Talmor D. Risk factors for ARDS in patients receiving mechanical ventilation for > 48 h. *Chest.* 2008;133:853-861.
3. Sheu CC, Gong MN, Zhai R, et al. Clinical characteristics and outcomes of sepsis-related vs non-sepsis-related ARDS. *Chest.* 2010;138:559-567.

Efficacy and economic assessment of conventional ventilatory support versus extracorporeal membrane oxygenation for severe adult respiratory failure (CESAR): a multicentre randomised controlled trial
Peek GJ, for the CESAR trial collaboration (Glenfield Hosp, Leicester, UK; et al)
Lancet 374:1351-1363, 2009

Background.—Severe acute respiratory failure in adults causes high mortality despite improvements in ventilation techniques and other treatments (eg, steroids, prone positioning, bronchoscopy, and inhaled nitric oxide). We aimed to delineate the safety, clinical efficacy, and cost-effectiveness of extracorporeal membrane oxygenation (ECMO) compared with conventional ventilation support.

Methods.—In this UK-based multicentre trial, we used an independent central randomisation service to randomly assign 180 adults in a 1:1 ratio to receive continued conventional management or referral to consideration for treatment by ECMO. Eligible patients were aged 18–65 years and had severe (Murray score > 3·0 or pH < 7·20) but potentially reversible respiratory failure. Exclusion criteria were: high pressure (>30 cm

H_2O of peak inspiratory pressure) or high FiO_2 (>0·8) ventilation for more than 7 days; intracranial bleeding; any other contraindication to limited heparinisation; or any contraindication to continuation of active treatment. The primary outcome was death or severe disability at 6 months after randomisation or before discharge from hospital. Primary analysis was by intention to treat. Only researchers who did the 6-month follow-up were masked to treatment assignment. Data about resource use and economic outcomes (quality-adjusted life-years) were collected. Studies of the key cost generating events were undertaken, and we did analyses of cost-utility at 6 months after randomisation and modelled lifetime cost-utility. This study is registered, number ISRCTN47279827.

Findings.—766 patients were screened; 180 were enrolled and randomly allocated to consideration for treatment by ECMO (n = 90 patients) or to receive conventional management (n = 90). 68 (75%) patients actually received ECMO; 63% (57/90) of patients allocated to consideration for treatment by ECMO survived to 6 months without disability compared with 47% (41/87) of those allocated to conventional management (relative risk 0·69; 95% CI 0·05–0·97, p = 0·03). Referral to consideration for treatment by ECMO treatment led to a gain of 0·03 quality-adjusted life-years (QALYs) at 6-month follow-up. A lifetime model predicted the cost per QALY of ECMO to be £19 252 (95% CI 7622–59 200) at a discount rate of 3·5%.

Interpretation.—We recommend transferring of adult patients with severe but potentially reversible respiratory failure, whose Murray score exceeds 3·0 or who have a pH of less than 7·20 on optimum conventional management, to a centre with an ECMO-based management protocol to significantly improve survival without severe disability. This strategy is also likely to be cost effective in settings with similar services to those in the UK.

▶ Our understanding of support to survival of patients with severe respiratory insufficiency has progressed significantly in the last decade. Unfortunately, we are not always successful in being able to support all patients from the pulmonary defect (eg, hypoxia), and they succumb. A variety of reasons exists for this untoward outcome that include the severity of illness, the inability to identify or eliminate the inciting event/agent, and at times the lack of compliance with accepted approaches to care. This trial, the CESAR trial. evaluates extracorporeal membrane oxygenation (ECMO) in patients with severe respiratory failure. Table 3 shows that the risk of death or disability at 6 months was lower in the ECMO group as compared with conventional management. This finding at first seems surprising given the concerns about ECMO-induced harm, and at first it seems consistent with the expansion of this methodology in these extremely ill patients. However, when one looks closer one notices that there is no difference in mortality between the groups, and a single severely disabled patient is driving the combined event rate, thus calling the significance of these findings into significant question. In addition, the patients were not truly randomized but cared for at different centers. Some patients in the

TABLE 3.—Death and Severe Disability

	ECMO Group (n = 90)*	Conventional Management Group (n = 90)	Relative Risk (95% CI, p Value)
Death or severe disability at 6 months	NA	NA	0·69 (0·05–0·97, 0·03)[†]
No	57 (63%)	41 (47%)[‡]	NA
Yes	33 (37%)	46 (53%)[‡]	NA
No information about severe disability	0	3 (3%)[§]	NA
Died at ≤6 months or before discharge	NA	NA	0·73 (0·52–1·03, 0·07)
No	57 (63%)	45 (50%)	NA
Yes	33 (37%)	45 (45%)	NA
Severe disability			
No	57 (63%)	41 (46%)	NA
Yes	0	1 (1%)	NA
Cause of death			
Respiratory failure	8 (9%)	24 (27%)	NA
Multiorgan failure	14 (16%)	15 (17%)	NA
Neurological disorder	4 (4%)	2 (2%)	NA
Cardiovascular disorder	1 (1%)	3 (3%)	NA
Related to ECMO	1 (1%)	0	NA
Other	1 (1%)	0	NA
Unknown	4 (4%)	1 (1%)	NA
Time between randomisation and death (days)	15 (3–41)	5 (2–14)	NA

Data are number (%) or median (IQR), unless otherwise indicated. ECMO = extracorporeal membrane oxygenation. NA = not applicable.

*Patients were randomly allocated to consideration for treatment by ECMO, but did not necessarily receive this treatment.

[†]Based on 177 patients with known primary outcome. Assuming that the three patients in the conventional management group who had no information about disability had all been severely disabled, or had not been severely disabled, relative risk of the primary outcome would be 0·67 (95% CI 0·48–0·94, p = 0·017), and 0·72 (0·51–1·01, p = 0·051), respectively.

[‡]Percentage calculated with denominator of 87 patients to exclude those with no information about severe disability.

[§]Patients had been discharged from hospital 1–3 months after randomisation, and were known to be alive at 6 months.

ECMO arm even died in transport to an ECMO center. Furthermore, the patients who were to be treated by conventional management appear to have received less than optimal care as measured by compliance with lung protective strategies. Given that there is no clear clinical benefit, the financial analysis is a moot point. What is an important finding is that the mortality rate in the group that was severely ill and received ECMO is lower than many would have projected; thus, these findings could be utilized in combination with other recently released observational data on ECMO in support of a true randomized clinical trial.

T. Dorman, MD

Neuromuscular Blockers in Early Acute Respiratory Distress Syndrome

Papazian L, for the ACURASYS Study Investigators (Université de la Méditerranée Aix-Marseille II, Marseille, France; et al)
N Engl J Med 363:1107-1116, 2010

Background.—In patients undergoing mechanical ventilation for the acute respiratory distress syndrome (ARDS), neuromuscular blocking agents may improve oxygenation and decrease ventilator-induced lung injury but may also cause muscle weakness. We evaluated clinical outcomes after 2 days of therapy with neuromuscular blocking agents in patients with early, severe ARDS.

Methods.—In this multicenter, double-blind trial, 340 patients presenting to the intensive care unit (ICU) with an onset of severe ARDS within the previous 48 hours were randomly assigned to receive, for 48 hours, either cisatracurium besylate (178 patients) or placebo (162 patients). Severe ARDS was defined as a ratio of the partial pressure of arterial oxygen (PaO_2) to the fraction of inspired oxygen (FiO_2) of less than 150, with a positive end-expiratory pressure of 5 cm or more of water and a tidal volume of 6 to 8 ml per kilogram of predicted body weight. The primary outcome was the proportion of patients who died either before hospital discharge or within 90 days after study enrollment (i.e., the 90-day in-hospital mortality rate), adjusted for predefined covariates and baseline differences between groups with the use of a Cox model.

Results.—The hazard ratio for death at 90 days in the cisatracurium group, as compared with the placebo group, was 0.68 (95% confidence interval [CI], 0.48 to 0.98; P = 0.04), after adjustment for both the baseline PaO_2:FiO_2 and plateau pressure and the Simplified Acute Physiology II score. The crude 90-day mortality was 31.6% (95% CI, 25.2 to 38.8) in the cisatracurium group and 40.7% (95% CI, 33.5 to 48.4) in the placebo group (P = 0.08). Mortality at 28 days was 23.7% (95% CI, 18.1 to 30.5) with cisatracurium and 33.3% (95% CI, 26.5 to 40.9) with placebo (P = 0.05). The rate of ICU-acquired paresis did not differ significantly between the two groups.

Conclusions.—In patients with severe ARDS, early administration of a neuromuscular blocking agent improved the adjusted 90-day survival and increased the time off the ventilator without increasing muscle weakness. (Funded by Assistance Publique–Hôpitaux de Marseille and the Programme Hospitalier de Recherche Clinique Régional 2004-26 of the French Ministry of Health; ClinicalTrials.gov number, NCT00299650.) (Table 2).

▶ "Neuromuscular blockers are dead! Long live neuromuscular blockers!" So after years of decreasing use of neuromuscular blockers (NMBs) because of concern for persistent severe muscle weakness after discontinuation, a randomized prospective study in severe acute respiratory distress syndrome (ARDS) suggests benefit.

TABLE 2.—Baseline Characteristics of the Patients, According to Study Group*

Characteristic[†]	Cisatracurium (N = 177)	Placebo (N = 162)	P Value
Age — yr	58±16	58±15	0.70
Tidal volume — ml/kg of predicted body weight	6.55±1.12	6.48±0.92	0.52
Minute ventilation — liters/min	10.0±2.5	10.1±2.2	0.83
PEEP applied — cm of water	9.2±3.2	9.2±3.5	0.87
Plateau pressure — cm of water	25.0±5.1	24.4±4.7	0.32
Respiratory-system compliance — ml/cm of water	31.5±11.6	31.9±10.7	0.71
FiO_2	0.79±0.19	0.77±0.20	0.33
$PaO2:FiO_2$[‡]	106±36	115±41	0.03
pH	7.31±0.10	7.32±0.10	0.11
PaO_2 — mm Hg	80±24	85±28	0.09
$PaCO_2$ — mm Hg	47±11	47±11	0.62
Prone position or inhaled nitric oxide or almitrine mesylate — no. (%)	33 (18.6)	23 (14.2)	0.31
SAPS II[§]	50±16	47±14	0.15
Nonfatal condition according to McCabe–Jackson score — no. (%)[¶]	133 (75.1)	125 (77.2)	0.66
Main reason for ICU admission — no. (%)			
Medical	129 (72.9)	113 (69.8)	0.52
Surgical, emergency	27 (15.3)	31 (19.1)	0.34
Surgical, scheduled	21 (11.9)	18 (11.1)	0.83
Corticosteroids for septic shock — no. (%)	70 (39.5)	73 (45.1)	0.30
Direct lung injury — no. (%)	142 (80.2)	123 (75.9)	0.34

*Plus–minus values are means ±SD. FiO_2 denotes fraction of inspired oxygen, ICU intensive care unit, PaCO2 partial pressure of arterial carbon dioxide, PEEP positive end-expiratory pressure, and SpO2 saturation of peripheral oxygen as measured by means of pulse oximetry.
[†]All variables listed except age, nonfatal condition according to McCabe–Jackson score, and main reason for ICU admission were inclusion criteria.
[‡]Partial pressure of arterial oxygen (PaO2) was measured in millimeters of mercury.
[§]The Simplified Acute Physiology Score (SAPS) II is calculated from 12 physiological measurements during a 24-hour period, information about previous health status, and some information obtained at admission. Scores can range from 0 to 163, with higher scores indicating more severe disease.
[¶]Possible McCabe–Jackson scores for medical condition are 1 (nonfatal), 2 (ultimately fatal), and 3 (fatal).

How can we reconcile the old thought with the new evidence?

1. Use was only in severe ARDS.
2. Use was limited to 48 hours.
3. There was preclinical rationale that spontaneous breathing (eliminated) with NMB could detrimentally increase transpulmonary pressures.

I have personally witnessed marked improvement in oxygenation following institution of NMB in ARDS patients with severe hypoxemia and ventilation dyssynchrony, despite application of state-of-the-art ventilation techniques. Of interest, over a third of patients were receiving steroids for septic shock. A final note related to personal preference: I would use a twitch monitor (not used in this study) targeting presentation of asserted breathing with highest twitch responses achieving that goal.

R. P. Dellinger, MD

Plateau and Transpulmonary Pressure With Elevated Intra-Abdominal Pressure or Atelectasis

Kubiak BD, Gatto LA, Jimenez EJ, et al (Upstate Med Univ, Syracuse, NY; Dept of Biological Sciences SUNY Cortland, NY; Orlando Regional Med Ctr, FL)
J Surg Res 159:e17-e24, 2010

Background.—ARDSnet standards limit plateau pressure (Pplat) to reduce ventilator induced lung injury (VILI). Transpulmonary pressure (Ptp) [Pplat–pleural pressure (Ppl)], not Pplat, is the distending pressure of the lung. Lung distention can be affected by increased intra-abdominal pressure (IAP) and atelectasis. We hypothesized that the changes in distention caused by increases in IAP and atelectasis would be reflected by Ptp but independent of Pplat.

Methods.—In Yorkshire pigs, esophageal pressure (Pes) was measured with a balloon catheter as a surrogate for Ppl under two experimental conditions: (1) high IAP group ($n = 5$), where IAP was elevated by CO_2 insufflation in 5mm Hg steps from 0 to 30mm Hg; and (2) Atelectasis group ($n = 5$), where a double lumen endotracheal tube allowed clamping and degassing of either lung by O_2 absorption. Lung collapse was estimated by increases in pulmonary shunt fraction.

Results.—High IAP: Sequential increments in IAP caused a linear increase in Pplat ($r^2 = 0.754$, $P < 0.0001$). Ptp did not increase ($r^2 = 0.014$, $P = 0.404$) with IAP due to the concomitant increase in Pes ($r^2 = 0.726$, $P < 0.0001$). Partial Lung Collapse: There was no significant difference in Pplat between the atelectatic (21.83 ± 0.63 cm H_2O) and inflated lung (22.06 ± 0.61 cmH$_2$O, $P < 0.05$). Partial lung collapse caused a significant decrease in Pes (11.32 ± 1.11 mm Hg) compared with inflation (15.89 ± 0.72mm Hg, $P < 0.05$) resulting in a significant increase in Ptp (inflated $= 5.97 \pm 0.72$mm Hg; collapsed $= 10.55 \pm 1.53$mm Hg, $P < 0.05$).

Conclusions.—Use of Pplat to set ventilation may under-ventilate patients with intra-abdominal hypertension and over-distend the lungs of patients with atelectasis. Thus, Ptp must be used to accurately set mechanical ventilation in the critically ill (Fig 2).

▶ In managing patients with acute lung injury (ALI) and the acute respiratory distress syndrome (ARDS), it is important to avoid alveolar overdistention and use a lung protective ventilatory support strategy to improve outcome and possibly avoid ventilator-induced lung injury.[1,2] Recently, there has been controversy over what parameter (volume or pressure) is the best target to ensure lung protection and obtain the best survival.[3] This experimental animal study evaluates the use of transpulmonary pressure as a better indicator of alveolar distention compared with simply using the end-inspiratory plateau pressure. To bring out potential problems with just relying on the end-inspiratory plateau pressure, the investigators used an experimental model with elevated intra-abdominal pressure to mimic patients with abdominal compartment syndrome.

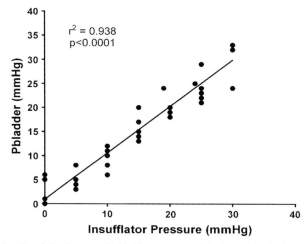

FIGURE 2.—Correlation between the bladder pressure and the intra-abdominal pressure measured with the CO_2 insufflator pressure. (Reprinted from Kubiak BD, Gatto LA, Jimenez EJ, et al. Plateau and transpulmonary pressure with elevated intra-abdominal pressure or atelectasis. *J Surg Res.* 2010;159:e17-e24, with permission from Elsevier.)

Several important observations come from this trial. The use of transplulmonary pressure appeared to outperform just the end-inspiratory plateau pressure as a measure of alveolar over- or underdistention. This finding would support further clinical research to determine if ALI-ARDS survival can be further improved using a similar approach. In addition, the investigators demonstrated that measuring bladder pressure as we typically do when we suspect intra-abdominal hypertension correlates very well with measured intra-abdominal pressure (Fig 2).

Further clinical efforts are warranted to determine if the transpulmonary pressure is a better target to guide our ventilatory management of patients with ALI and ARDS.

R. A. Balk, MD

References

1. Ventilation with lower tidal volumes as compared with traditional tidal volumes for acute lung injury and the acute respiratory distress syndrome. The Acute Respiratory Distress Syndrome Network. *N Engl J Med.* 2000;342:1301-1308.
2. Pinhu L, Whitehead T, Evans T, Griffiths M. Ventilator-associated lung injury. *Lancet.* 2003;361:332-340.
3. Talmor D, Sarge T, Malhotra A, et al. Mechanical ventilation guided by esophageal pressure in acute lung injury. *N Engl J Med.* 2008;359:2095-2104.

The Measure of Treatment Agreement Between Portable and Laboratory Blood Gas Measurements in Guiding Protocol-Driven Ventilator Management

Thomas FO, Hoffman TL, Handrahan DL, et al (Univ of Utah, Salt Lake City; Intermountain Life Flight, Salt Lake City, UT; Intermountain Healthcare Urban Central Region Statistical Data Ctr, Salt Lake City, UT)
J Trauma 67:303-314, 2009

Background.—Portable blood gas analyzer and monitor devices are increasingly being used to direct ventilator therapy. The purpose of this study was to evaluate the "measure of treatment agreement" between portable and laboratory blood gas measurements used in guiding protocol-driven ventilator management.

Materials and Methods.—Using National Institutes of Health Acute Respiratory Distress Syndrome network ventilator management guidelines to manage patient care, measurements taken from the Nonin 8500 M pulse oximeter (SpO_2), the Novametrix-610 end-tidal CO_2 ($ETCO_2$) detector, and the i-STAT 1 (SaO_2, PO_2, pH, PCO_2) were compared with the recommended treatment from paired laboratory ABL-725 ($SaCO_2$, PO_2, pH, PCO_2) measurements.

Results.—Four hundred forty-six intubated adult intensive care unit patients were studied prospectively. Except for the $ETCO_2$ ($R^2 = 0.460$), correlation coefficients between portable and laboratory measurements were high ($R^2 \geq 0.755$). Testing for equivalence, the Nonin-SpO_2, iSTAT-PO_2, iSTAT-pH, and iSTAT-PCO_2 were deemed "equivalent" surrogates to paired ABL measurements. Testing for the limits of agreement found only the iSTAT-PCO_2 to be an acceptable surrogate measurement. The measure of treatment agreement between the portable and paired laboratory blood gas measurements were Nonin-SpO_2 (68%), iSTAT-SaO_2 (73%), iSTAT-PO_2 (97%), iSTAT-pH (88%), iSTAT-PCO_2 (95%), and Novametrix-$ETCO_2$ (60%). Only the iSTAT-PO_2 and the iSTAT-PCO_2 achieved the $\geq 95\%$ treatment agreement threshold to be considered as acceptable surrogates to laboratory measurements.

Conclusions.—The iSTAT-PO_2 and -PCO_2 were portable device measurements acceptable as surrogates to standard clinical laboratory blood gas measurements in guiding protocol-directed ventilator management. The "measure of treatment agreement," based on standardized decisions and measurement thresholds of a protocol, provides a simple method for assessing clinical validity of surrogate measurements.

▶ The use of lung-protective ventilatory support to improve outcome in patients with acute respiratory distress syndrome (ARDS) and acute lung injury has gained widespread acceptance and is in use in most institutions.[1] The titration of positive end-expiratory pressure (PEEP) and FiO_2 is dependent on results of arterial blood gas analysis and maintaining defined targets. The authors of the study have been among the pioneers in developing computer-based treatment algorithms that use data to guide therapeutic management.[2]

The natural tendency is to find substitutes for frequent arterial blood gas analysis to help guide the titration of ventilatory support. This article reports on a large number of patients with ARDS who were evaluated with standard laboratory arterial blood gases (ABGs) and point-of-care ABG determinations and noninvasive monitors of oxygenation and ventilation. The authors present an excellent discussion on how to evaluate surrogate tests for their ability to substitute for the more standard clinical tests. The authors thoroughly review the methods to evaluate different tests to determine if they are equivalent, if they serve as appropriate measures of treatment agreement, and finally, if substituting one of these tests for another will result in the same outcome benefit. The accompanying editorial by Dr David Dries also emphasizes the importance of evaluating the outcome from a treatment strategy when different parameters are used to guide the management. In this study, the clear result was that there is no substitute for an arterial blood gas determination, but a point-of-care ABG is likely sufficient to guide the lung-protective ventilatory support strategy PEEP/FiO_2 nomogram.

R. A. Balk, MD

References

1. Ventilation with lower tidal volumes as compared with traditional tidal volumes for acute lung injury and the acute respiratory distress syndrome. The Acute Respiratory Distress Syndrome Network. *N Engl J Med.* 2000;342:1301-1308.
2. Morris AH, Wallace CJ, Menlove RL, et al. Randomized clinical trial of pressure-controlled inverse ratio ventilation and extracorporeal CO2 removal for adult respiratory distress syndrome. *Am J Respir Crit Care Med.* 1994;149:295-305.

Airway

Effect of Just-in-time Simulation Training on Tracheal Intubation Procedure Safety in the Pediatric Intensive Care Unit

Nishisaki A, Donoghue AJ, Colborn S, et al (The Children's Hosp of Philadelphia, PA; Univ of Pennsylvania, Philadelphia; et al)

Anesthesiology 113:214-223, 2010

Background.—Tracheal intubation-associated events (TIAEs) are common (20%) and life threatening (4%) in pediatric intensive care units. Physician trainees are required to learn tracheal intubation during intensive care unit rotations. The authors hypothesized that "just-in-time" simulation-based intubation refresher training would improve resident participation, success, and decrease TIAEs.

Methods.—For 14 months, one of two on-call residents, nurses, and respiratory therapists received 20-min multidisciplinary simulation-based tracheal intubation training and 10-min resident skill refresher training at the beginning of their on-call period in addition to routine residency education. The rate of first attempt and overall success between refresher-trained and concurrent non–refresher-trained residents (controls) during the intervention phase was compared. The incidence of TIAEs between preintervention and intervention phase was also compared.

Results.—Four hundred one consecutive primary orotracheal intubations were evaluated: 220 preintervention and 181 intervention. During intervention phase, neither first-attempt success nor overall success rate differed between refresher-trained residents *versus* concurrent non–refresher-trained residents: 20 of 40 (50%) *versus* 15 of 24 (62.5%), $P = 0.44$ and 23 of 40 (57.5%) *versus* 18 of 24 (75.0%), $P = 0.19$, respectively. The resident's first attempt and overall success rate did not differ between preintervention and intervention phases. The incidence of TIAE during preintervention and intervention phases was similar: 22.0% preintervention *versus* 19.9% intervention, $P = 0.62$, whereas resident participation increased from 20.9% preintervention to 35.4% intervention, $P = 0.002$. Resident participation continued to be associated with TIAE even after adjusting for the phase and difficult airway condition: odds ratio 2.22 (95% CI 1.28–3.87, $P = 0.005$).

Conclusions.—Brief just-in-time multidisciplinary simulation-based intubation refresher training did not improve the resident's first attempt or overall tracheal intubation success.

▶ Improving provider competency in a manner that translates into higher quality and/or safer care is important to providers and patients. Simple didactic education can be effective, although it has been shown to be less effective than strategies that use interactive methodologies and those that assess metric-based outcomes. Simulation education involves both interactive education and assessment and so will likely be a significant component of competency-based education in the future. There are several concerns regarding simulation education, and these include the physical overhead and costs associated with simulation as well as the fact that frequently simulation training occurs remotely from the incident requiring translation of that skill. For instance, simulation

TABLE 1.—Tracheal Intubation-Associated Events

Severe TIAE	Minor TIAE
Hypotension requiring treatment	Esophageal intubation with immediate recognition
Vomit with aspiration	Mainstem bronchial intubation with delayed recognition
Cardiac arrest (patient survived)	Dental/lip trauma
Cardiac arrest (patient died)	Vomit without aspiration
Esophageal intubation without immediate recognition	Hypertension requiring treatment
Laryngospasm	Epistaxis
Malignant hyperthermia	Medication error
Pneumothorax pneumomediastinum	Dysrhythmia
Direct airway injury	Pain/agitation requiring additional medication and delaying intubation

TIAE = tracheal intubation-associated event.

TABLE 3.—Patient Demographics (401 Oral Intubations)

Phase	Preintervention (December 23, 2004 to June 11, 2007)	Intervention (June 12, 2007 to August 31, 2008)	P Value
Intubation, n	220	181	
Age			
< 12 mo	49 (22.2)	46 (25.4)	1.00
1–7 yr	82 (37.3)	75 (41.4)	
≥ 8 yr	62 (28.2)	57 (31.5)	
Unknown	27 (12.3)	3 (1.7)	
Weight, kg*	14.5 (3.7–70)	15 (4–76)	0.30
Indication of primary intubation			
Oxygen failure	111 (50.5)	74 (40.9)	0.057
Ventilation failure	80 (36.4)	52 (28.7)	0.11
Elective procedure	33 (15.0)	49 (27.1)	0.004[†]
Upper-airway obstruction	22 (10.0)	17 (9.4)	0.87
Shock/CPR	20 (9.1)	9 (5.0)	0.13
Weakness, decreased protective reflex	12 (5.5)	6 (3.3)	0.34
Pulmonary toilet	7 (3.2)	8 (4.4)	0.60
Therapeutic hyperventilation	5 (2.3)	4 (2.2)	1.00
Emergency drug administration	1 (0.5)	1 (0.6)	1.00
History of DA	18 (8.2)	20 (11.5)	0.019[†]
Sign of potential DA by examination			
Limited mouth opening	44 (20.0)	45 (24.9)	0.04[†]
Small thyromental space	19 (8.6)	21 (11.6)	0.089
Upper airway obstruction	25 (11.4)	21 (11.6)	0.95
Limited neck extension	17 (7.7)	20 (11.1)	0.30
Any sign of potential DA by examination	102 (46.4)	78 (43.1)	0.55
Difficult airway (defined by ≥ 3 providers, or ≥ 3 attempts by nonresident provider)	12 (5.5)	11 (6.1)	0.83

Data are presented as n (%) or median (interquartile range).
CPR = cardiopulmonary resuscitation; DA = difficult airway.
*Wilcoxon rank-sum test.
[†]$P < 0.05$, Fisher exact test.

TABLE 4.—Explanatory Factors for Tracheal Intubation-Associated Events (Multivariate Analysis)

	Odds Ratio (95% CI)	P Value
Resident participation	2.22 (1.28–3.87)	0.005*
Simulation intervention period	0.68 (0.40–1.15)	0.15
Difficult airway (defined by ≥ 3 providers, or ≥ 3 attempts by nonresident provider)	9.37 (3.39–25.93)	< 0.0001*
Patient age		
Infant (< 12 mo)	Reference	
Child (1–7 yr)	1.55 (0.80–3.03)	0.20
Older child (≥ 8 yr)	1.12 (0.54–2.31)	0.76

Number of observations = 369; likelihood ratio (chi-square test, $df = 5$) = 27.26; $P = 0.0001$; Pseudo-R^2 = 0.07.
CI = confidence interval.
*$P < 0.05$.

training on anaphylaxis may occur weeks, months, or years before clinicians find themselves at bedside having to manage a patient with such a disease. This study, recognizing this latter concern, used a model of just-in-time training occurring during a resident's month in the intensive care unit. The results of this just-in-time airway training can be seen in Fig 1 in the original article. There was no benefit of this approach when assessed by success rates or complication rates (see Table 1 for complications). Furthermore, resident participation in the airway management remained a significant explanatory factor for the occurrence of a complication (Table 4). What should be noted, however, is that more residents were deemed appropriate to attempt to manage airways secondary to the just-in-time training and this despite there being a great percentage of patients with known difficult airways in the study group (Table 3). Thus, it is not so clear that the training was ineffective, especially because the only complications seen were considered minor. In addition, because the resident who did not receive the training was on call with a resident who did receive the training, there could have been some transfer of information as well as even skill discussion or practice, thus polluting the results in a manner toward the null. Consequently, studies like this should be repeated with a more concealed study group.

T. Dorman, MD

Endotracheal Tube Intracuff Pressure During Helicopter Transport

Bassi M, Zuercher M, Erne J-J, et al (Univ Hosp Basel, Switzerland; Swiss Air Rescue Organisation, Zurich, Switzerland)
Ann Emerg Med 56:89-93, 2010

Study Objective.—We evaluate changes in endotracheal tube intracuff pressures among intubated patients during aeromedical transport. We determine whether intracuff pressures exceed 30 cm H_2O during aeromedical transport.

Methods.—During a 12-month period, a helicopter-based rescue team prospectively recorded intracuff pressures of mechanically ventilated patients before takeoff and as soon as the maximum flight level was reached. With a commercially available pressure manometer, intracuff pressure was adjusted to ≤ 25 cm H_2O before loading of the patient. The endpoint of our investigation was the increase of endotracheal tube cuff pressure during helicopter transport.

Results.—Among 114 intubated patients, mean altitude increase was 2,260 feet (95% confidence interval [CI] 2,040 to 2,481 feet; median 2,085 feet; interquartile range [IQR] 1,477.5 to 2,900 feet). Mean flight time was 14.8 minutes (95% CI 13.1 to 16.4 minutes; median 13.5 minutes; IQR 10 to 16.1 minutes). Intracuff pressure increased from 28.7 cm H_2O (95% CI 27.0 to 30.4 cm H_2O [median 25 cm H_2O; IQR 25 to 30 cm H_2O]) to 62.6 cm H_2O (95% CI 58.8 to 66.5 cm H_2O; median 58; IQR 48 to 72 cm H_2O). At cruising altitude, 98% of patients

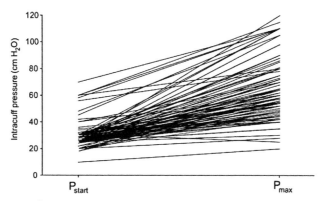

FIGURE 2.—Cuff pressure increase from takeoff (P_{start}) to maximum flight level (P_{max}). $\Delta P=33.9$ cm H_2O; 95% CI 30.6 to 37.3 cm H_2O (median 30 cm H_2O; IQR 20.9 to 44 cm H_2O). (Reprinted from Bassi M, Zuercher M, Erne J-J, et al. Endotracheal tube intracuff pressure during helicopter transport. *Ann Emerg Med.* 2010;56:89-93, with permission from the American College of Emergency Physicians.)

had intracuff pressures $\geq$30 cm H_2O, 72% had intracuff pressures $\geq$50 cm H_2O, and 20% even had intracuff pressures $\geq$80 cm H_2O.

Conclusion.—Endotracheal cuff pressure during transport frequently exceeded 30 cm H_2O during aeromedical transport. Hospital and out-of-hospital practitioners should measure and adjust endotracheal cuff pressures before and during flight (Fig 2).

▶ Transporting critically ill and injured patients is known to be associated with complications. This article evaluates a simple concept: Does the pressure within the cuff of an endotracheal tube increase at altitude as one would predict and if so by how much? As can be easily seen in Fig 2, the pressure indeed increased in essentially every single patient evaluated. This finding, although not surprising, given predicted expansion secondary to decreased ambient barometric pressure, is important unto itself as even short periods of elevated cuff pressure in animal models has been associated with tracheal mucosal lesions. What was most surprising was the magnitude of elevation despite ensuring that the cuff was not overinflated before helicopter liftoff. The intracuff pressure seemed to increase by more than 100% on average with > 70% increasing to > 50 cm H_2O and 20% increasing to > 80 cm H_2O. Given mucosal compromise is thought to occur around 30 cm H_2O, these pressure elevations are clearly concerning clinically. The major limitations in this work include: (1) the study is done in a helicopter to an altitude of about 2300 feet, and thus, the findings may not mirror lower altitude or changes during transport in a fixed wing barometrically controlled environment; (2) the device used to measure pressure may not be calibrated or validated at altitude so the pressure at altitude may not have been as elevated or possibly could have been even higher than measured; (3) patients with missing data were just eliminated and no information provided; and (4) intermediate- and long-term impact not evaluated. Despite these limitations, it seems extremely prudent to consider iterative cuff pressure monitoring during helicopter transport. Future studies should include a clinical impact evaluation.

T. Dorman, MD

Early vs Late Tracheotomy for Prevention of Pneumonia in Mechanically Ventilated Adult ICU Patients: A Randomized Controlled Trial
Terragni PP, Antonelli M, Fumagalli R, et al (Università di Torino, Turin, Italy; Università Cattolica del Sacro Cuore, Rome, Italy; Univ of Milano-Bicocca, Milan, Italy; et al)
JAMA 303:1483-1489, 2010

Context.—Tracheotomy is used to replace endotracheal intubation in patients requiring prolonged ventilation; however, there is considerable variability in the time considered optimal for performing tracheotomy. This is of clinical importance because timing is a key criterion for performing a tracheotomy and patients who receive one require a large amount of health care resources.

Objective.—To determine the effectiveness of early tracheotomy (after 6-8 days of laryngeal intubation) compared with late tracheotomy (after 13-15 days of laryngeal intubation) in reducing the incidence of pneumonia and increasing the number of ventilator-free and intensive care unit (ICU)-free days.

Design, Setting, and Patients.—Randomized controlled trial performed in 12 Italian ICUs from June 2004 to June 2008 of 600 adult patients enrolled without lung infection, who had been ventilated for 24 hours, had a Simplified Acute Physiology Score II between 35 and 65, and had a sequential organ failure assessment score of 5 or greater.

Intervention.—Patients who had worsening of respiratory conditions, unchanged or worse sequential organ failure assessment score, and no pneumonia 48 hours after inclusion were randomized to early tracheotomy (n = 209; 145 received tracheotomy) or late tracheotomy (n = 210; 119 received tracheotomy).

Main Outcome Measures.—The primary endpoint was incidence of ventilator-associated pneumonia; secondary endpoints during the 28 days immediately following randomization were number of ventilator-free days, number of ICU-free days, and number of patients in each group who were still alive.

Results.—Ventilator-associated pneumonia was observed in 30 patients in the early tracheotomy group (14%; 95% confidence interval [CI], 10%-19%) and in 44 patients in the late tracheotomy group (21%; 95% CI, 15%-26%) ($P=.07$). During the 28 days immediately following randomization, the hazard ratio of developing ventilator-associated pneumonia was 0.66 (95% CI, 0.42-1.04), remaining connected to the ventilator was 0.70 (95% CI, 0.56-0.87), remaining in the ICU was 0.73 (95% CI, 0.55-0.97), and dying was 0.80 (95% CI, 0.56-1.15).

Conclusion.—Among mechanically ventilated adult ICU patients, early tracheotomy compared with late tracheotomy did not result in statistically significant improvement in incidence of ventilator-associated pneumonia.

Trial Registration.—clinicaltrials.gov Identifier: NCT00262431.

▶ While many clinicians would support a tracheotomy in patients who are receiving mechanical ventilatory support for more than 7 to 10 days, its use earlier in the course of respiratory failure management remains controversial. Advocates for early performance of a tracheotomy emphasize that it may be more comfortable for the patient with respiratory failure, will facilitate weaning from ventilatory support, may allow ventilated patients to more effectively communicate, and even permit oral nutrition in some ventilated patients. Others will point out that a tracheotomy is an invasive procedure that requires anesthesia and increases the risk of bleeding and possibly infection. This randomized study attempted to answer the question of whether an early tracheotomy (after 6-8 days of ventilatory support) would decrease lung infections and improve weaning and reduce intensive care unit stay in comparison with a tracheotomy performed after 13 to 15 days of intubation.

I applaud the authors for trying to conduct a controlled trial to answer these important questions. Unfortunately, they were unable to find any significant difference and had to contend with the fact that approximately one-third of the patients in the early tracheotomy group did not receive an early tracheotomy, and 45% of the late tracheotomy group did not undergo the procedure. For now, we will continue with business as usual, with wide variation in the time for tracheotomy between individuals and institutions. We are in need of an updated consensus statement but can also use additional randomized controlled clinical trials to provide guidance for an updated consensus statement.

R. A. Balk, MD

Mechanical Ventilation/Weaning

High-frequency percussive ventilation improves perioperatively clinical evolution in pulmonary resection

Lucangelo U, Antonaglia V, Zin WA, et al (Univ School of Medicine, Trieste, Italy; Federal Univ of Rio de Janeiro, Brazil; et al)
Crit Care Med 37:1663-1669, 2009

Objective.—During thoracotomy, positive end-expiratory pressure is applied to the dependent lung and continuous positive airway pressure (CPAP) inflates the nondependent lung to avoid hypoxemia. These methods do not allow the removal of produced secretions. We hypothesized that high-frequency percussive ventilation (HFPV) can improve both conditions and reduce hospital length of stay in these patients.

Design.—Randomized prospective study.

Setting.—University Hospital.

Patients.—Fifty-three consecutive patients undergoing elective pulmonary partial resection were enrolled. Nine were excluded because of surgical reasons.

Interventions.—The nondependent lung was ventilated with HFPV in 22 patients and other 22 received CPAP. In both groups, the dependent lung was ventilated with continuous mechanical ventilation.

Measurement and Main Results.—Cardiocirculatory variables and blood gas analysis were measured during surgery. Postoperatively, all patients underwent chest physiotherapy, and Spo_2, body temperature, the amount of sputum produced, and chest radiography were recorded. Before nondependent lung re-expansion, HFPV patients presented higher Pao_2 than CPAP group ($p = 0.020$). The amount of secretions was higher in chronic obstructive pulmonary disease patients treated with HFPV than in those who received CPAP (199 and 64 mL, respectively, $p = 0.028$). HFPV increased by 5.28 times the chance of sputum production by chronic obstructive pulmonary disease patients ($\chi^2 = 46.66$, $p < 0.0001$; odds ratio = 5.28). A patient treated with HFPV had a 3.14-fold larger chance of being discharged earlier than a CPAP-treated subject (likelihood ratio = 11.5, $p = 0.0007$).

Conclusions.—Under the present settings, HFPV improved oxygenation in one-lung ventilation during pulmonary resection. Postoperatively, it decreased the length of stay and increased the removal of secretions in comparison with CPAP.

▶ Preliminary observations suggest a relationship between inspiratory and expiratory airflow based on inspiratory flow setting, respiratory frequency, and tidal volume. Mechanical ventilation patterns can encourage mouthward migration of secretions and fluids, if expiratory flow exceeds an effective threshold value relative to debris volume and consistency. For example, larger tidal volumes and lower values of positive end-expiratory pressure (PEEP) in conjunction with low airway resistance allow passive lung deflation to eliminate secretions.[1] Mouthward migration of secretions and mucus may benefit or harm a patient depending on whether the noxious materials are eliminated or propagated. In this setting, the authors have clearly instituted an aggressive suctioning program to remove unwanted secretions.

These authors demonstrate in a carefully controlled trial the value of optimizing mouthward migration of secretions. Patients have shorter hospital stay and improved physiologic parameters. These data further argue the value of mechanical interventions if optimally selected, as a means to control secretion movement.

I offer 1 final anatomic note. We typically place the diseased lung in a dependent position to minimize transfer of secretions. In this setting, the lung that is the presumed secretion source is in the nondependent position, but secretions are freed and aggressively controlled by the suctioning protocol used by this management team.

D. J. Dries, MSE, MD

Reference

1. Dries DJ. Key questions in ventilator management of the burn injured patient (second of two parts). *J Burn Care Res.* 2009;30:211-220.

Meta-analysis: Noninvasive Ventilation in Acute Cardiogenic Pulmonary Edema

Weng C-L, Zhao Y-T, Liu Q-H, et al (Peking Univ, Beijing, China; Beijing Chaoyang Hosp Affiliate of Capital Med Univ, China; Tsinghua Univ, Beijing, China; et al)
Ann Intern Med 152:590-600, 2010

Background.—Noninvasive ventilation (NIV) is commonly used to treat patients with acute cardiogenic pulmonary edema (ACPE), but the findings of a recent large clinical trial suggest that NIV may be less effective for ACPE than previously thought.

Purpose.—To provide an estimate of the effect of NIV on clinical outcomes in patients with ACPE that incorporates recent trial evidence and explore ways to interpret that evidence in the context of preceding evidence that favors NIV.

Data Sources.—PubMed and EMBASE from 1966 to December 2009, Cochrane Central Register of Controlled Trials and conference proceedings through December 2009, and reference lists, without language restriction.

Study Selection.—Randomized trials that compared continuous positive airway pressure and bilevel ventilation with standard therapy or each other.

Data Extraction.—Two independent reviewers extracted data. Outcomes examined were mortality, intubation rate, and incidence of new myocardial infarction (MI).

Data Synthesis.—Compared with standard therapy, continuous positive airway pressure reduced mortality (relative risk [RR], 0.64 [95% CI, 0.44 to 0.92]) and need for intubation (RR, 0.44 [CI, 0.32 to 0.60]) but not incidence of new MI (RR, 1.07 [CI, 0.84 to 1.37]). The effect was more prominent in trials in which myocardial ischemia or infarction caused ACPE in higher proportions of patients (RR, 0.92 [CI, 0.76 to 1.10] when 10% of patients had ischemia or MI vs. 0.43 [CI, 0.17 to 1.07] when 50% had ischemia or MI). Bilevel ventilation reduced the need for intubation (RR, 0.54 [CI, 0.33 to 0.86]) but did not reduce mortality or new MI. No differences were detected between continuous positive airway pressure and bilevel ventilation on any clinical outcomes for which they were directly compared.

Limitations.—The quality of the evidence base was limited. Definitions, cause, and severity of ACPE differed among the trials, as did patient characteristics and clinical settings.

Conclusion.—Although a recent large trial contradicts results from previous studies, the evidence in aggregate still supports the use of NIV for patients with ACPE. Continuous positive airway pressure reduces mortality more in patients with ACPE secondary to acute myocardial ischemia or infarction.

Primary Funding Source.—None.

▶ Despite a large number of clinical trials demonstrating the benefit of noninvasive positive pressure ventilatory support in the management of acute cardiogenic pulmonary edema, there continues to be some controversy surrounding its benefit, particularly in those patients with coronary artery disease. This large meta-analysis conducted by these investigators appears to support the benefit of using noninvasive positive pressure ventilation to decrease the need for intubation and to improve overall mortality in the setting of cardiogenic pulmonary edema. While we all recognize the potential problems with using a meta-analysis to settle clinical questions, the vast amount of data included in this analysis provides good support for both the efficacy and safety of noninvasive positive pressure ventilation in the setting of cardiogenic pulmonary edema.

R. A. Balk, MD

Monitoring of extubated patients: are routine arterial blood gas measurements useful and how long should patients be monitored in the intensive care unit?
See KC, Phua J, Mukhopadhyay A (Natl Univ Hosp, Singapore)
Anaesth Intensive Care 38:96-101, 2010

Restitution of respiratory support, which may include continuous positive airway pressure, non-invasive ventilation or reintubation, is needed in some patients post-extubation. We aimed to investigate whether serial arterial blood gas measurements done in the post-extubation period would help to identify such patients and to delineate the optimal post-extubation duration for close monitoring. We retrospectively analysed 115 consecutive adult patients who were extubated following successful spontaneous breathing trials in the medical intensive care unit, excluding patients who were extubated to immediate non-invasive ventilation. Arterial blood gases were measured at one and three hours post-extubation and patients were followed for any restitution of respiratory support for the remainder of their hospital stay. Restitution of respiratory support was required for 22 of 115 (19.1%) patients, of whom 20 were originally intubated for pneumonia. These patients could all be detected clinically from deteriorating pulse oximetry or increasing drowsiness. Performing serial arterial blood gas measurements following extubation did not improve the detection rate or allow earlier detection of patient deterioration. Among the patients with pneumonia, restitution of respiratory support was required within 24 hours of extubation for 16 patients (80%) and after more than 49 hours for four patients. Serial arterial blood gas measurements at one and three hours after a planned extubation are not useful and patients originally intubated for pneumonia should be monitored post-extubation for at least 24 hours in the intensive care unit.

▶ During weaning, clinicians would like to be able to predict which patients would fail extubation to minimize this complication, which is associated with a worse outcome. To risk assess patients, numerous studies have suggested a constellation of tests, none of which is fully predictive on its own. Thus, clinicians usually assess a battery of clinical and data elements before making the decision to liberate patients from mechanical ventilation. The clinical findings usually include wakefulness, ability to cough, general condition, and secretion color, viscosity, and quantity. Data elements might include minute ventilation, forced expiratory volume, negative inspiratory force, rapid shallow breathing index, net volume status, and vasopressor requirements to name a few. In addition, dynamic tests such as spontaneous breathing trial (SBT) have been advocated. This study attempts to answer 2 questions: are routine blood gases useful after extubation and how long should patients be monitored after extubation? The study is underpowered to adequately answer either question. The study

TABLE 3.—Baseline Patient Characteristics and Variables Assessed for the Spontaneous Breathing Trials

	Patients not Requiring RRS (n = 93)	Patients Requiring RRS (n = 22)	P Value
Baseline characteristics			
Age (y)	56.6 (±17.5)	61.3 (±19.6)	NS
Male (%)	53 (57.0)	17 (77.3)	NS
COPD (%)	3 (3.2)	1 (4.5)	NS
CCF (%)	7 (7.5)	4 (18.2)	NS
Intubation for pneumonia (%)	26 (28)	20 (90.9)	<0.001**
Day 1 APACHE II score	21 (±8.4)	25.5 (±7.8)	0.025*
Duration of intubation (h)	42.0 (IQR 17.6-64.4)	75.8 (IQR 37.6-185.3)	0.002*
Variables assessed just prior to the spontaneous breathing trial			
Absent/weak gag/cough (%)	6 (6.5)	3 (13.6)	NS
Moderate to large amount of secretions (%)	21 (22.6)	5 (22.7)	NS
Mean arterial pressure (mmHg)	89.1 (±17.8)	87.3 (±16.8)	NS
Vasopressor dependence during extubation (%)	23 (24.7)	9 (40.9)	NS
Fluid balance in last 24 h (ml)	336 (IQR -619-2068)	403 (IQR 781-1161)	NS
pH	7.46 (±0.05)	7.44 (±0.07)	NS
PCO$_2$ (mmHg)	38.7 (±8.5)	39.8 (±7.4)	NS
Base excess (mEq/l)	2.8 (±6.0)	3.4 (±6.7)	NS
PaO$_2$/FiO$_2$ ratio	312 (±149)	313 (±98)	NS
Rapid shallow breathing index	41 (IQR 30-51)	43 (IQR 36-67)	NS

RRS = restitution of respiratory support, NS = not significant, COPD = chronic obstructive pulmonary disease, CCF = congestive cardiac failure, APACHE II = Acute Physiology and Chronic Health Evaluation II score. Variables are expressed as absolute numbers (percentages), means (±standard deviation, SD), medians (interquartile range, IQR) as appropriate.
*Not significant on multivariate analysis.
**Significant on multivariate analysis.

is also contaminated by its design, which used a high-pressure support during the SBTs. The rescue rate (> 19%) was extremely high implying an inadequate assessment of readiness for extubation. The authors found (see Table 3) that the patients admitted with a diagnosis of pneumonia were more likely to fail extubation, and this may have been secondary to inadequate source control. Unfortunately, data are simply not presented to fully assess this aspect. Furthermore, the authors state that the initial blood gases were not useful but failed to recognize the benefit of knowing the pCO2, and the impact of this knowledge when subsequent gases show a significant increase as a marker of progressive hypercapneic failure. Finally, this study should be repeated and designed to evaluate only those with risk factors for failure as it is in that group that routine gases may be of benefit. Regarding the second question, it is duly noted that many patients fail extubation close to and beyond 24 hours after extubation. More robust clinical data are required to understand this observation as many of these patients were likely demonstrating progressive decline in numerous clinical signs and symptoms during this time frame.

T. Dorman, MD

Miscellaneous

Comparison of routine and on-demand prescription of chest radiographs in mechanically ventilated adults: a multicentre, cluster-randomised, two-period crossover study

Hejblum G, Chalumeau-Lemoine L, Ioos V, et al (Institut Natl de la Santé et de la Recherche Médicale, Paris, France; Hôpital Saint Antoine, Paris, France; et al)
Lancet 374:1687-1693, 2009

Background.—Present guidelines recommend routine daily chest radiographs for mechanically ventilated patients in intensive care units. However, some units use an on-demand strategy, in which chest radiographs are done only if warranted by the patient's clinical status. By comparison between routine and on-demand strategies, we aimed to establish which strategy was more efficient and effective for optimum patient care.

Methods.—In a cluster-randomised, open-label crossover study, we randomly assigned 21 intensive care units at 18 hospitals in France to use a routine or an on-demand strategy for prescription of chest radiographs during the first of two treatment periods. Units used the alternative strategy in the second period. Each treatment period lasted for the time taken for enrolment and study of 20 consecutive patients per intensive care unit; patients were monitored until discharge from the unit or for up to 30 days' mechanical ventilation, whichever was first. Units enrolled 967 patients, but 118 were excluded because they had been receiving mechanical ventilation for less than 2 days. The primary outcome measure was the mean number of chest radiographs per patient-day of mechanical ventilation. Analysis was by intention to treat. This study is registered with ClinicalTrials.gov, number NCT00893672.

Findings.—11 intensive care units were randomly allocated to use a routine strategy to order chest radiographs in the first treatment period, and 10 units to use an on-demand strategy. Overall, 424 patients had 4607 routine chest radiographs (mean per patient-day of mechanical ventilation $1 \cdot 09$, 95% CI $1 \cdot 05$–$1 \cdot 14$), and 425 had 3148 on-demand chest radiographs (mean $0 \cdot 75$, $0 \cdot 67$–$0 \cdot 83$), which corresponded to a reduction of 32% (95% CI 25–38) with the on-demand strategy ($p < 0 \cdot 0001$).

Interpretation.—Our results strongly support adoption of an on-demand strategy in preference to a routine strategy to decrease use of chest radiographs in mechanically ventilated patients without a reduction in patients' quality of care or safety.

▶ Management of the critically ill or injured and mechanically ventilated patient is quite complex. Many practitioners believe that such patients require a daily

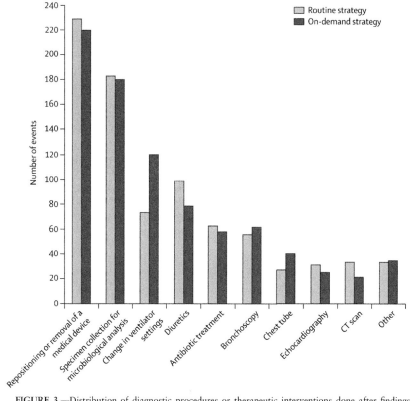

FIGURE 3.—Distribution of diagnostic procedures or therapeutic interventions done after findings from chest radiographs. (Reprinted from Hejblum G, Chalumeau-Lemoine L, Ioos V, et al. Comparison of routine and on-demand prescription of chest radiographs in mechanically ventilated adults: a multicentre, cluster-randomised, two-period crossover study. *Lancet.* 2009;374:1687-1693, with permission from Elsevier.)

TABLE 3.—Number of Chest Radiographs, Length of Stay, Duration of Mechanical Ventilation, and Mortality in Intensive Care Units

	Routine Strategy (n = 424)	On-Demand Strategy (n = 425)	p Value
Chest radiographs per patient-day of mechanical ventilation (total number; mean [95% CI])*	4607; 1·09 (1·05–1·14)	3148; 0·75 (0·67–0·83)	<0·0001
Morning rounds[†]	3779; 0·90 (0·86–0·93)	2224; 0·54 (0·47–0·60)	<0·0001
Unscheduled[†]	780; 0·18 (0·15–0·22)	893; 0·20 (0·16–0·25)	0·24
Days of mechanical ventilation (total number; mean [SD]; median [IQR])*	4172; 9·82 (8·24); 7 (4–13)	4226; 9·94 (8·75); 7 (3–14)	0·90
Length of stay (days; mean [SD]; median [IQR])	13·96 (11·61); 10 (5–19)	13·21 (11·01); 10 (5–19)	0·28
Mortality	131 (31%)	136 (32%)	0·79

Data are number (%) unless otherwise indicated.

*Data were censored to 30 days of mechanical ventilation; patients with more than 30 days of mechanical ventilation were regarded as having 30 days of mechanical ventilation in all calculations.

[†]For 48 chest radiographs done for patients on the routine strategy and 31 done for those on the on-demand strategy (p = 0·9), whether the chest radiograph was done during the morning round or was unscheduled was not recorded.

chest X-ray (CXR) while ventilated, and thus order a daily film usually obtained in the early AM so the image is available for review as part of morning rounds. These authors evaluated whether such an approach is equal to or better than an on-demand strategy. If an on-demand strategy remained at least equal to a routine strategy, then cost, patient pain related to movement and obtaining the film, and potential dislodgement of lines and artificial airways might all be prevented or saved. As can be seen in Table 3, there was indeed a significant reduction in the number of CXR obtained without a coincidental rise in the number of unscheduled/emergent films in a population of patients with equal numbers of days of mechanical ventilation, length of stay, and mortality. Fig 3 shows the numbers and the types of interventions done secondary to review of the films. There are some limitations to consider, and their impact on outcomes is not clear. These include that most patients are medical, the actual care ratios of providers to patients is not clear, and the use of respiratory therapist is quite low. The study is also likely underpowered for safety related to the interventions identified. This study does serve as the basis for a larger multi-centered trial. It would also be important to evaluate the first few days of intubation versus the days of mechanical ventilation that may occur after 2 weeks or a month of being supported. Even with these limitations in mind though, it would seem prudent to reconsider a daily routine CXR in all mechanically ventilated patients.

T. Dorman, MD

Confusion, Urea, Respiratory Rate and Shock Index or Adjusted Shock Index (CURSI or CURASI) criteria predict mortality in community-acquired pneumonia

Myint PK, Musonda P, Sankaran P, et al (Univ of East Anglia, Norwich, Norfolk, UK; James Paget Univ Hosp, Lowestoft, Norfolk, UK; et al)
Eur J Intern Med 21:429-433, 2010

Background.—Community-acquired pneumonia (CAP) is common and associated with a significant mortality. Shock index, heart rate divided by systolic blood pressure, has been shown to be associated with outcome in sepsis.

Objective.—To examine the usefulness of two new criteria CURSI (confusion, urea, respiratory rate and shock index), and CURASI where shock index is replaced by temperature adjusted shock index in mortality assessment of CAP.

Methods.—A prospective study was conducted in Norfolk and Suffolk, UK. We explored the usefulness of CURSI and CURASI which we derived and performed mapping exercise using a different cohort. In this study we compared these new indices with the CURB-65 criteria in correctly predicting mortality in CAP.

Results.—A total of 190 patients were included (males = 53%). The age range was 18–101 years (median = 76 years). There were a total of 54 deaths during a six-week follow-up. All died within 30-days. Sixty-five (34%) had severe pneumonia by CURB-65. Using CURSI and CURASI, 71(37%) and 69(36%) had severe pneumonia, respectively. The sensitivity, specificity, positive and negative predictive values in predicting death during six-week follow-up were comparable among three indices examined. The Receiver Operating Characteristic curve values (95%CI) for the criteria were 0.67(0.60–0.75) for CURB-65, 0.67(0.59–0.74) for CURSI and 0.66(0.58–0.74) for CURASI ($p>0.05$). There were strong agreements between these three indices (Kappa values ≥ 0.75 for all). Repeating analyses in those who were aged 65 years and over ($n = 135$) did not alter the results.

Conclusions.—Both CURSI and CURASI are similarly useful to CURB-65 in predicting deaths associated with CAP including older patients.

▶ Community-acquired pneumonia (CAP) is common and, when patients are admitted to the intensive care unit, carries significant mortality. Prediction tools for identifying high-risk patients with CAP have been validated in large clinical studies. CURB-65 score (confusion, serum urea nitrogen level > 19.6 mg/dL, respiratory rate ≥ 30/minute, low blood pressure [< 90 mm Hg systolic or ≤ 60 mm Hg diastolic], and age ≥ 65 years) is a commonly used score. With CURB-65, 1 point is assigned for each one of the components, and patients who have 3 or more points are identified as having high risk for death. In this study, the authors use a modified scoring tool in which they replace the blood pressure (B) and the age (65) from the CURB-65 with the shock index (SI). The SI is calculated as the ratio of the heart rate to systolic blood pressure. The authors propose that it might be easier to obtain and is more clinically relevant than either blood pressure or age. In addition, they use an Adjusted Shock Index (ASI), which corrects for increase in temperature related to the effect on heart rate. The authors tested these tools in a cohort of patients with CAP. With confusion, urea, respiratory rate and shock index (CURSI) and the confusion, urea, respiratory rate and adjusted shock index (CURASI), 1 point was given for the confusion, 1 point was given for the urea, 1 point for the respiratory rate over 30, and then 1 point for those patients who had an SI or ASI > 1. Patients who had 2 or more points were considered to be severe cases of CAP with a high risk of death. The authors compared the performance of the CURSI, the acute CURASI, and the CURB-65 in predicting mortality from pneumonia and found that they were all very similar. These simple scores can be calculated at the bedside and can be used by clinicians to identify high-risk patients. Whether one specific score has advantages over the other cannot be determined at this point.

S. L. Zanotti-Cavazzoni, MD

2 Cardiovascular

Cardiac Arrest

Significance of arterial hypotension after resuscitation from cardiac arrest

Trzeciak S, Jones AE, Kilgannon JH, et al (Cooper Univ Hosp, Camden, NJ; Carolinas Med Ctr, Charlotte, NC; et al)

Crit Care Med 37:2895-2903, 2009

Objective.—Expert guidelines advocate hemodynamic optimization after return of spontaneous circulation (ROSC) from cardiac arrest despite a lack of empirical data on prevalence of post-ROSC hemodynamic abnormalities and their relationship with outcome. Our objective was to determine whether post-ROSC arterial hypotension predicts outcome among postcardiac arrest patients who survive to intensive care unit admission.

Design.—Cohort study utilizing the Project IMPACT database (intensive care unit admissions from 120 U.S. hospitals) from 2001–2005.

Setting.—One hundred twenty intensive care units.

Patients.—Inclusion criteria were: 1) age ≥18 yrs; 2) nontrauma; and 3) received cardiopulmonary resuscitation before intensive care unit arrival.

Interventions.—None.

Measurements and Main Results.—Subjects were divided into two groups: 1) Hypotension Present-one or more documented systolic blood pressure <90 mm Hg within 1 hr of intensive care unit arrival; or 2) Hypotension Absent-all systolic blood pressure ≥90 mm Hg. The primary outcome was in-hospital mortality. The secondary outcome was functional status at hospital discharge among survivors. A total of 8736 subjects met the inclusion criteria. Overall mortality was 50%. Post-ROSC hypotension was present in 47% and was associated with significantly higher rates of mortality (65% vs. 37%) and diminished discharge functional status among survivors (49% vs. 38%), $p < .001$ for both. On multivariable analysis, post-ROSC hypotension had an odds ratio for death of 2.7 (95% confidence interval, 2.5–3.0).

Conclusions.—Half of postcardiac arrest patients who survive to intensive care unit admission die in the hospital. Post-ROSC hypotension is common, is a predictor of in-hospital death, and is associated with diminished functional status among survivors. These associations indicate that arterial hypotension after ROSC may represent a potentially treatable target to improve outcomes from cardiac arrest.

▶ Managing patients after cardiac arrest can be quite difficult. While trying to manage a potentially unstable patient, one is also iteratively assessing neurologic status to help predict outcome because guiding the family through this period is extremely important. This study opens our eyes to the fact there may be a difference between patients who have ongoing hypotension after arrest as compared with those that are normotensive. On examination of Table 2 it is clear that patients, who were subsequently hypotensive after arrest started off as a sicker population of patients, as measured by independence and chronic comorbidities. This confounder needs to be evaluated in a future study. Table 4 shows the utilization of vasoactive substances and demonstrates that despite the use of these agents some patients still had very low mean arterial pressures. This is concerning because it raises the question of adequacy of resuscitation and ongoing support. One must wonder, if given the concerns for neurologic outcome, if some patients remain underresuscitated. Fig 1 clearly shows that those remained hypotensive suffered a worse outcome. Interestingly, this figure also shows that if the outcome variable were survival at a time point 6 months or greater after arrest that the difference may disappear as the larger difference in

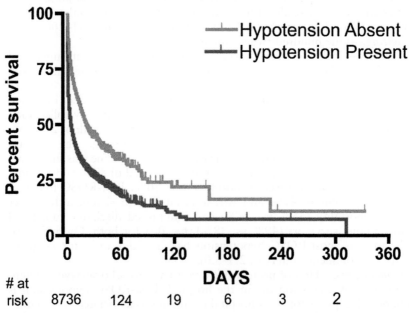

FIGURE 1.—Kaplan-Meier survival curves for patients with Hypotension Present and Hypotension Absent after return of spontaneous circulation from cardiac arrest (with censoring). The survival fractions diverged significantly by log-rank test ($p < .001$). (Courtesy of Trzeciak S, Jones AE, Kilgannon JH, et al. Significance of arterial hypotension after resuscitation from cardiac arrest. *Crit Care Med.* 2009;37: 2895-2903.)

TABLE 2.—Baseline Characteristics of the Study Subjects and Hospital Characteristics

	All Subjects (n = 8736)	Hypotension Present (n = 4092)	Hypotension Absent (n = 4644)	p^a
Age, yrs (mean ± SD)	64 ± 16	66 ± 16	63 ± 16	<.01
Gender, female, n (%)	4015 (46)	1874 (46)	2141 (46)	.80
Race, n (%)				
White/caucasian	6581 (75)	3060 (75)	3521 (76)	.29
Black/African-American	1376 (16)	695 (17)	681 (15)	<.01
Latino/Hispanic	330 (4)	155 (4)	175 (4)	.96
Asian/Pacific Islander	71 (1)	28 (<1)	43 (<1)	.21
Other	378 (4)	154 (4)	224 (5)	.02
Preadmission functional status,[b] n (%)				
Independent	5882 (67)	2562 (63)	3320 (71)	<.01
Partially dependent	1814 (21)	981 (24)	833 (18)	<.01
Fully dependent	1040 (12)	549 (13)	491 (11)	<.01
Chronic comorbidities, n (%)				
Severe cardiovascular disease[c]	1000 (11)	541 (13)	459 (10)	<.01
End-stage renal disease	707 (8)	394 (10)	313 (7)	<.01
Hepatic cirrhosis (with portal hypertension)	198 (2)	121 (3)	77 (2)	<.01
Cancer with metastatic disease	363 (4)	226 (6)	137 (3)	<.01
Active chemotherapy	181 (2)	122 (3)	59 (1)	<.01
Hematologic malignancy	37 (<1)	22 (<1)	15 (<1)	.12
Acquired immune deficiency syndrome	52 (<1)	21 (<1)	31 (<1)	.35
Site of origin immediately before ICU arrival, n (%)				
Emergency department	3792 (43)	1481 (36)	2311 (50)	<.01
Inpatient	4944 (57)	2611 (64)	2333 (50)	<.01
Admitted to ICU at night (11 PM–6:59 AM), n (%)	2184 (25)	1053 (26)	1131 (24)	.14
Hospital characteristics, n (%)				
Hospital size[d]				
Small to medium (≤300 beds)	1455 (17)	630 (15)	825 (18)	<.01
Large (301–500 beds)	3615 (41)	1790 (44)	1825 (39)	<.01
Extra large (>500 beds)	3666 (42)	1672 (41)	1994 (43)	.05
Hospital type				
Community, nonacademic	6939 (79)	3228 (79)	3711 (80)	.24
Academic, university-based	1561 (19)	749 (18)	812 (18)	.32
Public	178 (2)	88 (2)	90 (2)	.48
Military	58 (<1)	27 (<1)	31 (<1)	.97
Hospital location				
Urban	4616 (53)	2070 (51)	2546 (55)	<.01
Suburban	2765 (32)	1280 (31)	1485 (32)	.49
Rural	1355 (15)	742 (18)	613 (13)	<.01
On-site cardiac catheterization laboratory	8342 (95)	3940 (96)	4402 (95)	<.01

ICU, intensive care unit.
[a]Comparing Hypotension Present and Hypotension Absent groups;
[b]As defined in Table 1;
[c]Defined as baseline symptoms, such as angina or shortness of breath at rest or on minimal exertion (New York Heart Association Class IV) plus one or more of the following diagnoses: severe coronary artery disease; severe valvular heart disease; or severe cardiomyopathy;
[d]As defined according to the criteria from Halpern et al (41).

TABLE 4.—Outcomes

	All Subjects (n = 8736)	Hypotension Present (n = 4092)	Hypotension Absent (n = 4644)	p[a]
In-hospital mortality, n (%)	4375 (50)	2672 (65)	1703 (37)	<.001
Survivors, n	4361	1420	2941	
Functional status of survivors at hospital discharge, n (%)				
Independent	1840 (42)	460 (32)	1380 (47)	<.001
Partially dependent	1652 (38)	616 (44)	1036 (35)	<.001
Fully dependent	869 (20)	344 (24)	525 (18)	<.001
Decline in functional status on discharge compared with preadmission, n (%)[b]	1653 (42)	627 (49)	1026 (38)	<.001

[a]Comparing Hypotension Present and Hypotension Absent groups;
[b]Determined for all survivors who were not classified as fully dependent before admission (Hypotension Present, n = 1288; Hypotension Absent, n = 2688).

outcome seen up to about 180 days after arrest appears to significantly diminish over time after 180 days.

T. Dorman, MD

Cardiopulmonary Resuscitation/Other

Chest-compression-only versus standard cardiopulmonary resuscitation: a meta-analysis
Hüpfl M, Selig HF, Nagele P (Med Univ of Vienna, Austria)
Lancet 376:1552-1557, 2010

Background.—In out-of-hospital cardiac arrest, dispatcher-assisted chest-compression-only bystander CPR might be superior to standard bystander CPR (chest compression plus rescue ventilation), but trial findings have not shown significantly improved outcomes. We aimed to establish the association of chest-compression-only CPR with survival in patients with out-of-hospital cardiac arrest.

Methods.—Medline and Embase were systematically reviewed for studies published between January, 1985, and August, 2010, in which chest-compression-only bystander CPR was compared with standard bystander CPR for adult patients with out-of-hospital cardiac arrest. In the primary meta-analysis, we included trials in which patients were randomly allocated to receive one of the two CPR techniques, according to dispatcher instructions; and in the secondary meta-analysis, we included observational cohort studies of chest-compression-only CPR. All studies had to supply survival data. The primary outcome was survival to hospital discharge. A fixed-effects model was used for both meta-analyses because of an absence of heterogeneity among the studies ($I^2=0\%$).

Findings.—In the primary meta-analysis, pooled data from three randomised trials showed that chest-compression-only CPR was associated with improved chance of survival compared with standard CPR (14% [211/1500] *vs* 12% [178/1531]; risk ratio 1·22, 95% CI 1·01–1·46). The absolute increase in survival was $2 \cdot 4$ (95% CI $0 \cdot 1$–$4 \cdot 9$), and the number needed to treat was 41 (95% CI 20–1250). In the secondary meta-analysis of seven observational cohort studies, no difference was recorded between the two CPR techniques (8% [223/2731] *vs* 8% [863/11 152]; risk ratio $0 \cdot 96$, 95% CI $0 \cdot 83$–$1 \cdot 11$).

Interpretation.—For adults with out-of-hospital cardiac arrest, instructions to bystanders from emergency medical services dispatch should focus on chest-compression-only CPR.

▶ This meta-analysis pooled data for clinical studies of chest-compression-only cardiopulmonary resuscitation (CPR) versus standard CPR. The study proceeded in 2 phases. The first was a conventional meta-analysis based on randomized controlled trials of compression-only CPR. In the second phase, observational cohort studies were included. In these studies, instructions for compression-only CPR were administered by emergency medical services dispatchers. The primary outcome measure for both of the analyses was survival at hospital discharge. The authors found a signal of benefit in the 3 randomized trials of compression-only CPR. In the secondary meta-analysis of the observational cohort studies, they found no difference in the primary outcome. The authors conclude that compression-only CPR should be used.

The rationale behind compression-only CPR is that rescue breaths are unnecessary. It is now well accepted that quality of CPR is a critical determinant of outcome, and compression-only CPR can increase the effective chest compressions that are delivered to the patient (ie, CPR does not need to be interrupted for rescue breaths). Another attractive factor associated with compression-only CPR is that it does not require mouth-to-mouth ventilation at the scene of cardiac arrest. This may reduce the perceived barriers to CPR and result in an increase in bystander CPR in the community. It is important to recognize that the available data show that compression-only CPR is not inferior to CPR with rescue breaths, and therefore, it can be concluded that compression-only CPR is at least safe if not more efficacious. Therefore, compression-only CPR appears to be the preferred technique to teach the public.

S. Trzeciak, MD, MPH

Conventional and chest-compression-only cardiopulmonary resuscitation by bystanders for children who have out-of-hospital cardiac arrests: a prospective, nationwide, population-based cohort study
Kitamura T, for the implementation working group for All-Japan Utstein Registry of the Fire and Disaster Management Agency (Kyoto Univ Health Service, Japan; et al)
Lancet 375:1347-1354, 2010

Background.—The American Heart Association recommends cardiopulmonary resuscitation (CPR) by bystanders with chest compression only for adults who have cardiac arrests, but not for children. We assessed the effect of CPR (conventional with rescue breathing or chest compression only) by bystanders on outcomes after out-of-hospital cardiac arrests in children.

Methods.—In a nationwide, prospective, population-based, observational study, we enrolled 5170 children aged 17 years and younger who had an out-of-hospital cardiac arrest from Jan 1, 2005, to Dec 31, 2007. Data collected included age, cause, and presence and type of CPR by bystander. The primary endpoint was favourable neurological outcome 1 month after an out-of-hospital cardiac arrest, defined as Glasgow-Pittsburgh cerebral performance category 1 or 2.

Findings.—3675 (71%) children had arrests of non-cardiac causes and 1495 (29%) cardiac causes. 1551 (30%) received conventional CPR and 888 (17%) compression-only CPR. Data for type of CPR by bystander were not available for 12 children. Children who were given CPR by a bystander had a significantly higher rate of favourable neurological outcome than did those not given CPR (4·5% [110/2439] vs 1·9% [53/2719]; adjusted odds ratio [OR] 2·59, 95% CI 1·81–3·71). In children aged 1–17 years who had arrests of non-cardiac causes, favourable neurological outcome was more common after bystander CPR than no CPR (5·1% [51/1004] vs 1·5% [20/1293]; OR 4·17, 2·37–7·32). However, conventional CPR produced more favourable neurological outcome than did compression-only CPR (7·2% [45/624] vs 1·6% [six of 380]; OR 5·54, 2·52–16·99). In children aged 1–17 years who had arrests of cardiac causes, favourable neurological outcome was more common after bystander CPR than no CPR (9·5% [42/440] vs 4·1% [14/339]; OR 2·21, 1·08–4·54), and did not differ between conventional and compression-only CPR (9·9% [28/282] vs 8·9% [14/158]; OR 1·20, 0·55–2·66). In infants (aged <1 year), outcomes were uniformly poor (1·7% [36/2082] with favourable neurological outcome).

Interpretation.—For children who have out-of-hospital cardiac arrests from non-cardiac causes, conventional CPR (with rescue breathing) by bystander is the preferable approach to resuscitation. For arrests of cardiac causes, either conventional or compression-only CPR is similarly effective.

▶ In adult patients with out-of-hospital cardiac arrest, the current recommendation is for compression-only cardiopulmonary resuscitation (CPR) as opposed to conventional CPR with rescue breathing. Whether or not this is the optimal technique for children who suffer cardiac arrest was unclear. The investigators performed a prospective observational study for more than 5000 children, who had an out-of-hospital cardiac arrest over a 2-year period. The primary outcome measure was favorable neurological outcome as defined by a well-accepted neurological scale. Because this was an observational study, there was heterogeneity in the type of CPR performed, ranging from no bystander CPR to compression-only CPR to conventional CPR with rescue breathing. As expected, those who received CPR had better neurological outcomes compared with those without any CPR. However, they found a higher proportion of favorable neurological outcomes in those who received conventional CPR compared with compression-only CPR. Among those with presumed cardiac etiology of the arrest, the 2 techniques were not significantly dissimilar in the proportion of favorable neurological outcomes. The authors concluded that for out-of-hospital cardiac arrest from noncardiac causes (which is most pediatric cardiac arrest, eg, primary respiratory arrest), conventional CPR should be used rather than compression-only CPR.

Typically, we reserve treatment recommendations for studies with an experimental design. This observational study shows that conventional CPR is associated with more favorable outcomes. Causality is plausible because children who suffer from cardiac arrest may benefit from rescue breathing, especially those with primary respiratory arrest. In contrast, in adults with sudden cardiac death and out-of-hospital cardiac arrest, most of these events are cardiac in nature. Therefore, compression-only CPR may be more efficacious.

S. Trzeciak, MD, MPH

Induction of Therapeutic Hypothermia by Paramedics After Resuscitation From Out-of-Hospital Ventricular Fibrillation Cardiac Arrest: A Randomized Controlled Trial

Bernard SA, for the Rapid Infusion of Cold Hartmanns (RICH) Investigators (Ambulance Victoria, Melbourne, Australia; et al)
Circulation 122:737-742, 2010

Background.—Therapeutic hypothermia is recommended for the treatment of neurological injury after resuscitation from out-of-hospital cardiac arrest. Laboratory studies have suggested that earlier cooling may be associated with improved neurological outcomes. We hypothesized that induction of therapeutic hypothermia by paramedics before hospital arrival would improve outcome.

Methods and Results.—In a prospective, randomized controlled trial, we assigned adults who had been resuscitated from out-of-hospital cardiac arrest with an initial cardiac rhythm of ventricular fibrillation to either prehospital cooling with a rapid infusion of 2 L of ice-cold lactated Ringer's solution or cooling after hospital admission. The primary outcome measure was functional status at hospital discharge, with a favorable outcome defined as discharge either to home or to a rehabilitation facility. A total of 234 patients were randomly assigned to either paramedic cooling (118 patients) or hospital cooling (116 patients). Patients allocated to paramedic cooling received a median of 1900 mL (first quartile 1000 mL, third quartile 2000 mL) of ice-cold fluid. This resulted in a mean decrease in core temperature of 0.8°C ($P = 0.01$). In the paramedic-cooled group, 47.5% patients had a favorable outcome at hospital discharge compared with 52.6% in the hospital-cooled group (risk ratio 0.90, 95% confidence interval 0.70 to 1.17, $P = 0.43$).

Conclusions.—In adults who have been resuscitated from out-of-hospital cardiac arrest with an initial cardiac rhythm of ventricular fibrillation, paramedic cooling with a rapid infusion of large-volume, ice-cold intravenous fluid decreased core temperature at hospital arrival but was not shown to improve outcome at hospital discharge compared with cooling commenced in the hospital.

▶ This was a large randomized trial testing the hypothesis that out-of-hospital induction of therapeutic hypothermia with ice-cold lactated Ringer's solution would be associated with improved outcome compared with therapeutic hypothermia initiated in the emergency department after arrival at the hospital. Essentially, this clinical trial was testing whether or not faster initiation of hypothermia would improve the proportion of favorable outcomes. There was no control arm in this study (ie, no normothermia group). The authors randomized 234 patients to paramedic cooling versus cooling at the hospital. They found no significant difference in the incidence of a favorable outcome at hospital discharge between the 2 groups.

One potential interpretation of the study results is that the early initiation of hypothermia was not clinically meaningful. However, inspection of the data reveals that the temperature of the patients in both arms had essentially the same body temperature 60 minutes after arrival in the hospital. There are 2 possibilities. One is that the out-of-hospital cooling efforts were not particularly effective. Another possibility is that the in-hospital cooling efforts were so effective that they resulted in similar temperature drops in both arms, regardless of the treatment allocation. Another important consideration is that the mean body temperature was relatively hypothermic at the scene of arrest. This latter factor probably played a large role in the equivalence of the temperatures at the 1-hour mark.

Therapeutic hypothermia is the only proven treatment for anoxic brain injury associated with cardiac arrest, and it should be initiated as soon as possible after the return of spontaneous circulation in patients who do not follow commands after the pulse is restored. Whether or not the prehospital time interval is critical to the efficacy of therapeutic hypothermia remains unclear.

S. Trzeciak, MD, MPH

The effect of transplant center volume on survival after heart transplantation: A multicenter study
Shuhaiber JH, Moore J, Dyke DB (Harvard Med School, Boston, MA; Univ of Michigan Health System, Ann Arbor)
J Thorac Cardiovasc Surg 139:1064-1069, 2010

Objective.—Few studies have examined the association between procedural volume and clinical outcomes in heart transplantation. This retrospective study was performed on a contemporary cohort of heart transplant recipients to better elucidate the effect of transplant center volume on 1-year mortality.

Methods.—Data from the Scientific Registry of Transplant Recipients were used to analyze the relationship between transplant center volume and short-term survival. Center volume designation (very low, low, medium, and high) was assigned on the basis of quartiles with approximately equal numbers of patients per group. Survival differences were explored using Cox proportional hazards modeling to adjust for differences in variables between volume groups and to determine variables associated with 1-year mortality.

Results.—Between January 1, 1999, and May 31, 2005, 13,230 heart transplantations were performed at 147 transplant centers in the United States. Although most recipient and donor characteristics were similar across quartiles, larger volume centers were more likely to perform transplantations in older candidates and accept organs from older donors with longer cold ischemia times. A statistically significant relationship between transplant center volume and 1-year mortality was observed. Compared with the reference group (very low volume), the hazard ratios for the low, medium, and high-volume quartiles were 0.71, 0.64, and 0.56, respectively ($P < .001$ for each group compared with the reference).

Conclusion.—There was a significant association between transplant center volume and 1-year survival. Patients who undergo cardiac transplantation at very low-volume centers are at higher risk for early mortality than those who undergo transplantation in higher-volume centers.

▶ The volume-outcome relationship continues to be a debate in discussions about the quality of care delivery of different patient populations. Early data supported that centers performing higher volumes of coronary artery bypass procedures had better outcomes (lower mortality). Recent studies that used different statistical tools refute these findings;however, they still report variations in outcomes. Despite this, the question of the volume-outcome relationship remains active. A preliminary look at lung transplant performance suggests that this difference in outcomes is dependent on center volume when risk adjusted.[1] The authors of this article evaluate the effect of center volume on survival after heart transplantation. In a cohort of over 13 000 patients at 147 centers, Shuhaiber and colleagues assessed the impact of center volume on 1-year mortality following heart transplantation. Using data from the Scientific Registry of Transplant Recipients, they captured relevant patient risk factors and surgical factors in addition to outcomes. After adjusting for donor and recipient variables, they demonstrated that the very low-volume centers, with a mean annual volume of 5 cases, were associated with a significant (29%-44%) increased relative risk of mortality at 1-year posttransplant compared with low-volume, medium-volume, and high-volume centers. There did not seem to be a statistical difference between the low-volume, medium-volume, and high-volume centers. The volume strata were determined statistically by dividing total number of patients equally across the quartiles, as opposed to defining a volume cutoff (Table 1).

While this study gives us some insight into the variation in outcomes for heart transplant centers, it has important limitations that should be acknowledged.

TABLE 1.—Heart Transplant Center Characteristics by Volume Quartile

	Volume Quartile			
	Very Low	Low	Medium	High
No. of transplants	3089	3546	3370	3225
No. of centers	84	35	19	9
Median annual volume per center	5	16	28	48
Median years experience per center	5.9	6.3	6.4	6.4

Given its retrospective nature, there is a risk of unmeasured confounders, and there may be some important information that could be gleaned from adjusting for surgeon and surgeon volume. Furthermore, their lack of incorporating a hierarchical statistical model may have significant impact. Hierarchical modeling takes into account that patients undergoing a surgical intervention within the same hospital may be correlated, violating one of the basic assumptions of traditional regression analysis.[2] Many of the early studies of the coronary artery bypass grafting volume-outcome relationship that demonstrated a significant inverse relationship between volume and mortality did not use hierarchical modeling, whereas those that used more advanced statistical modeling (hierarchical) did not show a significant association. It would be important to perform a similar analysis to evaluate this relationship after heart transplantation. However, even if the volume-outcome relationship holds true with hierarchical statistical modeling, we are still left with the question of what the mechanism of this association is. Is it just center experience or something else that has not been identified? This is extremely important because, as the authors note, one-quarter of all heart transplants are performed in low-volume centers. It is imperative that we identify what structures and processes of care delivery, that are present at high-volume or high-performing centers, contribute to this mortality difference, and we evaluate whether outcomes can be improved if these practices are implemented in low-performing centers.

E. A. Martinez, MD, MHS

References

1. Weiss ES, Allen JG, Meguid RA, et al. The impact of center volume on survival in lung transplantation: an analysis of more than 10,000 cases. *Ann Thorac Surg.* 2009;88:1062-1070.
2. D'Errigo P, Tosti ME, Fusco D, et al. Use of hierarchical models to evaluate performance of cardiac surgery centres in the Italian CABG outcome study. *BMC Med Res Methodol.* 2007;7:29.

Myocardial Infarction/Cardiogenic Shock/Cardiogenic Pulmonary Edema

Atrial fibrillation management strategies and early mortality after myocardial infarction: results from the Valsartan in Acute Myocardial Infarction (VALIANT) Trial

Nilsson KR Jr, Al-Khatib SM, Zhou Y, et al (Duke Univ Med Ctr, Durham, NC; et al)

Heart 96:838-842, 2010

Objective.—The management of patients with atrial fibrillation (AF) following a myocardial infarction (MI) remains uncertain. This study compared a rate control strategy to an anti-arrhythmic-based rhythm control strategy for the treatment of AF following myocardial infarction.

Design, Setting and Patients.—We studied 1131 patients with AF after MI who were enrolled in the Valsartan in Acute Myocardial Infarction Trial (VALIANT). We classified patients into those treated with a rhythm control strategy (n=371) and those treated with a rate control strategy (n=760).

Main Outcomes Measures.—Using Cox models, we compared the two groups with respect to both death and stroke during two different time periods after randomisation for which data collection had been prespecified: 0–45 days and 45–1096 days.

Results.—After adjustment, a rhythm control strategy was found to be associated with increased early mortality (0–45 days: HR: 1.9, 95% CI 1.2 to 3.0, p=0.004) but not late mortality (45–1096 days: HR 1.1, 95% CI 0.9 to 1.4, p=0.45). No difference was observed in the incidence of stroke (0–45 days: HR 1.2, 95% CI 0.4 to 3.7, p=0.73; 45–1096 days: HR 0.6, 95% CI 0.3 to 1.3, p=0.21).

Conclusions.—In patients with AF after an MI, an antiarrhythmic drug-based rhythm control strategy is associated with excess 45-day mortality compared with a rate control strategy, but is not associated with increased mortality outside of the immediate peri-infarct period. These results potentially identify a patient population in whom the use of anti-arrhythmic drug therapy may portend an increased risk of death.

▶ Both atrial and ventricular arrhythmias are common in patients with acute myocardial infarction (MI). The incidence of atrial fibrillation (AF) was 10.4% among 40 891 patients with ST-segment elevation MI (STEMI) who received fibrinolytic therapy.[1] Patients who developed AF after admission were more likely to have a stroke or die within 30 days after acute MI. Among 13 858 patients with STEMI who received fibrinolytic therapy and had sinus rhythm on the baseline electrocardiogram (ECG), 906 patients developed AF or atrial flutter during hospitalization.[2] The median time from presentation to the onset of AF or atrial flutter was 2 days.[2] AF or flutter during hospitalization for acute MI is an independent predictor of increased in-hospital mortality and mortality at 30 days, 1 year, and 5 years.[1-6]

The management of new-onset AF in the setting of an acute MI represents a significant challenge. There are conflicting data regarding the effect of antiarrhythmic agents on the outcomes of patients with MI and AF. Wong et al[7] described the management and outcome of 1138 patients with acute MI complicated by AF. Three hundred and seventeen patients received an antiarrhythmic drug: 132 (12%) a class I agent, 55 (5%) sotalol, and 168 (15%) amiodarone. Sinus rhythm was restored in 72% of patients who received class I agents, 67% of those who received sotalol, and 79% of those who received amiodarone. There was a strong trend toward lower mortality associated with the use of sotalol or class I antiarrhythmic agents.

Nilsson et al analyzed the management and outcomes of 1131 patients with AF after MI who were enrolled in the Valsartan in Acute Myocardial Infarction (VALIANT) trial. An antiarrhythmic drug-based rhythm control strategy was associated with a higher rate of death than a rate control strategy in the first 45 days post-MI. The VALIANT investigators have attributed the excess mortality among patients who were treated with antiarrhythmic drugs to amiodarone.[8] This conclusion differs from the results of a previous randomized trial that did not observe increased all-cause or cardiac mortality among patients with left ventricular dysfunction post-MI who were randomized to amiodarone.[9]

Randomized clinical trials have demonstrated that several antiarrhythmic drugs increase mortality in patients with a history of MI, including encainide,[10] flecainide,[10] moricizine,[11] and d-sotalol.[12] Compared with the placebo arms of each trial, there were 37 excess deaths among the patients who were randomized to encainide and flecainide, 18 extra deaths among the patients who were randomized to moricizine, and 30 excess deaths among the patients who were randomized to d-sotalol.[13] Long-term treatment with dofetilide, a class III antiarrhythmic agent, did not increase cardiac or all-cause mortality among patients with a recent MI and left ventricular dysfunction.[14] Torsade de pointes, a proarrhythmia that is observed in patients who are treated with a class III antiarrhythmic agent, occurred in 7 patients treated with dofetilide, 5 within the first several days after treatment was initiated.[14] In patients with AF or flutter, dofetilide was better than placebo in restoring sinus rhythm.[14]

The alternative to antiarrhythmic therapy in patients with acute MI and AF is rate control and chronic anticoagulation. Intravenous β-adrenergic blockade is the preferred therapy to control the ventricular rate in patients with sustained AF or atrial flutter that is not associated with hemodynamic compromise, while sustained AF or atrial flutter that is associated with hemodynamic compromise is an indication for synchronized cardioversion. Intravenous amiodarone is indicated for treatment of AF that does not respond to electrical cardioversion or recurs after cardioversion.

The options for chronic therapy to control the ventricular rate in patients with sustained AF after acute MI are somewhat problematic. Intravenous diltiazem is useful to control the ventricular rate in patients with acute AF, but chronic oral diltiazem has been shown to increase mortality in patients with acute MI associated with pulmonary congestion on chest X-ray.[15,16] The safety of chronic digoxin therapy after acute MI is uncertain.[17] The safest approach is probably β-blockade because β-blockers have been shown to reduce long-term mortality in patients with acute MI.[18,19]

Both individual randomized trials and a meta-analysis of randomized trials have demonstrated that oral anticoagulation therapy, with adjusted-dose warfarin or other vitamin K antagonists, is superior to antiplatelet therapy, including the combination of aspirin and clopidogrel, for prevention of vascular events in patients with AF at high risk of stroke.[20,21] Therefore, chronic anticoagulation has become the standard of care to reduce the risk of stroke in patients with AF.[22]

Unfortunately, studies have demonstrated that dual antiplatelet therapy is superior to the combination of aspirin and a vitamin K antagonist for the prevention of MI and stent thrombosis after coronary artery stenting.[23,24] A drug-eluting stent is a class I indication for dual antiplatelet therapy (aspirin plus a thienopyridine) for a minimum of 12 months.[25] A bare-metal stent is a class I indication for dual antiplatelet therapy for a minimum of 1 month, but 12 months is recommended.[25] Irrespective of whether a patient has received a coronary stent, an acute MI is a class I indication for dual antiplatelet therapy with aspirin and a thienopyridine.[25] Aspirin should be continued indefinitely, and the recommended dose depends on whether the patient received a stent and the type of stent.[25] A minimum of 14 days of clopidogrel is recommended for patients who have not received a coronary stent.[25]

Thus, patients with acute MI complicated by AF have class I indications for so-called triple antithrombotic therapy with aspirin, a thienopyridine, and a vitamin K antagonist. A Swedish cohort study of patients with both acute MI and AF provided somewhat reassuring evidence that oral anticoagulant therapy, compared with antiplatelet therapy, was associated with a reduction in death due to stroke or ischemic heart disease, but there were no data regarding the effects of triple antithrombotic therapy on outcomes.[26] Compared with monotherapy or dual therapy, triple therapy with aspirin, clopidogrel, and a vitamin K antagonist poses an increased risk of bleeding complications.[27] The annual incidence of hospitalization for bleeding was 12% among a registry of 40 812 patients who were followed up for a mean of 476.5 days post-MI.[27] The corresponding rates of hospitalization for bleeding were 3.7% for aspirin plus clopidogrel and 4.3% for a vitamin K antagonist alone.[27] The current American College of Cardiology/American Heart Association guidelines for the management of acute MI recommend lower doses of aspirin (75-81 mg) and warfarin (target international normalized ratio of 2.0-2.5) when triple antithrombotic therapy is indicated.[25] Future studies will be needed to address the risk-benefit ratio of combining aspirin, a thienopyridine, and an oral direct thrombin inhibitor, such as dabigatran,[28,29] in patients with acute MI and AF.

S. W. Werns, MD

References

1. Crenshaw BS, Ward SR, Granger CB, Stebbins AL, Topol EJ, Califf RM. Atrial fibrillation in the setting of acute myocardial infarction: the GUSTO-I experience. Global Utilization of Streptokinase and TPA for Occluded Coronary Arteries. *J Am Coll Cardiol.* 1997;30:406-413.

2. Wong CK, White HD, Wilcox RG, et al. New atrial fibrillation after acute myocardial infarction independently predicts death: the GUSTO-III experience. *Am Heart J.* 2000;140:878-885.

3. Pederson OD, Baggert H, Kober L, Torp-Pedersen C. The occurrence and prognostic significance of atrial fibrillation/-flutter following acute myocardial infarction. TRACE Study group. TRAndolapril Cardiac Evalution. *Eur Heart J.* 1999; 20:748-754.

4. Lehto M, Snapinn S, Dickstein K, Swedberg K, Nieminen MS. Prognostic risk of atrial fibrillation in acute myocardial infraction complicated by left ventricular dysfunction: the OPTIMAAL experience. *Eur Heart J.* 2005;26:350-356.

5. Schmitt J, Duray G, Gersh BJ, Hohnloser SH. Atrial fibrillation in acute myocardial infarction: a systematic review of the incidence, clinical features and prognostic implications. *Eur Heart J.* 2009;30:1038-1045.

6. Lopes RD, Elliott LE, White HD, et al. Antithrombotic therapy and outcomes of patients with atrial fibrillation following primary percutaneous coronary intervention: result from the APEX-AMI trial. *Eur Heart J.* 2009;30:2019-2028.

7. Wong C-K, White HD, Wilcox RG, et al. Management and outcome of patients with atrial fibrillation during acute myocardial infarction: the GUSTO-III experience. Global use of strategies to open occluded coronary arteries. *Heart.* 2002;88: 357-362.

8. Thomas KL, Al-Khatib SM, Lokhnygina Y, et al. Amiodarone use after acute myocardial infarction complicated by heart failure and/or left ventricular dysfunction may be associated with excess mortality. *Am Heart J.* 2008;155: 87-93.

9. Julian DG, Camm AJ, Frangin G, et al. Randomized trial of effect of amiodarone on mortality in patients with left-ventricular dysfunction after recent myocardial infarction: EMIAT. European Myocardial Infarct Amiodarone Trial Investigators. *Lancet.* 1997;349:667-674.

10. Echt DS, Liebson PR, Mitchell LB, et al. Mortality and morbidity in patients receiving encainide, flecainide, or placebo. The Cardiac Arrhythmia Suppression Trial. *N Engl J Med.* 1991;324:781-788.

11. Effect of the antiarrhythmic agent moricizine on survival after myocardial infarction. The Cardiac Arrhythmia Suppression Trial II Investigators. *N Engl J Med.* 1992;327:227-233.

12. Waldo AL, Camm AJ, deRuyter H, et al. Effect of d-sotalol on mortality in patients with left ventricular dysfunction after recent and remote myocardial infarction. The SWORD Investigators. Survival With Oral d-Sotalol. *Lancet.* 1996;348:7-12.

13. Sanderson J. The SWORD of Damocles. *Lancet.* 1996;348:2-3.

14. Kober L, Thomsen PE, Møller M, et al. Effect of dofetilide in patients with recent myocardial infarction and left-ventricular dysfunction: a randomized trial. *Lancet.* 2000;356:2052-2058.

15. Siu C-W, Lau C-P, Lee W-L, Lam K-F, Tse H-F. Intravenous diltiazem is superior to intravenous amiodarone or digoxin for achieving ventricular rate control in patients with acute uncomplicated atrial fibrillation. *Crit Care Med.* 2009;37: 2174-2179.

16. The effect of diltiazem on mortality and reinfarction after myocardial infarction. The Multicenter Diltiazem Postinfarction Trial Research Group. *N Engl J Med.* 1988;319:385-392.

17. Spargias KS, Hall AS, Ball SG. Safety concerns about digoxin after acute myocardial infarction. *Lancet.* 1999;354:391-392.

18. Freemantle N, Cleland J, Young P, Mason J, Harrison J. β Blockade after myocardial infarction: systematic review and meta regression analysis. *BMJ.* 1999;318: 1730-1737.

19. Dargie HJ. Effect of carvedilol on outcome after myocardial infarction in patients with left-ventricular dysfunction: the CAPRICORN randomised trial. *Lancet.* 2001;357:1385-1390.

20. The ACTIVE Writing Group on behalf of the ACTIVE Investigators. Clopidogrel plus aspirin versus oral anticoagulation for atrial fibrillation in the Atrial fibrillation Clopidogrel Trial with Irbesartan for prevention of Vascular Events (ACTIVE W): a randomised controlled trial. *Lancet.* 2006;367:1903-1912.
21. Hart RG, Pearce LA, Aguilar MI. Meta-analysis: antithrombotic therapy to prevent stroke in patients who have nonvalvular atrial fibrillation. *Ann Intern Med.* 2007;146:857-867.
22. Fuster V, Ryden LE, Cannom DS, et al. ACC/AHA/ESC 2006 guidelines for the management of patients with atrial fibrillation-executive summary: a report of the American College of Cardiology/American Heart Association Task Force on Practice Guidelines and the European Society of Cardiology Committee for Practice Guidelines. *Circulation.* 2006;114:700-752.
23. Schömig A, Neumann F-J, Kastrati A, et al. A randomized comparison of antiplatelet and anticoagulant therapy after the placement of coronary-artery stents. *N Engl J Med.* 1996;334:1084-1089.
24. Leon MB, Baim DS, Popma JJ, et al. A clinical trial comparing three antithrombotic-drug regimens after coronary-artery stenting. Stent Anticoagulation Restenosis Study Investigators. *N Engl J Med.* 1998;339:1665-1671.
25. Antman EM, Hand M, Armstrong PW, et al. 2007 focused update of the ACC/AHA 2004 guidelines for the management of patients with ST-elevation myocardial infarction: a report of the American College of Cardiology/American Heart Association Task Force on Practice Guidelines. *J Am Coll Cardiol.* 2008; 51:210-247.
26. Stenestrand U, Lindbäck J, Wallentin L, RIKS-HIA Registry. Anticoagulation therapy in atrial fibrillation in combination with acute myocardial infarction influences long-term outcome. a prospective cohort study from the Register of Information and Knowledge About Swedish Heart Intensive Care Admissions (RIKS-HIA). *Circulation.* 2005;112:3225-3231.
27. Sørensen R, Hansen ML, Abildstrom SZ, et al. Risk of bleeding in patients with acute myocardial infarction treated with different combinations of aspirin, clopidogrel, and vitamin K antagonists in Denmark: a retrospective analysis of nationwide registry data. *Lancet.* 2009;374:1967-1974.
28. Connolly SJ, Ezekowitz MD, Yusuf S, et al. Dabigatran versus warfarin in patients with atrial fibrillation. *N Engl J Med.* 2009;361:1139-1151.
29. Wallentin L, Yusuf S, Ezekowitz MD, et al. Efficacy and safety of dabigatran compared with warfarin at different levels of international normalised ratio control for stroke prevention in atrial fibrillation: an analysis of the RE-LY trial. *Lancet.* 2010;376:975-983.

aVR ST elevation: an important but neglected sign in ST elevation acute myocardial infarction

Wong C-K, for the HERO-2 Investigators (Univ of Otago, Dunedin, New Zealand; et al)
Eur Heart J 31:1845-1853, 2010

Aim.—This study evaluated the prognostic implications of aVR ST elevation during ST elevation acute myocardial infarction (AMI).

Methods and Results.—The Hirulog and Early Reperfusion/Occlusion-2 study randomized 17 073 patients with acute ST elevation AMI within 6 h of symptom onset to receive either bivalirudin or heparin, in addition to streptokinase and aspirin. The treatments had no effect on the primary endpoint of 30-day mortality. Electrocardiographic recordings were performed at randomization and at 60 min after commencing streptokinase. aVR ST elevation ≥1 mm was associated with higher 30-day mortality in 15 315 patients with normal intraventricular conduction regardless of AMI location (14.7% vs. 11.2% for anterior AMI, $P = 0.0045$ and 16.0% vs. 6.4% for inferior AMI, $P < 0.0001$). After adjusting for summed ST elevation and ST depression in other leads, associations with higher mortality were found with aVR ST elevation of ≥1.5 mm for anterior [odds ratio 1.69 (95% CI 1.16 to 2.45)] and of ≥1 mm for inferior AMI [odds ratio 2.41 (95% CI 1.76 to 3.30)]. There was a significant interaction between aVR ST elevation and infarct location. Thirty-day mortality was similar with anterior and inferior AMI when aVR ST elevation was present (11.5% vs. 13.2%, respectively, $P = 0.51$ with 1 mm and 23.5% vs. 22.5% respectively, $P = 0.84$ with ≥ 1.5 mm ST elevation). After fibrinolytic therapy, resolution of ST elevation in aVR to <1 mm was associated with lower mortality, while new ST elevation ≥1 mm was associated with higher mortality.

Conclusion.—aVR ST elevation is an important adverse prognostic sign in AMI.

▶ The 12-lead electrocardiogram (ECG) provides a variety of diagnostic and prognostic information in patients with acute coronary syndrome (ACS) or acute myocardial infarction (MI).[1] The presence of Q waves in the infarct territory on the initial ECG is an independent predictor of greater 30-day and 90-day mortality, even in patients without a previous MI.[2,3] The number of leads with ST-segment elevation correlates with in-hospital mortality.[4] The degree that ST-segment elevation resolves after either fibrinolytic therapy or primary percutaneous coronary intervention (PCI) correlates with the extent of microvascular perfusion and myocardial salvage, the recovery of regional wall motion, and both short-term and long-term mortality.[5-9] Less than 50% resolution of ST-segment elevation (in the lead showing the worst initial elevation) 90 minutes after fibrinolytic therapy is a class IIa indication for coronary angiography with intent to perform PCI.[10]

The location and magnitude of ST-segment depression or elevation are important determinants of risk assessment and management in patients with ST-segment elevation MI (STEMI). According to the current American College of Cardiology/American Heart Association practice guidelines for STEMI, ≥2 mm of ST elevation in ≥2 leads in patients with anterior MI is a class IIa indication to transfer patients to a PCI-capable facility after administration of fibrinolytic therapy at a non–PCI-capable facility.[11] Among patients with an acute inferior STEMI, ST-segment depression in the precordial leads is associated with larger infarctions, more frequent complications, and a higher mortality rate.[12] ST-segment elevation in lead V4R is diagnostic of right ventricular MI and an independent predictor of major complications and in-hospital death among patients with acute inferior MI.[13] Therefore, the presence of ≥2 mm of ST depression in the anterior leads or ≥1 mm of ST elevation in V4R in patients with an inferior MI are class IIa indications to transfer patients to a PCI-capable facility after administration of fibrinolytic therapy at a non–PCI-capable facility.[11]

The study by Wong et al is an important reminder that ST-segment elevation in lead aVR, a lead that is frequently overlooked, carries important prognostic information. An earlier study by Engelen et al[14] concluded that ST-elevation in lead aVR is one of several electrocardiographic indicators of occlusion of the left anterior descending coronary artery proximal to the first septal branch in patients with acute anterior MI. A subsequent study found that ST elevation in aVR equal to or greater than ST elevation in V1 is associated with acute occlusion of the left main coronary artery.[15] Barrabes et al[16] analyzed the ECGs of 775 patients with a first acute MI and either no ST-segment elevation or ST-segment elevation confined to leads aVR and/or V1. ST-segment elevation in lead aVR on the initial ECG was the only independent electrocardiographic predictor of in-hospital death.[16] The adjusted odds ratio for in-hospital death was 6.6 (95% confidence interval 2.5-17.6) for the patients with ≥0.1 mV of ST-segment elevation in aVR (n = 134) compared with the patients without ST-segment elevation in aVR (n = 525). The prevalence of left main or 3-vessel disease was 66% among patients with ≥0.1 mV of ST-segment elevation in aVR, compared with 22% among patients without ST-segment elevation in aVR ($P < .001$).[16] Thus, patients with an ACS or an acute MI who have ST-segment elevation in aVR represent a high-risk group that should be managed accordingly.

S. W. Werns, MD

References

1. Zimetbaum PJ, Josephson ME. Use of the electrocardiogram in acute myocardial infarction. *N Engl J Med*. 2003;348:933-940.
2. Wong C-K, Gao W, Raffel OC, French JK, Stewart RA, White HD. Initial Q waves accompanying ST-segment elevation at presentation of acute myocardial infarction and 30-day mortality in patients given streptokinase therapy: an analysis from HERO-2. *Lancet*. 2006;367:2061-2067.
3. Armstrong PW, Fu Y, Westerhout CM, et al. Baseline Q-wave surpasses time from symptom onset as a prognostic marker in ST-segment elevation myocardial infarction patients treated with primary percutaneous coronary intervention. *J Am Coll Cardiol*. 2009;53:1503-1509.
4. Mauri F, Gasparini M, Barbonaglia L, et al. Prognostic significance of the extent of myocardial injury in acute myocardial infarction treated by streptokinase (the GISSI trial). *Am J Cardiol*. 1989;63:1291-1295.
5. Andrews J, Straznicky IT, French JK, et al. ST-Segment recovery adds to the assessment of TIMI 2 and 3 flow in predicting infarct wall motion after thrombolytic therapy. *Circulation*. 2000;101:2138-2143.
6. Dong J, Ndrepepa G, Schmitt C, et al. Early resolution of ST-segment elevation correlates with myocardial salvage assessed by Tc-99m sestamibi scintigraphy in patients with acute myocardial infarction after mechanical or thrombolytic reperfusion therapy. *Circulation*. 2002;105:2946-2949.
7. Santoro GM, Valenti R, Bounamici P, et al. Relation between ST-segment changes and myocardial perfusion evaluated by myocardial contrast echocardiography in patients with acute myocardial infarction treated with direct angioplasty. *Am J Cardiol*. 1998;82:932-937.
8. van't Hof AW, Liem A, de Boer MJ, Zijlstra F. Clinical value of 12-lead electrocardiogram after successful reperfusion therapy for acute myocardial infarction. Zwolle Myocardial Infarction Study Group. *Lancet*. 1997;350:615-619.
9. Anderson RD, White HD, Ohman EM, et al. Predicting outcome after thrombolysis in acute myocardial infarction according to ST-segment resolution at

90 minutes: a substudy of the GUSTO-III trial. Global Use of Strategies To Open occluded coronary arteries. *Am Heart J.* 2002;144:81-88.

10. Antman EM, Hand M, Armstrong PW, et al. 2007 focused update of the ACC/AHA 2004 guidelines for the management of patients with ST-elevation myocardial infarction: a report of the American College of Cardiology/American Heart Association Task Force on Practice Guidelines. *J Am Coll Cardiol.* 2008; 51:210-247.

11. Kushner FG, Hand M, Smith SC Jr, et al. 2009 Focused Updates: ACC/AHA guidelines for the management of patients with ST-elevation myocardial infarction (updating the 2004 guideline and 2007 focused update) and ACC/AHA/SCAI guidelines on percutaneous coronary intervention (updating the 2005 guidelines and 2007 focused update): a report of the American College of Cardiology Foundation/American Heart Association Task Force on Practice Guidelines. *Circulation.* 2009;120:2271-2306.

12. Peterson ED, Hathaway WR, Zabel KM, et al. Prognostic significance of precordial ST segment depression during inferior myocardial infarction in the thrombolytic era: results in 16,521 patients. *J Am Coll Cardiol.* 1996;28:305-312.

13. Zehender M, Kasper W, Kauder E, et al. Right ventricular infarction as an independent predictor of prognosis after acute inferior myocardial infarction. *N Engl J Med.* 1993;328:981-988.

14. Engelen DJ, Gorgels AP, Cheriex EC, et al. Value of the electrocardiogram in localizing the occlusion site in the left anterior descending coronary artery in acute anterior myocardial infarction. *J Am Coll Cardiol.* 1999;34:389-395.

15. Yamaji H, Iwasaki K, Kusachi S, et al. Prediction of acute left main coronary artery obstruction by 12-lead electrocardiography: ST segment elevation in lead aVR with less ST segment elevation in lead (V1). *J Am Coll Cardiol.* 2001;38: 1348-1354.

16. Barrabés JA, Figueras J, Moure C, Cortadellas J, Soler-Soler J. Prognostic value of lead aVR in patients with a first non-ST-segment elevation acute myocardial infarction. *Circulation.* 2003;108:814-819.

Contraindicated Medication Use in Dialysis Patients Undergoing Percutaneous Coronary Intervention

Tsai TT, for the National Cardiovascular Data Registry (Denver VA Med Ctr, CO; et al)
JAMA 302:2458-2464, 2009

Context.—The US Food and Drug Administration guides clinicians through drug labeling of medications that are contraindicated or not recommended for use in specific patient groups. Little is known about the use of such medications and their effects on outcomes in clinical practice.

Objective.—To investigate the use of the contraindicated/not-recommended agents enoxaparin and eptifibatide among dialysis patients undergoing percutaneous coronary intervention (PCI) and their association with outcomes.

Design, Setting, and Participants.—Data from 829 US hospitals on 22 778 dialysis patients who underwent PCI between January 1, 2004, and August 31, 2008.

Main Outcome Measures.—In-hospital bleeding and death.

Results.—Five thousand eighty-four patients (22.3%) received a contraindicated antithrombotic; of these patients, 2375 (46.7%) received enoxaparin, 3261 (64.1%) received eptifibatide, and 552 (10.9%) received both. Compared with patients who did not receive a contraindicated antithrombotic, patients who did had higher rates of in-hospital bleeding (5.6% vs 2.9%; odds ratio [OR], 1.93; 95% confidence interval [CI], 1.66-2.23) and death (6.5% vs 3.9%; OR, 1.68; 95% CI, 1.46-1.95). After multivariable adjustment, patients receiving contraindicated antithrombotics had significantly higher risks of in-hospital bleeding (OR, 1.66; 95% CI, 1.43-1.92) and death (OR, 1.24; 95% CI, 1.04-1.48). In 10 158 patients matched by propensity scores, receipt of contraindicated antithrombotics remained significantly associated with in-hospital bleeding (OR, 1.63; 95% CI, 1.35-1.98) but not in-hospital death (OR, 1.15; 95% CI, 0.97-1.36).

Conclusions.—In a sample of dialysis patients undergoing PCI, 22.3% received a contraindicated antithrombotic medication. In propensity-matched analysis, receipt of these medications was significantly associated with an increased risk of in-hospital major bleeding.

▶ Patients who have an acute coronary syndrome (ACS) and patients who undergo percutaneous coronary intervention (PCI) are routinely treated with a combination of antiplatelet and antithrombin agents.[1,2] The antiplatelet agents include aspirin, thienopyridines, for example, clopidogrel and prasugrel, and glycoprotein IIb/IIIa inhibitors, for example, eptifibatide, tirofiban, or abciximab. The antithrombin agents include unfractionated heparin, low-molecular weight heparin, for example, enoxaparin, and bivalirudin.

Patients with chronic kidney disease (CKD) have an increased risk of bleeding after PCI,[3,4] an independent risk factor for death.[5,6] Creatinine clearance < 70 mL/min was associated with increased rates of minor and major bleeding and transfusion compared with creatinine clearance ≥70 mL/min among 4623 patients who were treated with a glycoprotein IIb/IIIa inhibitor during PCI.[4]

The elevated risk of bleeding is exacerbated by the increased frequency of excessive dosing of antithrombotic drugs in patients with CKD who undergo PCI.[7,8] Among 33 patients with a creatinine clearance < 50 mL/min who were enrolled in a PCI study, the maintenance infusion of eptifibatide was not adjusted appropriately in 15 patients (45%).[7] Renal insufficiency, defined as a serum creatinine > 2.0 mg/dL, creatinine clearance < 30 mL/min, or need for dialysis, was associated with excess dosing of antiplatelet and antithrombin agents among 30 136 patients who were enrolled in a registry of patients hospitalized for ACS.[8]

Clinical trials have demonstrated that eptifibatide and enoxaparin, either alone or in combination, are safe and effective in patients with ACS and in patients who undergo PCI.[9-12] Both enoxaparin and eptifibatide are cleared from the circulation by the kidneys. Therefore, the doses must be adjusted in patients with CKD, and they are contraindicated or not recommended in patients undergoing dialysis. Nevertheless, among 22 778 patients undergoing dialysis who were enrolled in a PCI registry, 2375 patients (10.4%) received enoxaparin, 3261 (14.3%) received eptifibatide, and 552 (2.4%) received both drugs. After risk adjustment, there was a significant association of enoxaparin with in-hospital major bleeding and death.

It is critical to recognize that enoxaparin and eptifibatide require dose adjustment in patients with CKD and should not be used in patients undergoing dialysis. Bivalirudin was found to cause less bleeding than unfractionated heparin in patients with CKD and may be a better option.[3]

S. W. Werns, MD

References

1. Bonaca MP, Steg PG, Feldman LJ, et al. Antithrombotics in acute coronary syndromes. *J Am Coll Cardiol.* 2009;54:969-984.
2. Desai NR, Bhatt DL. The state of periprocedural antiplatelet therapy after recent trials. *JACC Cardiovasc Interv.* 2010;3:571-583.
3. Chew DP, Bhatt DL, Kimball W, et al. Bivalirudin provides increasing benefit with decreasing renal function: a meta-analysis of randomized trials. *Am J Cardiol.* 2003;92:919-923.
4. Berger PB, Best PJ, Topol EJ, et al. The relation of renal function to ischemic and bleeding outcomes with 2 different glycoprotein IIb/IIIa inhibitors: the do Tirofiban and ReoPro Give Similar Efficacy Outcome (TARGET) trial. *Am Heart J.* 2005;149:869-875.
5. Budaj A, Eikelboom JW, Mehta SR, et al. Improving clinical outcomes by reducing bleeding in patients with non-ST-elevation acute coronary syndromes. *Eur Heart J.* 2009;30:655-661.
6. Mehran R, Pocock SJ, Stone GW, et al. Associations of major bleeding and myocardial infarction with the incidence and timing of mortality in patients presenting with non-ST-elevation acute coronary syndromes: a risk model from the ACUITY trial. *Eur Heart J.* 2009;30:1457-1466.
7. Kirtane AJ, Piazza G, Murphy SA, et al. Correlates of bleeding events among moderate-to high-risk patients undergoing percutaneous coronary intervention and treated with eptifibatide: observations from the PROTECT-TIMI-30 Trial. *J Am Coll Cardiol.* 2006;47:2374-2379.
8. Alexander KP, Chen AY, Roe MT, et al. Excess dosing of antiplatelet and antithrombin agents in the treatment of non-ST-segment elevation acute coronary syndromes. *JAMA.* 2005;294:3108-3116.
9. Bhatt DL, Topol EJ. Current role of platelet glycoprotein IIb/IIIa inhibitors in acute coronary syndromes. *JAMA.* 2000;284:1549-1558.
10. Dumaine R, Borentain M, Bertel O, et al. Intravenous low-molecular-weight heparins compared with unfractionated heparin in percutaneous coronary intervention: quantitative review of randomized trials. *Arch Intern Med.* 2007;167: 2423-2430.
11. Murphy SA, Gibson CM, Morrow DA, et al. Efficacy and safety of the low-molecular weight heparin enoxaparin compared with unfractionated heparin across the acute coronary syndrome spectrum: a meta-analysis. *Eur Heart J.* 2007;28:2077-2086.
12. Goodman SG, Fitchett D, Armstrong PW, Tan M, Langer A. Randomized evaluation of the safety and efficacy of enoxaparin versus unfractionated heparin in high-risk patients with non-ST-segment elevation acute coronary syndromes receiving the glycoprotein IIb/IIIa inhibitor eptifibatide. *Circulation.* 2003;107: 238-244.

Dose Comparisons of Clopidogrel and Aspirin in Acute Coronary Syndromes
The CURRENT–OASIS 7 Investigators (McMaster Univ and Hamilton Health Sciences, Ontario, Canada; Univ Hosp Jean Minjoz, Besançon, France; et al)
N Engl J Med 363:930-942, 2010

Background.—Clopidogrel and aspirin are widely used for patients with acute coronary syndromes and those undergoing percutaneous coronary intervention (PCI). However, evidence-based guidelines for dosing have not been established for either agent.

Methods.—We randomly assigned, in a 2-by-2 factorial design, 25,086 patients with an acute coronary syndrome who were referred for an invasive strategy to either double-dose clopidogrel (a 600-mg loading dose on day 1, followed by 150 mg daily for 6 days and 75 mg daily thereafter) or standard-dose clopidogrel (a 300-mg loading dose and 75 mg daily thereafter) and either higher-dose aspirin (300 to 325 mg daily) or lower-dose aspirin (75 to 100 mg daily). The primary outcome was cardiovascular death, myocardial infarction, or stroke at 30 days.

Results.—The primary outcome occurred in 4.2% of patients assigned to double-dose clopidogrel as compared with 4.4% assigned to standard-dose clopidogrel (hazard ratio, 0.94; 95% confidence interval [CI], 0.83 to 1.06; $P = 0.30$). Major bleeding occurred in 2.5% of patients in the double-dose group and in 2.0% in the standard-dose group (hazard ratio, 1.24; 95% CI, 1.05 to 1.46; $P = 0.01$). Double-dose clopidogrel was associated with a significant reduction in the secondary outcome of stent thrombosis among the 17,263 patients who underwent PCI (1.6% vs. 2.3%; hazard ratio, 0.68; 95% CI, 0.55 to 0.85; $P = 0.001$). There was no significant difference between higher-dose and lower-dose aspirin with respect to the primary outcome (4.2% vs. 4.4%; hazard ratio, 0.97; 95% CI, 0.86 to 1.09; $P = 0.61$) or major bleeding (2.3% vs. 2.3%; hazard ratio, 0.99; 95% CI, 0.84 to 1.17; $P = 0.90$).

Conclusions.—In patients with an acute coronary syndrome who were referred for an invasive strategy, there was no significant difference between a 7-day, double-dose clopidogrel regimen and the standard-dose regimen, or between higher-dose aspirin and lower-dose aspirin, with respect to the primary outcome of cardiovascular death, myocardial infarction, or stroke. (Funded by Sanofi-Aventis and Bristol-Myers Squibb; ClinicalTrials.gov number, NCT00335452.)

▶ The American College of Cardiology/American Heart Association (ACC/AHA) 2007 guidelines for the management of unstable angina/non-ST-elevation myocardial infarction include numerous recommendations regarding antiplatelet therapy.[1] They include class I recommendations to prescribe dual-antiplatelet therapy with both aspirin and clopidogrel, irrespective of whether an initial invasive or initial conservative management strategy is selected. The guidelines do not specify the maintenance dose of aspirin or loading dose of clopidogrel, presumably because there is uncertainty regarding the optimal doses of either drug. The Clopidogrel and Aspirin Optimal Dose Usage to Reduce Recurrent Events-Seventh Organization to Assess Strategies in Ischemic Syndromes (CURRENT-OASIS 7) Trial, the first randomized trial to compare 2 different doses of aspirin in patients with acute coronary syndrome (ACS), was designed to plug this gap in the evidence base.[2,3]

The primary results have been published in 2 complementary articles in the September 2, 2010 issue of *The New England Journal of Medicine* (NEJM) and the October 9, 2010 issue of *Lancet*.[3] The NEJM article presents an analysis of the entire enrollment of 25 086 patients, including patients who did not undergo coronary angiography or percutaneous coronary intervention (PCI), while the *Lancet* article describes a prespecified analysis of the 17 263 patients who underwent PCI.

Among the entire cohort of 25 086 patients, there was no significant difference between the higher dose of aspirin (300-325 mg daily) and the lower dose of aspirin (75-100 mg daily) with respect to the primary composite end point of cardiovascular death, myocardial infarction (MI), or stroke at 30 days. Although the rates of major bleeding were 2.3% for both doses of aspirin, there was significantly less minor bleeding among the patients who received the lower dose of aspirin (4.4% vs 5.0%; hazard ratio 1.13; $P = .04$).

Previously published analyses of the Clopidogrel in Unstable Angina to Prevent Recurrent Events (CURE) trial, however, concluded that lower doses of aspirin are associated with significantly less major bleeding than higher doses.[4-6] The CURE trial randomized 12 562 patients with ACS to aspirin plus clopidogrel 75 mg daily or aspirin plus placebo.[4] The study protocol recommended an aspirin dose of 75 to 325 mg, and the dose was left to the discretion of the local investigator. In both arms of the study, higher doses of aspirin were associated with an increased risk of major bleeding, but clinical event rates were not reduced by higher doses of aspirin. PCI-CURE was a substudy of the CURE trial that consisted of the 2658 patients who underwent PCI.[5,6] A post hoc analysis of the patients who were enrolled in PCI-CURE found that the moderate-dose (101-199 mg) and high-dose ($\geq$200 mg) aspirin groups had similar rates of cardiovascular death, MI, or stroke compared with the low-dose ($\leq$100 mg) aspirin group, but the high-dose aspirin was associated with an increased risk of major bleeding.[5,6]

Four randomized trials of aspirin in patients with non-ST-segment elevation ACS demonstrated a 50% or greater reduction in the risk of death or MI by aspirin doses ranging from 75 mg daily to 1200 mg daily. A prospective, randomized, double-blinded, placebo-controlled multicenter trial demonstrated that an aspirin dose of 75 mg daily significantly reduced the risk of death or MI after 1 year in men with unstable angina or non-Q-wave MI (risk ratio 0.52; 95% confidence interval [CI] 0.37-0.72; $P = .0001$).[7] Coronary angiography was performed only if a patient had incapacitating angina despite antianginal medications. Nevertheless, after follow-up for 12 months, a revascularization procedure was performed less often among patients who were treated with aspirin than among patients who received placebo (43 vs 65; $P = .03$). Among 20 521 patients with ACS who were enrolled in the Global Utilization of Streptokinase and Tissue Plasminogen Activator for Occluded Coronary Arteries IIb and Platelet Glycoprotein IIb/IIIa in Unstable Angina: Receptor

Suppression Using Integrilin Therapy trials, an aspirin dose of 150 mg or greater was associated with a lower risk of MI at 6 months compared with an aspirin dose less than 150 mg (hazard ratio 0.79; 95% CI 0.64-0.98; $P = .03$).[8]

The ACC/AHA/Society for Cardiac Angiography and Interventions 2007 Focused Update for PCI recommended the following aspirin regimens after PCI: 162-325 mg daily for at least 1 month after a bare-metal stent, 3 months after a sirolimus-eluting stent, and 6 months after a paclitaxel-eluting stent, followed by 75-162 mg/day dose indefinitely.[9] The evidence base discussed above suggests that any benefit of higher doses of aspirin remains unproven, while it is clear that higher doses confer an increased risk of bleeding. Bleeding is an independent risk factor for death in patients with ACS.[10-12] Therefore, it is reasonable to conclude that there is no justification to prescribe more than 162 mg of aspirin in patients with ACS who undergo PCI and no more than 75 mg of aspirin in patients who do not undergo PCI.

The enzymatic activities that convert clopidogrel from an inactive prodrug to an active metabolite are reduced in patients with loss-of-function cytochrome P450 alleles, resulting in increased risk of cardiovascular events, including stent thrombosis and death.[13] Also, on November 17, 2009, the Food and Drug Administration issued a public health advisory that concomitant therapy with proton-pump inhibitors may reduce the efficacy of clopidogrel. Increasing the dose is one potential approach to overcoming hyporesponsiveness to clopidogrel. Numerous studies have found that a 600-mg loading dose, compared with a 300-mg loading dose, reduces the risk of major adverse cardiovascular events after PCI without increasing the risk of major bleeding.[14] Therefore, it is uncertain whether the higher maintenance dose of clopidogrel that was administered for 6 days in the CURRENT-OASIS 7 trial provided any additional benefit beyond the 600-mg loading dose. The frequency of major bleeding was greater among the patients who were randomized to the higher dose of clopidogrel. Therefore, it is reasonable to conclude that a 600-mg loading dose of clopidogrel is appropriate in patients with ACS who may undergo PCI, while the 150-mg maintenance dose cannot be recommended. Cytochrome P450 genetic polymorphisms do not affect drug metabolite concentrations, inhibition of platelet aggregation, or clinical event rates in patients treated with prasugrel, another thienopyridine.[15,16] Thus, prasugrel is an alternative to double-dose clopidogrel in patients with ACS who undergo PCI.

S. W. Werns, MD

References

1. Anderson JL, Adams CD, Antman EM, et al. ACC/AHA 2007 guidelines for the management of patients with unstable angina/non-ST-elevation myocardial infarction: a report of the American College of Cardiology/American Heart Association Task Force on Practice Guidelines (Writing Committee to Revise the 2002 Guidelines for the Management of Patients With Unstable Angina/Non ST-Elevation Myocardial Infarction): developed in collaboration with the American College of Emergency Physicians, the Society for Cardiovascular Angiography and Interventions, and the Society of Thoracic Surgeons: endorsed by the American Association of Cardiovascular and Pulmonary Rehabilitation and the Society for Academic Emergency Medicine. *Circulation.* 2007;116:e148-e304.

2. Mehta SR, Bassand JP, Chrolavicius S, et al. Design and rationale of CURRENT-OASIS 7: a randomized, 2 × 2 factorial trial evaluating optimal dosing strategies for clopidogrel and aspirin in patients with ST and non-ST-elevation acute coronary syndromes managed with an early invasive strategy. *Am Heart J.* 2008;156:1080-1088.

3. Mehta SR, Tanguay J-F, Eikelboom JW, et al. Double-dose versus standard-dose clopidogrel and high-dose versus low-dose aspirin in individuals undergoing percutaneous coronary intervention for acute coronary syndromes (CURRENT-OASIS 7): a randomised factorial trial. *Lancet.* 2010;376:1233-1243.

4. Peters RJG, Mehta SR, Fox KA, et al. Effects of aspirin dose when used alone or in combination with clopidogrel in patients with acute coronary syndromes. observations from the Clopidogrel in Unstable angina to prevent Recurrent Events (CURE) study. *Circulation.* 2003;108:1682-1687.

5. Mehta SR, Yusuf S, Peters RJ, et al. Effects of pretreatment with clopidogrel and aspirin followed by long-term therapy in patients undergoing percutaneous coronary intervention: the PCI-CURE study. *Lancet.* 2001;358:527-533.

6. Jolly SS, Pogue J, Haladyn K, et al. Effects of aspirin dose on ischaemic events and bleeding after percutaneous coronary intervention: insights from the PCI-CURE study. *Eur Heart J.* 2009;30:900-907.

7. Wallentin LC. Aspirin (75 mg/day) after an episode of unstable coronary artery disease: long-term effects on the risk for myocardial infarction, occurrence of severe angina and the need for revascularization. Research Group on Instability in Coronary Artery Disease in Southeast Sweden. *J Am Coll Cardiol.* 1991;18:1587-1593.

8. Quinn MJ, Aronow HD, Califf RM, et al. Aspirin dose and six-month outcome after an acute coronary syndrome. *J Am Coll Cardiol.* 2004;43:972-978.

9. King SB III, Smith SC Jr, Hirshfeld JW Jr. 2007 focused update of the ACC/AHA/SCAI 2005 Guideline Update for Percutaneous Coronary Intervention: a report of the American College of Cardiology/American Heart Association Task Force on Practice Guidelines: 2007 Writing Group to Review New Evidence and Update the ACC/AHA/SCAI 2005 Guideline Update for Percutaneous Coronary Intervention, Writing on Behalf of the 2005 Writing Committee. *Circulation.* 2008;117:261-295.

10. Yan AT, Yan RT, Huynh T, et al. Bleeding and outcome in acute coronary syndrome: insights from continuous electrocardiogram monitoring in the Integrilin and Enoxaparin Randomized Assessment of Acute Coronary Syndrome Treatment (INTERACT) trial. *Am Heart J.* 2008;156:769-775.

11. Budaj A, Eikelboom JW, Mehta SR, et al. Improving clinical outcomes by reducing bleeding in patients with non-ST-elevation acute coronary syndromes. *Eur Heart J.* 2009;30:655-661.

12. Mehran R, Pocock SJ, Stone GW, et al. Associations of major bleeding and myocardial infarction with the incidence and timing of mortality in patients presenting with non-ST-elevation acute coronary syndromes: a risk model from the ACUITY trial. *Eur Heart J.* 2009;30:1457-1466.

13. Hulot J-S, Collet J-P, Silvain J, et al. Cardiovascular risk in clopidogrel-treated patients according to cytochrome P450 2C19*2 loss-of-function allele or proton pump inhibitor coadministration: a systematic meta-analysis. *J Am Coll Cardiol.* 2010;56:134-143.

14. Siller-Matula JM, Huber K, Christ G, et al. Impact of clopidogrel loading dose on clinical outcome in patients undergoing percutaneous coronary intervention: a systematic review and meta-analysis. *Heart.* 2010 [published online ahead of print August 23, 2010].

15. Varenhorst C, James S, Erlinge D, et al. Genetic variation of CYP2C19 affects both pharmacokinetic and pharmacodynamic responses to clopidogrel but not prasugrel in aspirin-treated patients with coronary artery disease. *Eur Heart J.* 2009;30:1744-1752.

16. Mega JL, Close SL, Wiviott SD, et al. Cytochrome P450 genetic polymorphisms and the response to prasugrel: relationship to pharmacokinetic, pharmacodynamic, and clinical outcomes. *Circulation.* 2009;119:2553-2560.

Effect of Narcotic Treatment on Outcomes of Acute Coronary Syndromes
Iakobishvili Z, Porter A, Battler A, et al (Tel Aviv Univ, Israel; et al)
Am J Cardiol 105:912-916, 2010

Current guidelines have recommended intravenous narcotics (IVNs) for patients with ST-segment elevation acute coronary syndromes (STEACS) and patients with non-STEACS (NSTEACS), although the safety of IVNs has been challenged. We performed a retrospective analysis of the 30-day outcomes stratified by IVN use among patients enrolled in a national survey, using logistic regression and propensity score analysis. Of the 765 patients with STEACS and 993 patients with NSTEACS, 261 (34.1%) and 97 (9.8%) had received IVNs, respectively. The patients with STEACS who received IVNs were more likely to undergo reperfusion (79.7% vs 55.2%, p <0.0001), received it more rapidly (median 59 minutes vs 70 minutes, p = 0.02), and were more likely to undergo coronary angiography and revascularization. No difference was found in hemodynamic status. The patients with NSTEACS who received IVNs were more likely to present with Killip class II-IV (39.2% vs 10.0%, p <0.001) and to have left ventricular systolic dysfunction (39.0% vs 17.0%, p <0.001). No difference was found in the use of invasive procedures. Using propensity score analysis, of 249 matched STEACS pairs, the rate of 30-day death was lower in the group that had received IVNs (2.4% vs 6.2%, p = 0.04), and this trend persisted after logistic regression analysis (odds ratio 0.40, 95% confidence interval 0.14 to 1.14, p = 0.09). Using propensity score analysis, of 95 matched NSTEACS pairs, no difference was found in the 30-day death rate (2.2% for patients receiving IVNs vs 6.3%, p = 0.16), even after logistic regression analysis (odds ratio 0.56, 95% confidence interval 0.14 to 2.33, p = 0.43). In conclusion, IVNs were commonly used in different scenarios—patients with STEACS were more likely to receive IVNs in the context of prompt reperfusion, and patients with NSTEACS were more likely to receive IVNs in the context of heart failure. In both scenarios, IVN use did not adversely affect the outcomes.

▶ Pain relief is an important goal in patients with acute coronary syndrome (ACS) or acute myocardial infarction (MI). According to the American College of Cardiology/American Heart Association guidelines for the management of patients with ST-elevation MI (STEMI), pain associated with STEMI is a class I indication for intravenous morphine sulfate.[1] Unstable angina or non-ST-segment elevation MI is a class IIa indication for intravenous morphine "if there is uncontrolled ischemic chest discomfort despite NTG, provided that additional therapy is used to manage the underlying ischemia."[2] Although there are no published randomized trials of morphine therapy in patients with ACS or acute MI, registry data have been analyzed and reported.[3,4] Among patients with non-ST-segment elevation ACS who were enrolled in the Can Rapid Risk Stratification of Unstable Angina Patients Suppress Adverse Outcomes with Early Implementation of the ACC and AHA Guidelines registry, the administration of morphine, alone or in combination with nitroglycerin, was associated with an increased in-hospital mortality (odds ratio 1.41, 95% confidence interval 1.26-1.57).[3] The study by Iakobishvili et al[4] is a retrospective analysis of narcotic use in patients with ACS or acute MI, but it provides welcome evidence that intravenous narcotics may not adversely affect outcomes.

S. W. Werns, MD

References

1. Antman EM, Hand M, Armstrong PW, et al. 2007 focused update of the ACC/AHA 2004 Guidelines for the management of patients with ST-elevation myocardial infarction: a report of the American College of Cardiology/American Heart Association Task Force on Practice Guidelines. *J Am Coll Cardiol.* 2008; 51:210-247.
2. Anderson HL, Adams CD, Antman EM, et al. ACC/AHA 2007 guidelines for the management of patients with unstable angina/non-ST-elevation myocardial infarction: a report of the American College of Cardiology/American Heart Association Task Force on Practice Guidelines (Writing Committee to Revise the 2002 Guidelines for the Management of Patients With Unstable Angina/Non ST-Elevation Myocardial Infarction): developed in collaboration with the American College of Emergency Physicians, the Society for Cardiovascular Angiography and Interventions, and the Society of Thoracic Surgeons: endorsed by the American Association of Cardiovascular and Pulmonary Rehabilitation and the Society for Academic Emergency Medicine. *Circulation.* 2007;116:e148-e304.
3. Meine TJ, Roe MT, Chen AY, et al. Association of intravenous morphine use and outcomes in acute coronary syndromes: results from the CRUSADE Quality Improvement Initiative. *Am Heart J.* 2005;149:1043-1049.
4. Iakobishvili Z, Porter A, Battler A, et al. Effect of narcotic treatment on outcomes of acute coronary syndromes. *Am J Cardiol.* 2010;105:912-916.

Impact of Delay to Angioplasty in Patients With Acute Coronary Syndromes Undergoing Invasive Management: Analysis From the ACUITY (Acute Catheterization and Urgent Intervention Triage strategY) Trial

Sorajja P, Gersh BJ, Cox DA, et al (Mayo Clinic and Mayo Foundation, Rochester, MN; Mid Carolina Cardiology, Charlotte, NC; et al)

J Am Coll Cardiol 55:1416-1424, 2010

Objectives.—The aim of this study was to determine the impact of delay to angioplasty in patients with acute coronary syndromes (ACS).

Background.—There is a paucity of data on the impact of delays to percutaneous coronary intervention (PCI) in patients with non–ST-segment elevation acute coronary syndromes (NSTE-ACS) undergoing an invasive management strategy.

Methods.—Patients undergoing PCI in the ACUITY (Acute Catheterization and Urgent Intervention Triage strategY) trial were stratified according to timing of PCI after clinical presentation for outcome analysis.

Results.—Percutaneous coronary intervention was performed in 7,749 patients (median age 63 years; 73% male) with NSTE-ACS at a median of 19.5 h after presentation (<8 h [n = 2,197], 8 to 24 h [n = 2,740], and

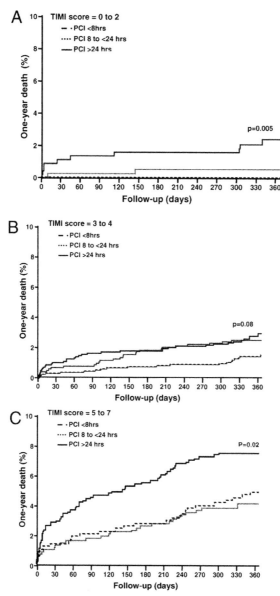

FIGURE 5.—1-Year mortality by patient risk and timing of PCI. Risk for each patient was classified according to Thrombolysis In Myocardial Infarction (TIMI) score (0 to 2 = low, 3 to 4 = intermediate, 5 to 7 = high). **(A)** Low-risk; **(B)** intermediate-risk; **(C)** high-risk. PCI = percutaneous coronary intervention. (Reprinted from Sorajja P, Gersh BJ, Cox DA, et al. Impact of delay to angioplasty in patients with acute coronary syndromes undergoing invasive management. analysis from the ACUITY (Acute Catheterization and Urgent Intervention Triage strategY) Trial. *J Am Coll Cardiol*. 2010;55:1416-1424, with permission from the American College of Cardiology Foundation.)

>24 h [n = 2,812]). Delay to PCI >24 h after clinical presentation was significantly associated with increased 30-day mortality, myocardial infarction (MI), and composite ischemia (death, MI, and unplanned revascularization). By multivariable analysis, delay to PCI of >24 h was a significant independent predictor of 30-day and 1-year mortality. The incremental risk of death attributable to PCI delay >24 h was greatest in those patients presenting with high-risk features.

Conclusions.—In this large-scale study, delaying revascularization with PCI >24 h in patients with NSTE-ACS was an independent predictor of early and late mortality and adverse ischemic outcomes. These findings suggest that urgent angiography and triage to revascularization should be a priority in NSTE-ACS patients (Fig 5).

▶ Early percutaneous coronary intervention (PCI) as an invasive strategy for management of patients with non–ST-segment elevation acute coronary syndromes (NSTE-ACSs) has been shown to improve outcomes and is currently widely accepted as the standard of care.[1] The current recommendations are that angiography be performed within 48 to 72 hours of hospital admission. This is in contrast to the 90-minute standard of care for patients presenting with an ST-segment elevation myocardial infarction (MI). Given that there are little data on exactly when this intervention should take place for the NSTE-ACS patient population, the authors of this article sought to understand the impact of delayed angioplasty and to gain better insight into a more precise time frame for intervention. They assessed the impact of timing of PCI on outcomes in a cohort of patients who were included in a randomized controlled trial (RCT) evaluating the impact of 3 different antithrombotic regimens.[2] The authors provide evidence suggesting that a delay to PCI of > 24 hours in the NSTE-ACS population is associated with increased 30-day and 1-year mortality and combined death or MI and that this hazard of death is greatest in the highest risk patients independent of the antithrombin randomization (Fig 5). It is very important to note that the groups (based on timing of PCI) varied significantly at baseline and with respect to the antithrombin intervention they received. While the authors performed a robust regression analysis to account for the measured differences, there are likely unmeasured confounders as well. For example, the captured baseline characteristics do not tell the whole story as to why a cardiologist elected to perform an early versus late PCI. Perhaps those who had delayed PCI were perceived to be more ill and thus at higher risk of a worse outcome. The authors acknowledge this limitation, in addition to the fact that this was a post hoc analysis of the parent RCT. We agree with the authors that these findings are important and should be considered as hypothesis generating. Based on this study, the current accepted practice of intervention within 72 hours of presentation is potentially putting many patients at increased risk. Future research needs to address the question of the timing of PCI using a well-designed RCT to guide further refinement of care of these high-risk patients.

E. A. Martinez, MD, MHS

References

1. Anderson JL, Adams CD, Antman EM, et al. ACC/AHA 2007 guidelines for the management of patients with unstable angina/non-ST-Elevation myocardial infarction: a report of the American College of Cardiology/American Heart Association Task Force on Practice Guidelines (Writing Committee to Revise the 2002 Guidelines for the Management of Patients With Unstable Angina/Non-ST-Elevation Myocardial Infarction) developed in collaboration with the American College of Emergency Physicians, the Society for Cardiovascular Angiography and Interventions, and the Society of Thoracic Surgeons endorsed by the American Association of Cardiovascular and Pulmonary Rehabilitation and the Society for Academic Emergency Medicine. *J Am Coll Cardiol.* 2007;50:e1-e157.
2. Stone GW, Bertrand M, Colombo A, et al. Acute Catheterization and Urgent Intervention Triage strategY (ACUITY) trial: study design and rationale. *Am Heart J.* 2004;148:764-775.

Incidence and Predictors of Postoperative Deep Vein Thrombosis in Cardiac Surgery in the Era of Aggressive Thromboprophylaxis

Schwann TA, Kistler L, Engoren MC, et al (Mercy Saint Vincent Med Ctr, Toledo, OH; Univ of Toledo – College of Medicine, OH)
Ann Thorac Surg 90:760-768, 2010

Background.—Deep venous thrombosis (DVT) is a well-known complication of surgery but its significance in cardiac surgery is not well defined. We reviewed the results of a prospective observational protocol for repeated postoperative lower extremity duplex venous scans (DVS) screening starting on postoperative day 3-4 through hospital discharge.

Methods.—A total of 1,070 (88%) of the 1,219 overall unique adult cardiac surgery patients at our institution (August 2005 to December 2007) underwent DVS screening. The 149 exclusions included 15 due to early death (1.2%); 39 with a history of preoperative DVT (3.2%) and 93 missed patients (7.6%). All patients underwent maximally aggressive thromboprophylaxis as stipulated by the American College of Chest Physicians Evidence-Based Clinical Practice Guidelines (8th Edition), and complemented with postoperative clopidogrel in coronary artery bypass grafting patients.

Results.—A positive DVS (within 30 days of surgery) for at least 1 lower extremity DVT was observed in 139 of 1,070 eligible patients (DVT: 13.0%). Incidence of DVT was similar in coronary artery bypass grafting (118 of 948; 12.4%) and valve (33 of 237; 13.9%) patients. Hemorrhagic complication requiring reexploration occurred in only 19 patients (1.8%) despite thromboprophylaxis. The DVT cohort showed significantly worse operative (in-hospital or <30 days) mortality (DVT: 9 [6.5%] vs no DVT: 16 [1.7%]; $p < 0.003$), postoperative hospital stay (14.4 ± 12.9 vs 8.3 ± 7.3 days; $p < 0.001$), and 30-day hospital readmissions (20.9% vs 10.3%; $p = 0.001$). Multivariate logistic regression predictors for developing DVT were increased age (odds ratio [OR; 95% confidence interval = 1.24 (1.07 to 1.41) per 10-year increments]), blood transfusion

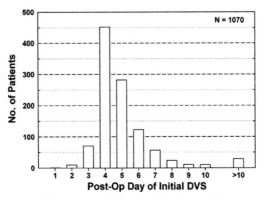

FIGURE 1.—Histogram of the postoperative day at which the initial duplex venous scan (DVS) was performed. (Reprinted from Schwann TA, Kistler L, Engoren MC, et al. Incidence and predictors of postoperative deep vein thrombosis in cardiac surgery in the era of aggressive thromboprophylaxis. *Ann Thorac Surg.* 2010;90:760-768, with permission from The Society of Thoracic Surgeons.)

TABLE 1.—Incidence of DVT and Type of Operation Performed

Operation	Patients N	DVT n	n/N (%)
Overall (N_{ALL})	1,070	139	13.0%
CABG surgery (any)	948	102	10.8%
Isolated CABG	648	77	11.9%
Valve surgery (any)	237	33	13.9%
Isolated valve	75	15	20.0%
CABG + valve (any)	129	16	12.4%
Other surgery	14	4	28.6%

CABG = coronary artery bypass grafting; DVT = deep venous thrombosis.

(OR = 2.24 [1.49 to 3.39]), initial time on the ventilator/prolonged mechanical ventilation (OR = 1.02 [1.01 to 1.04] per 10-hour increments), and need for reintubation (OR = 2.57 [1.48 to 4.47]).

Conclusions.—A considerable number (13%) of cardiac surgery patients develop otherwise silent DVT despite maximal thromboprophylaxis. Aggressive mechanical and pharmacologic thromboprophylaxis in this population appears safe and indicated. Whether routine postoperative DVS screening alters patients' outcomes and is cost effective remains undefined, but should be considered in case of a complicated-prolonged postoperative course (Fig 1, Table 1).

▶ "Thomboprophylaxis often and early!"

The risk is low and the benefit is substantial. Mechanical ventilation time and reintubation offer significant risks for pulmonary embolism. Furthermore, when considering the significant false-negative rate of postoperative leg ultrasound to detect deep venous thrombosis, the take-home message here is even stronger.

R. P. Dellinger, MD

Meta-analysis: Noninvasive Ventilation in Acute Cardiogenic Pulmonary Edema

Weng C-L, Zhao Y-T, Liu Q-H, et al (Peking Univ, Beijing, China; Tsinghua Univ, Beijing, China; First Affiliated Hosp of Xiamen Univ, China)
Ann Intern Med 152:590-600, 2010

Background.—Noninvasive ventilation (NIV) is commonly used to treat patients with acute cardiogenic pulmonary edema (ACPE), but the findings of a recent large clinical trial suggest that NIV may be less effective for ACPE than previously thought.

Purpose.—To provide an estimate of the effect of NIV on clinical outcomes in patients with ACPE that incorporates recent trial evidence and explore ways to interpret that evidence in the context of preceding evidence that favors NIV.

Data Sources.—PubMed and EMBASE from 1966 to December 2009, Cochrane Central Register of Controlled Trials and conference proceedings through December 2009, and reference lists, without language restriction.

Study Selection.—Randomized trials that compared continuous positive airway pressure and bilevel ventilation with standard therapy or each other.

Data Extraction.—Two independent reviewers extracted data. Outcomes examined were mortality, intubation rate, and incidence of new myocardial infarction (MI).

Data Synthesis.—Compared with standard therapy, continuous positive airway pressure reduced mortality (relative risk [RR], 0.64 [95% CI, 0.44 to 0.92]) and need for intubation (RR, 0.44 [CI, 0.32 to 0.60]) but not incidence of new MI (RR, 1.07 [CI, 0.84 to 1.37]). The effect was more prominent in trials in which myocardial ischemia or infarction caused ACPE in higher proportions of patients (RR, 0.92 [CI, 0.76 to 1.10] when 10% of patients had ischemia or MI vs. 0.43 [CI, 0.17 to 1.07] when 50% had ischemia or MI). Bilevel ventilation reduced the need for intubation (RR, 0.54 [CI, 0.33 to 0.86]) but did not reduce mortality or new MI. No differences were detected between continuous positive airway pressure and bilevel ventilation on any clinical outcomes for which they were directly compared.

Limitations.—The quality of the evidence base was limited. Definitions, cause, and severity of ACPE differed among the trials, as did patient characteristics and clinical settings.

Conclusion.—Although a recent large trial contradicts results from previous studies, the evidence in aggregate still supports the use of NIV for patients with ACPE. Continuous positive airway pressure reduces mortality more in patients with ACPE secondary to acute myocardial ischemia or infarction.

▶ Why would continuous positive airway pressure (CPAP) positive end-expiratory pressure (PEEP) be a good therapeutic match for the pathophysiology of acute cardiac pulmonary edema?

1. Increases in intrathoracic pressure will:
   a. Decrease venous return, decrease pulmonary capillary pressure, and decrease lung water and hypoxemia.
   b. Decrease left ventricular afterload thereby decreasing cardiac work and increasing stroke volume.
2. PEEP will present edematous lung from collapsing at end expiration and improve lung compliance and oxygenation.
3. Add noninvasive ventilation (NIV) and you decrease work of breathing.

Downsides of CPAP on NIV? I can't think of any. I use NIV as a personal preference with severe acute cardiac pulmonary edema.

R. P. Dellinger, MD

Transfusion and mortality in patients with ST-segment elevation myocardial infarction treated with primary percutaneous coronary intervention

Jolicœur EM, for the APEX-AMI Investigators (Duke Clinical Res Inst, Durham, NC; et al)

Eur Heart J 30:2575-2583, 2009

Aims.—Red blood cell transfusion is associated with increased mortality among patients with acute coronary syndromes, but little is known about the consequences of transfusion in a contemporary setting of ST-segment elevation myocardial infarction. We describe the association between transfusion and 90-day mortality among patients with acute myocardial infarction treated with primary percutaneous coronary intervention.

Methods and Results.—Analyses were performed on 5532 patients with ST-elevation myocardial infarction from the Assessment of Pexelizumab in Acute Myocardial Infarction trial. The primary objective of this analysis was to ascertain the relation between red blood cell transfusion and 90-day mortality in patients with recent myocardial infarction. We initially determined the baseline and in-hospital predictors of transfusion (multivariable logistic regressions) and subsequently assessed the association between transfusion and mortality using a series of Cox proportional hazards regression combined to a landmark analyses. A total of 213 patients (3.9%) received a transfusion. Transfusion remained significantly associated with mortality [hazards ratio = 2.16 (1.20–3.88)], despite adjustment for baseline characteristics, in-hospital co-interventions, and for propensity of receiving a transfusion. Among patients who survived to hospital discharge, however, the hazard of death was not different in patients treated with transfusion.

Conclusion.—Transfusion is associated with 90-day mortality in acute myocardial infarction treated with primary percutaneous coronary intervention. Although transfusion may be causally related to mortality, it is likely that at least part of the association is due to confounding. This association illustrates the complex relationship between transfusion, bleeding, and mortality and underscores the need for further research to understand the relationship between transfusion and clinical outcomes.

▶ Anemia is common in patients with chronic heart failure, and it is associated with increased mortality.[1,2] A meta-analysis of 34 studies found that 37% of patients with chronic heart failure were anemic.[2] Patients with anemia had an increased risk of mortality (adjusted hazard ratio 0.46; 95% confidence interval [CI] 1.26-1.69; *P* < .001).[2] Among 5010 patients with acute myocardial infarction (MI) complicated by heart failure, 9.3% were anemic at baseline, and among patients who were not anemic at baseline, 10% were anemic after 1 year of follow-up.[3] A hematocrit of 39% or lower was present among 43.4% of 78 974 Medicare beneficiaries 65 years old or older, who were hospitalized with acute MI.[4] Both anemia[3,5,6] and bleeding[7-11] have been shown to be correlated with adverse events, including death, in patients with acute coronary syndromes (ACS) or MI.

Despite the evidence that anemia and bleeding are associated with adverse outcomes in patients with ischemic heart disease, the use of red blood cell transfusion is somewhat controversial because there are conflicting data regarding the impact of red blood cell transfusions on the outcomes of patients with ACS or MI.[12,13] Wu's[4] retrospective study of 78 974 Medicare beneficiaries with acute MI found that blood transfusion was associated with lower short-term mortality if the admission hematocrit was 30% or lower. Additional studies, however, have suggested that blood transfusion may have adverse effects in patients with ACS or MI.[14-18] Among 24 112 enrollees in 3 large clinical trials of patients with ACS, blood transfusion was associated with higher 30-day mortality.[14] Interestingly, an analysis of 39 922 patients with ACS concluded that transfusion was associated with opposite effects in patients with ST-segment elevation MI (STEMI) and patients with non-STEMI (NSTEMI).[5] Among patients with NSTEMI, transfusion was associated with an increased risk of a composite clinical end point (cardiovascular death, MI, and recurrent ischemia). Among patients with STEMI, however, transfusion was associated with a decreased risk of cardiovascular death when the baseline hemoglobin was < 12 g/dL (adjusted odds ratio 0.42; 95% CI 0.20-0.89) but not when the baseline hemoglobin was ≥12 g/dL (adjusted odds ratio 1.42; 95% CI 0.94-2.17).

Jolicoeur et al analyzed the relationship between red blood cell transfusion and 90-day mortality among 5532 patients who underwent primary percutaneous coronary intervention for STEMI. After multivariable adjustment, blood transfusion was an independent predictor of mortality at 90 days (hazard ratio 2.21; 95% CI 1.32-2.99).

Although the preponderance of evidence indicates that transfusion has an adverse effect on outcome in patients with ACS or MI, bleeding is a factor that confounds the association between transfusion and mortality. Therefore, a randomized controlled trial is needed to confirm that association between transfusion and mortality. Given the existing data regarding transfusions, strategies that reduce the risk of bleeding bear consideration. They include cardiac catheterization from the radial artery rather than the femoral artery and the use of bivalirudin or fondaparinux instead of unfractionated heparin.

S. W. Werns, MD

References

1. Anand IS. Anemia and chronic heart failure: implications and treatment options. *J Am Coll Cardiol.* 2008;52:501-511.
2. Groenveld HF, Januzzi JL, Damman K. Anemia and mortality in heart failure patients: a systematic review and meta-analysis. *J Am Coll Cardiol.* 2008;52:818-827.
3. Anker SD, Voors A, Okonko D, et al. Prevalence, incidence, and prognostic value of anaemia in patients after an acute myocardial infarction: data from the OPTI-MAAL trial. *Eur Heart J.* 2009;30:1331-1339.
4. Wu W-C, Rathore SS, Wang Y, Radford MJ, Krumholz HM. Blood transfusion in elderly patients with acute myocardial infarction. *N Engl J Med.* 2001;345:1230-1236.
5. Sabatine MS, Morrow DA, Giugliano RP, et al. Association of hemoglobin levels with clinical outcomes in acute coronary syndromes. *Circulation.* 2005;111:2042-2049.
6. Hasin T, Sorkin A, Markiewicz W, Hammerman H, Aronson D. Prevalence and prognostic significance of transient, persistent, and new-onset anemia after acute myocardial infarction. *Am J Cardiol.* 2009;104:486-491.
7. Rao SV, O'Grady K, Pieper KS, et al. Impact of bleeding severity on clinical outcomes among patients with acute coronary syndromes. *Am J Cardiol.* 2005;96:1200-1206.
8. Eikelboom JW, Mehta SR, Anand SS, Xie C, Fox KA, Yusuf S. Adverse impact of bleeding on prognosis in patients with acute coronary syndromes. *Circulation.* 2006;114:774-782.
9. Manoukian SV, Feit F, Mehran R, et al. Impact of major bleeding on 30-day mortality and clinical outcomes in patients with acute coronary syndromes: an analysis from the ACUITY Trial. *J Am Coll Cardiol.* 2007;49:1362-1368.
10. Budaj A, Eikelboom JW, Mehta SR, et al. Improving clinical outcomes by reducing bleeding in patients with non-ST-elevation acute coronary syndromes. *Eur Heart J.* 2009;30:655-661.
11. Mehran R, Pocock SJ, Stone GW, et al. Association of major bleeding and myocardial infarction with the incidence and timing of mortality in patients presenting with non-ST-elevation acute coronary syndromes: a risk model from the ACUITY trial. *Eur Heart J.* 2009;30:1457-1466.
12. Rao SV, Eikelboom JA, Granger CB, Harrington RA, Califf RM, Bassand JP. Bleeding and blood transfusion issues in patients with non-ST-segment elevation acute coronary syndromes. *Eur Heart J.* 2007;28:1193-1204.
13. Gerber DR. Transfusion of packed red blood cells in patients with ischemic heart disease. *Crit Care Med.* 2008;36:1068-1074.
14. Rao SV, Jollis JG, Harrington RA, et al. Relationship of blood transfusion and clinical outcomes in patients with acute coronary syndromes. *JAMA.* 2004;292:1555-1562.
15. Yang X, Alexander KP, Chen AY, et al. The implications of blood transfusions for patients with non-ST-segment elevation acute coronary syndromes: results from the CRUSADE National Quality Improvement Initiative. *J Am Coll Cardiol.* 2005;46:1490-1495.
16. Singla I, Zahid M, Good CB, Macioce A, Sonel AF. Impact of blood transfusions in patients presenting with anemia and suspected acute coronary syndrome. *Am J Cardiol.* 2007;99:1119-1121.

17. Shishehbor MH, Madhwal S, Rajagopal V, et al. Impact of blood transfusion on short and long-term mortality in patients with ST-segment elevation myocardial infarction. *JACC Cardiovasc Interv.* 2009;2:46-53.
18. Nikolsky E, Mehran R, Sadeghi HM, et al. Prognostic impact of blood transfusion after primary angioplasty for acute myocardial infarction: Analysis from CADILLAC (Controlled Abciximab and Device Investigation to Lower Late Angioplasty Complications) trial. *JACC Cardiovasc Interv.* 2009;2: 624-632.

Pulmonary Embolism/Pulmonary Artery Hypertension

Duration of deep vein thrombosis prophylaxis in the surgical patient and its relation to quality issues

Muntz J (Univ of Texas Health Ctr, Houston)
Am J Surg 200:413-421, 2010

Background.—Venous thromboembolism (VTE) is a major cause of mortality and morbidity in patients after major surgery. The US Acting Surgeon General issued a "call to action" to reduce the number of VTE cases nationwide.

Data Sources.—PubMed literature searches were performed to identify original studies.

Results and Conclusions.—Noncompliance with VTE guidelines is common in clinical practice. Thromboprophylaxis is frequently stopped on discharge, not meeting recommendations for standard-duration prophylaxis (7–10 days) because of shorter hospital stays or for extended-duration prophylaxis (10–35 days). Appropriate pharmacologic prophylaxis options for orthopedic surgery patients include the low–molecular-weight heparins (LMWHs), fondaparinux, or warfarin (10–35 days). For patients undergoing abdominal surgery for cancer, the LMWHs are recommended beyond hospitalization (up to 28 days). Performance measures should help establish VTE-prevention policies that close

TABLE 1.— Published Venous Thromboembolism Prophylaxis Rates Including Levels of Appropriate Prophylaxis in Different Surgical Groups[5,7]

Type of Surgery	Ref	N	Rate of any Prophylaxis, %	Rate of Appropriate Prophylaxis, %
Orthopedic surgery	5	2324	73.2	52.4
	7	4545	96.1	73.8
General surgery*	5	35,124	22.5	12.7
	7	73,921	71.9	31.0
Urologic surgery	5	1388	21.5	9.9
	7	3420	67.3	25.8
Gynecologic surgery	5	9175	8.5	6.7
	7	809	69.1	23.9
Neurosurgery	5	5768	7.1	2.8
	7	3275	74.2	12.4

Editor's Note: Please refer to original journal article for full references.
*At risk of venous thromboembolism (as defined in the 2001 ACCP guidelines).

TABLE 2.— Length of Hospital Stay and Duration of Prophylaxis Recommendations

Type of Surgery	Length of Hospital Stay, d[5]	ACCP-Recommended Duration of Prophylaxis[2]		Duration of Prophylaxis in RCTs Showing Efficacy/Safety of Prophylaxis*	
		Standard	Extended	Standard	Extended
Abdominal Surgery	4.4 ± 6.5	Until hospital discharge[†]	Up to 28 d (high-risk patients; cancer, previous VTE)[†]	7–10	25–31
Orthopedic Surgery	3.9 ± 2.3				
THA		≥10 d	10 d–35 d	7–10	30–42
TKA		≥10 d	10 d–35 d	7–10	30–42
HFS		≥10 d	10 d–35 d	7–10	25–31
Gynecologic surgery	2.0 ± 1.7	Until hospital discharge	Up to 28 d (high-risk patients; cancer, previous VTE)		
Urological surgery	3.9 ± 5.3	Not specified			
Neurosurgery	2.5 ± 4.0	Not specified			

ACCP = American College of Chest Physicians; HFS = hip fracture surgery; RCTs = randomized controlled trials; THA = total hip arthroplasty; TKA = total knee arthroplasty; VTE = venous thromboembolism.
Editor's Note: Please refer to original journal article for full references.
*As defined in references 9, 11, 12, and 25 to 38.
[†]For moderate and higher VTE-risk general surgery.

the gap between guideline recommendations and clinical practice in a greater number of hospitals (Tables 1 and 2).

▶ As individuals who assist in the postoperative management of surgical patients who pass through the intensive care unit (ICU), it is important that we, given the opportunity, assist in assuring that high-risk postoperative patients go home in deep vein thrombosis prophylaxis. This may be most important after major surgery for abdominal cancer because this patient group almost always passes through the ICU.

R. P. Dellinger, MD

Incidence and risk factors for fatal pulmonary embolism after major trauma: a nested cohort study
Ho KM, Burrell M, Rao S, et al (Univ of Western Australia, Australia; Royal Perth Hosp, Western Australia; et al)
Br J Anaesth 105:596-602, 2010

Background.—Venous thromboembolism is common after major trauma. Strategies to prevent fatal pulmonary embolism (PE) are widely utilized, but the incidence and risk factors for fatal PE are poorly understood.

Methods.—Using linked data from the intensive care unit, trauma registry, Western Australian Death Registry, and post-mortem reports, the incidence and risk factors for fatal PE in a consecutive cohort of major trauma patients, admitted between 1994 and 2002, were assessed. Non-linear relationships between continuous predictors and risk of fatal PE were modelled by logistic regression.

Results.—Of the 971 consecutive trauma patients considered in the study, 134 (13.8) died after their injuries. Fatal PE accounted for 11.9% of all deaths despite unfractionated heparin prophylaxis being used in

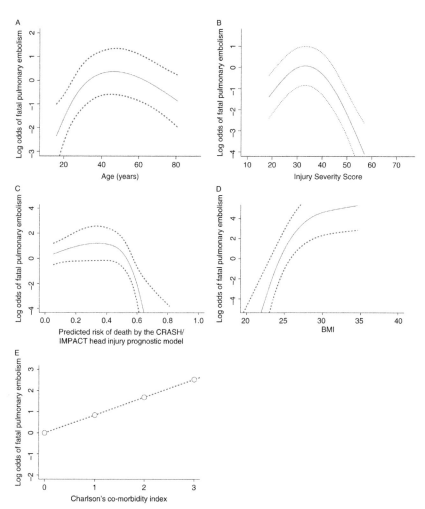

FIGURE 3.—Relationship between risk of fatal pulmonary embolism and (A) age, (B) Injury Severity Score, (C) severity of head injury, (D) BMI, and (E) Charlson's co-morbidity index after adjusting for other covariates (dotted lines signify CI). (Reprinted from Ho KM, Burrell M, Rao S, et al. Incidence and risk factors for fatal pulmonary embolism after major trauma: a nested cohort study. *Br J Anaesth.* 2010;105:596-602.)

44% of these patients. Fatal PE occurred in those who were older (mean age 51- *vs* 37-yr-old, *P*=0.01), with more co-morbidities (Charlson's co-morbidity index 1.1 *vs* 0.2, *P*=0.01), had a larger BMI (31.8 *vs* 24.5, *P*=0.01), and less severe head and systemic injuries when compared with those who died of other causes. Sites of injuries were not significantly related to the risk of fatal PE. Fatal PE occurred much later than deaths from other causes (median 18 *vs* 2 days, *P*=0.01), and the estimated attributable mortality of PE was 49 (95 confidence interval 36–62%).

Conclusions.—Fatal PE appeared to be a potential preventable cause of late mortality after major trauma. Severity of injuries, co-morbidity, and BMI were important risk factors for fatal PE after major trauma (Fig 3).

▶ The take-home message here is that although fatal pulmonary embolism (PE) after major trauma is infrequent, it remains high on the list for potentially preventable death. And at least in this study, it correlates with comorbidities by the Charlson's Index and body mass index. Although inferior vena cava filter might be argued to be a definitive presentation, it is still difficult to narrow target population for insertion. Heparin, intermittent compression (when not contraindicated), and early diagnosis of deep vein thrombosis/PE remain the cornerstones of successful management.

R. P. Dellinger, MD

Delay and misdiagnosis in sub-massive and non-massive acute pulmonary embolism

Alonso-Martínez JL, Sánchez FJA, Echezarreta MAU (Hosp of Navarra, Pamplona, Spain)
Eur J Intern Med 21:278-282, 2010

Background.—There is limited information about the extent and clinical importance of the delay in the diagnosis of acute pulmonary embolism.

Patients and Methods.—Between 1998 and 2009, all consecutive patients diagnosed of acute pulmonary embolism from a registry of a single department were evaluated. We recorded the start or shift in symptoms as the beginning of pulmonary embolism and the mistaken diagnosis for which the patients had been treated. We evaluated the factors associated with the delay and misdiagnosis and their relation with mortality.

Results.—Overall 375 patients were evaluated. Median age was 75 years, interquartile range (IQR) 15, and female 186 (49%). Median delay was 6 (IQR 12) days. Median Wells score was 4.5 (IQR 3).

Delay in diagnosis was longer than 6 days in 50% (95% CI 44–55) of patients, longer than 14 days in 25% (95% CI 21–30) and longer than 21 days in 10% (95% CI 7–13). Misdiagnosis occurred in 50% (95% CI 44–55) of patients. Higher age, more days of delay and the absence of syncope or sudden onset dyspnea were factors associated with misdiagnosis.

Follow-up was carried out in 331 patients during a median of 31 (IQR 45) months. 36% (95% CI 33–43) of patients died [median 8 (IQR 29) months]. Higher age, misdiagnosis and a history of cancer were factors associated with mortality. Days of delay were not associated with mortality.

Conclusions.—Delay and misdiagnosis of pulmonary embolism is frequent. Elderly patients and the absence of syncope or sudden onset dyspnea favour the misdiagnosis. Delay in diagnosis does not participate in mortality.

▶ Previous studies have shown that the underlying cause of the acute respiratory distress syndrome (ARDS) is the most common cause of death among patients who die early in the course of ARDS. In contrast, nosocomial pneumonia and sepsis are the most common causes of death among patients who die later in the clinical course of ARDS. Respiratory failure is an uncommon cause of mortality.[1] It is not surprising to find a higher mortality due to sepsis-induced ARDS, as mortality from severe sepsis is greater than mortality due to other causes of ARDS.

The results of this study are consistent with the observations above. However, this is the first study that gives a comprehensive, direct comparative assessment of mortality in sepsis-related versus nonsepsis-related ARDS.

R. P. Dellinger, MD

Reference

1. Bersten AD, Edibam C, Hunt T, Moran J. Incidence and mortality of acute lung injury and the acute respiratory distress syndrome in three Australian States. *Am J Respir Crit Care Med.* 2002;165:443-448.

Inflammation in right ventricular dysfunction due to thromboembolic pulmonary hypertension

von Haehling S, von Bardeleben RS, Kramm T, et al (Johannes Gutenberg-Univ, Mainz, Germany; Catholic Hosp, Mainz, Germany; et al)
Int J Cardiol 144:206-211, 2010

Objectives and Background.—Activation of the immune system is well established in patients with chronic heart failure (CHF) and impaired left ventricular function. High levels of pro-inflammatory cytokines are associated with a poor prognosis. Chronic thromboembolic pulmonary hypertension (CTEPH) frequently leads to impaired right ventricular function. It is not known whether such patients display chronic immune activation as well.

Methods and Results.—We studied 49 patients with CTEPH (50 ± 2 years, right ventricular ejection fraction [RVEF] 29 ± 2%, left ventricular ejection fraction [LVEF] 51 ± 3%, mean ± SEM) and compared their results with 17 patients with CHF (71 ± 2 years, LVEF

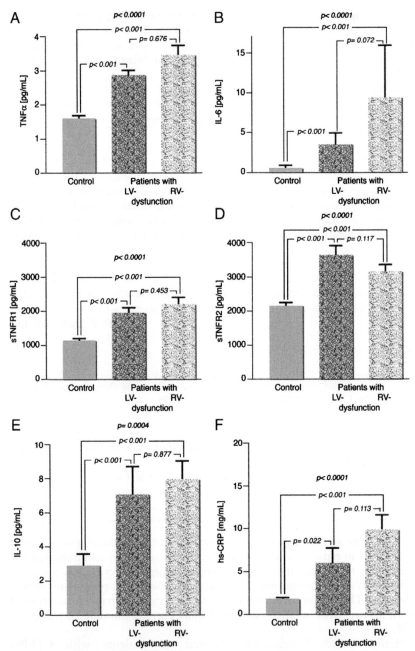

FIGURE 1.—(A–F): Serum levels of inflammatory and anti-inflammatory cytokines in patients with left ventricular (LV) and right ventricular (RV) dysfunction compared with controls. Data are expressed as mean ± SEM. (Reprinted from von Haehling S, von Bardeleben RS, Kramm T, et al. Inflammation in right ventricular dysfunction due to thromboembolic pulmonary hypertension. *Int J Cardiol.* 2010;144:206-211, with permission from Elsevier.)

23 ± 1%) and 34 age-matched control subjects (age 57 ± 2 years). We studied serum levels of tumor necrosis factor-α (TNFα), its soluble receptors 1 and 2 (sTNFR1 and 2), interleukin-10 (IL-10) and plasma N-terminal-pro-B-type natriuretic peptide (NT-proBNP). Serum TNFα was not different in CTEPH compared with CHF patients ($p = 0.67$) but both their levels were significantly higher than in controls (both $p < 0.001$). Similar results were obtained for sTNFR1, sTNFR2, and IL-10. Levels of NT-proBNP were not different in patients with CTEPH or CHF ($p = 0.54$), but significantly higher than in control subjects (both $p < 0.001$). There were significant correlations between RVEF as assessed by magnetic resonance imaging and sTNFR1, sTNFR2, IL-6, high sensitivity C-reactive protein, and NT-proBNP (all $p < 0.05$) in patients with CTEPH.

Conclusion.—Similar levels of immune activation as reflected by high levels of pro-inflammatory cytokines are present in patients with isolated right ventricular dysfunction due to CTEPH and patients with CHF and left ventricular dysfunction (Fig 1).

▶ When organ tissue is assaulted by injurious forces, it has 2 basic options, hibernate or fight. If the tissue chooses to fight and the insult is not amenable to reversal by a proinflammatory response, the end result is likely to be suboptimal. Tumor necrosis factor has long been identified as being associated with cardiac cachexia. This study adds significant elegance to our further understanding of right heart dysfunction due to chronic pulmonary embolism and proinflammation. More important questions are "How damaging is it?" and "Can we ameliorate it with improvement in function?"

R. P. Dellinger, MD

Preoperative Placement of Inferior Vena Cava Filters and Outcomes After Gastric Bypass Surgery

Birkmeyer NJO, for the Michigan Bariatric Surgery Collaborative (Univ of Michigan, Ann Arbor; et al)
Ann Surg 252:313-318, 2010

Objective.—To assess relationships between inferior vena cava (IVC) filter placement and complications within 30 days of gastric bypass surgery.

Summary of Background Data.—IVC filters are increasingly being used as prophylaxis against postoperative pulmonary embolism in patients undergoing bariatric surgery, despite a lack of evidence of effectiveness.

Methods.—On the basis of data from a prospective clinical registry involving 20 Michigan hospitals, we identified 6376 patients undergoing gastric bypass surgery between 2006 and 2008. We then assessed relationships between IVC filter placement and complications within 30 days of surgery. We used propensity scores and fixed effects logistic regression to control for potential selection bias.

Results.—A total of 542 gastric bypass patients (8.5%) underwent preoperative IVC filter placement, most of whom (65%) had no history of venous thromboembolism. The use of IVC filters for gastric bypass patients varied widely across hospitals (range, 0%–34%). IVC filter patients did not have reduced rates of postoperative venous thromboembolism (adjusted odds ratio [OR], = 1.28; 95% confidence interval [CI], 0.51–3.21), serious complications (adjusted OR, = 1.40; 95% CI, 0.91–2.16), or death/permanent disability (adjusted OR, = 2.49; 95% CI, 0.99–6.26). More than half (57%) of the IVC filter patients in the latter group had a fatal pulmonary embolism or complications directly related to the IVC filter itself, including filter migration or thrombosis of the vena cava. In subgroup analyses, we were unable to identify any patient group for whom IVC filters were associated with improved outcomes.

Conclusions.—Prophylactic IVC filters for gastric bypass surgery do not reduce the risk of pulmonary embolism and may lead to additional complications.

▶ This article offers both potentially clinically useful information and a definitely confusing conclusion. The clinically useful information is that there is no support from this registry that would allow hypostasis generation for "IVC filters reduce PE and improve outcome in post-operative bariatric surgery patients." The confusion enters the equation when this patient group still has pulmonary embolism (PE), despite filter placement preoperatively. This is counter to the current assumption that clinically significant PE would occur after filter placement. One must remember that only a prospective trial can truly answer this question. In the interim, with the exception of patients undergoing bariatric surgery with other pre-existing major risk factors for PE or diagnosed previously with PE, patients undergoing bariatric surgery should likely not get prophylaxis.

R. P. Dellinger, MD

Pulmonary Embolism at CT Angiography: Implications for Appropriateness, Cost, and Radiation Exposure in 2003 Patients
Mamlouk MD, vanSonnenberg E, Gosalia R, et al (Univ of California, Irvine, Orange; St Joseph's Hosp and Med Ctr, Phoenix, AZ; et al)
Radiology 256:625-632, 2010

Purpose.—To determine whether thromboembolic risk factor assessment could accurately indicate the pretest probability for pulmonary embolism (PE), and if so, computed tomographic (CT) angiography might be targeted more appropriately than in current usage, resulting in decreased costs and radiation exposure.

Materials and Methods.—Institutional review board approval was obtained. Electronic medical records of 2003 patients who underwent

TABLE 3.—Test Results According to Risk Factors

Total No. of Risk Factors	Total No. of Patients	No. of Patients with Positive CT Angiograms*	Percentage
0	520	5	0.96
1	837	47	5.62
2	484	96	19.83
3	140	39	27.86
4	21	10	47.62
5	1	0	0
6	0	0	...
7	0	0	...
Overall	2003	197	9.84

Note.—$\chi^2 = 202.75$, $df = 5$, $P < .001$.
*Positive CT angiograms are those positive for PE.

TABLE 6.—Multivariate Logistic Regression Analyses and PE Odds Ratios

Risk Factor	Lower 95% Confidence Limit	Odds Ratio Point Estimate*	Upper 95% Confidence Limit	P Value[†]
Immobilization	4.08	5.95	8.68	<.001
Hypercoagulable state	5.94	8.42	11.93	<.001
Malignancy	1.05	1.75	2.90	<.031
Prior PE and/or DVT	3.56	7.56	15.93	<.001
Excess estrogen state	1.77	3.63	7.45	<.001
Age[‡]	1.16	1.67	2.41	<.006
Sex[§]	0.95	1.33	1.86	<.1

*The point estimate is the odds ratio that determines how much more likely a PE is to occur.
[†]A difference with $P < .05$ was considered significant.
[‡]Coded with score 1 for age 65 years or older and score 0 for age younger than 65 years.
[§]Coded with score 1 for male sex and score 0 for female sex.

CT angiography for possible PE during $1\frac{1}{2}$ years (July 2004 to February 2006) were reviewed retrospectively for thromboembolic risk factors. Risk factors that were assessed included immobilization, malignancy, hypercoagulable state, excess estrogen state, a history of venous thromboembolism, age, and sex. Logistic regressions were conducted to test the significance of each risk factor.

Results.—Overall, CT angiograms were negative for PE in 1806 (90.16%) of 2003 patients. CT angiograms were positive for PE in 197 (9.84%) of 2003 patients; 6.36% were Emergency Department patients, and 13.46% were inpatients. Of the 197 patients with CT angiograms positive for PE, 192 (97.46%) had one or more risk factors, of which age of 65 years or older (69.04%) was the most common. Of the 1806 patients with CT angiograms negative for PE, 520 (28.79%) had no risk factors. The sensitivity and negative predictive value of risk factor assessment in all patients were 97.46% and 99.05%, respectively. All risk factors, except sex, were significant in the multivariate logistic regression ($P < .031$).

Conclusion.—In the setting of no risk factors, it is extraordinarily unlikely (0.95% chance) to have a CT angiogram positive for PE. This selectivity and triage step should help reduce current costs and radiation exposure to patients (Tables 3 and 6).

▶ Regardless of clinical presentation, the absence of pre-existing historical risk factors for pulmonary embolism (PE) lowers the chance of positive CT angiography to < 1%. The integration of treating physician pretest clinical probability based on the historical risk factors and clinical findings would either make the possibility of PE even more unlikely (low-risk) or higher (intermediate- or high-risk). Although an independent look at prediction scores based on risk factors only is of academic interest, composite risk scores using both historical risk factors and clinical presentation are likely more practical.

R. P. Dellinger, MD

Pulmonary Embolism in Pregnancy: CT Pulmonary Angiography Versus Perfusion Scanning

Shahir K, Goodman LR, Tali A, et al (Med College of Wisconsin, Milwaukee; et al)
AJR Am J Roentgenol 195:W214-W220, 2010

Objective.—The purpose of this study was to evaluate the equivalence of CT pulmonary angiography and perfusion scanning in terms of diagnostic quality and negative predictive value in the imaging of pulmonary embolism (PE) in pregnancy.

Materials and Methods.—Between 2000 and 2007 at a university hospital and a large private hospital, 199 pregnant patients underwent 106 CT pulmonary angiographic examinations and 99 perfusion scans. Image quality was evaluated, and the findings were reread by radiologists and compared with the original clinical readings. Three-month follow-up findings of PE and deep venous thrombosis were recorded.

Results.—PE was found in four of the 106 patients (3.7%) who underwent CT pulmonary angiography. The overall image quality was poor in 5.6% of cases, acceptable in 17.9%, and good in 76.4%. Fourteen CT and nine radiographic studies showed other clinically significant abnormalities. Six patients had indeterminate CT pulmonary angiographic findings, three had normal perfusion scans, and none underwent anticoagulation. All perfusion scan findings were normal. There was one incomplete study, and follow-up CT pulmonary angiography performed the same day showed PE. Two of 99 studies (2.02%) showed intermediate probability of the presence of PE; PE was not found at CT pulmonary angiography, but pneumonia was found. PE was found in one postpartum patient 9 weeks after she had undergone CT pulmonary angiography and ultrasound with normal findings. None of the patients died.

Conclusion.—CT pulmonary angiography and perfusion scanning have equivalent clinical negative predictive value (99% for CT pulmonary angiography; 100% for perfusion scanning) and image quality in the care of pregnant patients. Therefore, the choice of study should be based on other considerations, such as radiation concern, radiographic results, alternative diagnosis, and equipment availability. Reducing the amount of radiation to the maternal breast favors use of perfusion scanning when the radiographic findings are normal and there is no clinical suspicion of an alternative diagnosis.

▶ Decisions on choosing CT pulmonary angiography (CTPA) versus ventilation/perfusion (V/Q) scanning to diagnose or exclude pulmonary embolism in the pregnant patient are complex. This study supports excellent and similar negative study predictive capability. CTPA increases radiation risk to the breast and V/Q scanning to the fetus, although the fetal radiation exposure with both is very low.[1]

Radiation exposure increases with both procedures as the fetus rises toward the thorax in pregnancy. The incidence of inadequate CTPA studies increases with gestational time.

R. P. Dellinger, MD

Reference

1. Schembri GP, Miller AE, Smart R. Radiation dosimetry and safety issues in the investigation of pulmonary embolism. *Semin Nucl Med.* 2010;40:442-454.

Safety of withholding anticoagulant therapy in patients with suspected pulmonary embolism with a negative multislice computed tomography pulmonary angiography

Galipienzo J, García de Tena J, Flores J, et al (Hosp Universitario Príncipe de Asturias, Alcalá de Henares, Spain; Hosp Universitario de Guadalajara, Spain)
Eur J Intern Med 21:283-288, 2010

Background.—To assess the safety of withholding anticoagulant therapy in patients with clinically suspected pulmonary embolism with a negative multislice computed tomography pulmonary angiography (MCTPA).

Methods.—Three hundred and eighty six patients who were consecutively assessed in the emergency room of our institution for suspected pulmonary embolism were eligible for our study. Patients with either a low or an intermediate clinical probability of pulmonary embolism according to the Wells score and a negative MCTPA for pulmonary embolism were enrolled. Patients with anticoagulant therapy for other medical conditions were excluded from this study. We assessed the percentage of patients in whom venous thromboembolic events or death related to this condition within three months after the negative CT.

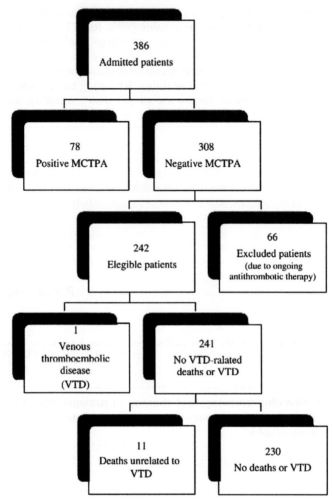

FIGURE 2.—Flow-chart showing the admitted patients, MCTPA findings, venous thromboembolic events and deaths during follow-up. (Reprinted from Galipienzo J, García de Tena J, Flores J, et al. Safety of withholding anticoagulant therapy in patients with suspected pulmonary embolism with a negative multislice computed tomography pulmonary angiography. *Eur J Intern Med.* 2010;21:283-288, with permission from European Federation of Internal Medicine.)

Results.—Two hundred and forty two patients were included in our series [mean age ± standard deviation (SD) (63.1 ± 18.1)]. Only one patient (0.41% [95% confidence interval −0.4%–1.22%]) showed a non-fatal pulmonary embolism during the three-month follow-up period after an initial negative CT scan (negative predictive value, 99.58%). Eleven patients died during the follow-up period due to conditions unrelated to venous thromboembolic disease (pneumonia [$n = 5$], lung cancer [$n = 2$], wasting syndrome [$n = 1$], acute myocardial infarction [$n = 1$], leiomyosarcoma [$n = 1$], and severe pulmonary hypertension [$n = 1$]).

Conclusions.—Withholding anticoagulant therapy in patients with suspected venous thromboembolic disease with a negative result on MCTPA seems to be safe in our clinical setting (Fig 2).

▶ This article adds to existing literature as to the clinical utility of using low-risk Wells score to enhance the sensitivity of a negative test for pulmonary embolism (PE). In this study, it was added to a negative multislice computed tomography pulmonary angiography in emergency department patient evaluations. A previous study demonstrates similar findings with low-risk Wells score combined with negative D-dimer.[1] What is an acceptable percentage of the incidence of false negatives? In this prospective study of 242 patients, less than 0.5% incidence of PE occurred through 3 months' follow-up (confidence interval 0.4-1.22).

R. P. Dellinger, MD

Reference

1. Anderson DR, Kahn SR, Rodger MA, et al. Computed tomographic pulmonary angiography vs ventilation-perfusion lung scanning in patients with suspected pulmonary embolism: a randomized controlled trial. *JAMA*. 2007;298:2743-2753.

3 Hemodynamics and Monitoring

Thenar oxygen saturation measured by near infrared spectroscopy as a noninvasive predictor of low central venous oxygen saturation in septic patients

Mesquida J, Masip J, Gili G, et al (Universitat Autonoma de Barcelona, Sabadell, Spain)
Intensive Care Med 35:1106-1109, 2009

Objective.—To validate thenar oxygen saturation (StO_2) measured by near-infrared spectroscopy (NIRS) as a noninvasive estimation of central venous saturation ($ScvO_2$) in septic patients.

Design.—Prospective observational study.

Setting.—A 26-bed medical-surgical intensive care unit at a university-affiliated hospital.

Patients.—Patients consecutively admitted to the ICU in the early phase of severe sepsis and septic shock, after normalization of blood pressure with fluids and/or vasoactive drugs.

Measurement.—We recorded demographic data, severity score, hemodynamic data, and blood lactate, as well as $ScvO_2$, and StO_2 measured simultaneously on inclusion. Patients were divided into two groups according to $ScvO_2$ values: group A, with $ScvO_2 < 70\%$, and group B, with $ScvO_2 \geq 70\%$.

Results.—Forty patients were studied. StO_2 was significantly lower in group A than in group B (74.7 ± 13.0 vs. 83.3 ± 6.2, P 0.018). No differences in age, severity score, hemodynamics, vasoactive drugs, or lactate were found between groups. Simultaneously measured $ScvO_2$ and StO_2 showed a significant Pearson correlation ($r = 0.39$, P 0.017). For a StO_2 value of 75%, sensitivity was 0.44, specificity 0.93, positive predictive value 0.92, and negative predictive value 0.52 for detecting $ScvO_2$ values lower than 70%.

Conclusions.—StO_2 correlates with $ScvO_2$ in normotensive patients with severe sepsis or septic shock. We propose a StO_2 cut-off value of 75% as a specific, rapid, noninvasive first step for detecting patients with

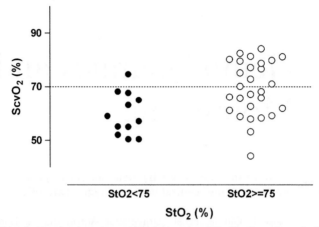

FIGURE 1.—ScvO$_2$ values in patients with high versus low StO$_2$. The figure shows ScvO$_2$ in patients divided into two groups according to the proposed StO$_2$ cut-off value of 75%. (With kind permission from Springer Science+Business Media: Mesquida J, Masip J, Gili G, et al. Thenar oxygen saturation measured by near infrared spectroscopy as a noninvasive predictor of low central venous oxygen saturation in septic patients. *Intensive Care Med* 2009;35:1106-1109.)

low ScvO$_2$ values. Further studies are necessary to analyze the role of noninvasive StO$_2$ measurement in future resuscitation algorithms.

▶ Use of central venous saturation as a measure of adequacy of resuscitation has grown in recent years. Given the invasive nature of such an approach these authors have evaluated a noninvasive approach to see if it correlates with central venous saturation; thus, patients could be spared the incumbent risks of a central line, and a more rapid assessment of adequacy of resuscitation could be obtained as the time to place a central line would be avoided. In addition, such an approach makes the assessment ubiquitously available in the field and limits cost. As can be seen in Fig 1, if the saturation as measured over the thenar eminence by near-infrared spectroscopy was less than 75%, then in (all but one) most patients studied, the central venous saturation was also less than 70%. Unfortunately, numerous limitations exists in this study that preclude extrapolation and thus utility in the clinical environment at present. The Pearson correlation is indeed statistically significant but with a r value of 0.39, significant concern remains. In addition, the poor negative predictive value (0.52) means that almost half of the patients that have a low central venous saturation would be missed by such a monitoring device. Furthermore, this study was conducted after the patients were felt to be adequately resuscitated (average MAP of 79 mmHg); thus, utility during resuscitation was not assessed.

T. Dorman, MD

Tracking Hypotension and Dynamic Changes in Arterial Blood Pressure with Brachial Cuff Measurements

Lakhal K, Ehrmann S, Runge I, et al (Hôpital Bichat-Claude Bernard, Paris, France; Hôpital Bretonneau, Tours, France; Hôpital de La Source, Orléans, France)
Anesth Analg 109:494-501, 2009

Background.—Arterial cannulation is strongly recommended during shock. Nevertheless, this procedure is associated with significant risks and may delay other emergent procedures. We assessed the discriminative power of brachial cuff oscillometric noninvasive blood pressure (NIBP) for identifying patients with an invasive mean arterial blood pressure (MAP) below 65 mm Hg or increasing their invasive MAP after cardiovascular interventions.

Methods.—This prospective study, conducted in three intensive care units, included adults in circulatory failure who underwent 45° passive leg raising, 300 mL fluid loading, and additional 200 mL fluid loading. The collected data were four invasive and noninvasive MAP measurements at each study phase.

Results.—Among 111 patients (50 septic, 15 cardiogenic, and 46 other source of shock), when averaging measurements of each study phase, NIBP measurements accurately predicted an invasive MAP lower than 65 mm Hg: area under the receiver operating characteristic curve 0.90 (95% CI: 0.71–1), positive and negative likelihood ratios 7.7 (95% CI: 5.4–11) and 0.31 (95% CI: 0.22–0.44) (cutoff 65 mm Hg).

For identifying patients increasing their invasive MAP by more than 10%, the area under the receiver operating characteristic curve was 0.95 (95% CI: 0.92–0.96); positive and negative likelihood ratios (cutoff 10%) were 25.7 (95% CI: 10.8–61.4) and 0.26 (95% CI: 0.2–0.34).

Conclusions.—NIBP measurements have a good discriminative power for identifying hypotensive patients and performed even better in tracking MAP changes, provided that one averages four NIBP measurements.

▶ Adequate resuscitation is critical for survival. At present, most of the algorithms for resuscitation focus at achieving a mean arterial pressure (MAP) of 65 mmHg or greater. Clinicians are left to decide if this should be measured invasively or invasively by a standard brachial cuff. This study attempts to address that concern. As can be seen in Fig 1, patients were studied at a variety of MAPs and under a variety of resuscitation conditions. In all cases the brachial cuff on average was sufficient for both basal measurement and measurement of responsivness to an intervention. This is quite comforting and supports using brachial cuff monitoring instead of arterial monitoring for those with no other indication for invasive monitoring. Although some of the patients evaluated were on pressors, many were not. The ability to adequately track pressure at much lower values is not evaluated and thus remains a concern. In addition, these authors studied 2 different invasive devices and compared it with brachial

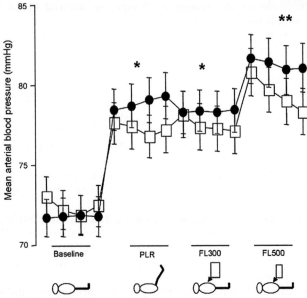

FIGURE 1.—Protocol-induced mean arterial blood pressure changes. Circles represent intraarterial pressure measurements. Squares represent noninvasive oscillometric blood pressure measurements. Bars represent standard errors. PLR = passive leg raising; FL300 = measurements after 300 mL rapid fluid loading; FL500 = measurements after additional 200 mL rapid fluid loading (total volume 500 mL). *$P < 0.05$ for invasive and oscillometric measurements compared with baseline; **$P < 0.05$ for invasive and oscillometric measurements compared with all other study phases. (Reprinted from Lakhal K, Ehrmann S, Runge I, et al. Tracking hypotension and dynamic changes in arterial blood pressure with brachial cuff measurements. *Anesth Analg.* 2009;109:494-501, with permission from the International Anesthesia Research Society.)

pressure in opposite arm and/or femoral arterial pressure. Consequently, the true ability for noninvasive meaurements taken at a variety of sites to track invasive monitoring remains unclear. Of note, the others did find that there is some variability in sequential measurement making averaging across 4 measurements necessary. The time delay in so doing may prove important in those patients with severe perfusion deficits and in those slow to respond to interventions. It would seem prudent to start with noninvasive monitoring for those with mild reductions in blood pressure and for those that respond fairly quickly to interventions to correct perfusion deficits. Thus, invasive monitoring could be avoided in some patients whereas others may very well proceed to invasive monitoring.

T. Dorman, MD

Ultrasound localization of central vein catheter and detection of postprocedural pneumothorax: An alternative to chest radiography

Vezzani A, Brusasco C, Palermo S, et al (Hosp of Parma, Italy; Univ of Genoa, Italy)

Crit Care Med 38:533-538, 2010

Objective.—To determine the usefulness of ultrasound to evaluate central venous catheter misplacements and detection of pneumothorax, thus obviating postprocedural radiograph. After the insertion of a central venous catheter, chest radiograph is usually obtained to ensure correct positioning of the catheter tip and detect postprocedural complications.

Design.—Prospective observational study.

Setting.—Adult intensive care unit.

Patients.—111 consecutive patients undergoing central venous catheter positioning, using a landmark technique and contrast-enhanced ultrasonography.

Measurements and Main Results.—A postprocedural chest radiograph was obtained for all patients and was considered as a reference technique. At the end of the procedure, a B-mode ultrasonography was first performed to assess catheter position and detect pneumothorax. Right atrium positioning was detected in 19 patients by ultrasonography, and an additional six by contrast enhanced ultrasonography. Combining ultrasonography and contrast enhanced ultrasonography yielded a 96% sensitivity and 93% specificity in detecting catheter misplacement. Concordance was 95% and κ value was 0.88 ($p < .001$). Pneumothorax was detected in four patients by ultrasonography and in two by chest radiograph (concordance = 98%). The mean time required to perform ultrasonography plus contrast enhanced ultrasonography was 10 ± 5 mins vs. 83 ± 79 mins for chest radiograph ($p < .05$).

Conclusions.—The close concordance between ultrasonography plus contrast enhanced ultrasonography and chest radiograph justifies the use of sonography as a standard technique to ensure the correct positioning of the catheter tip and to detect pneumothorax after central venous catheter cannulation to optimize use of hospital resources and minimize time consumption and radiation. Chest radiograph will be necessary when sonographic examination is impossible to perform by technical limitations.

▶ Use of ultrasound has become standard in many intensive care units (ICUs) and hospitals for the placement of central access devices. Furthermore, ultrasound is growing in its bedside utility. As this occurs, ultrasound courses are proliferating, and bedside ultrasound appears to be on a trajectory that will land it as one of the most commonly used devices/diagnostic approaches in the critically ill and injured. This study, surprisingly, does not use ultrasound to place central access devices but used it after placement to determine correctness of placement and to look for complications like pneumothorax. The total rate of complications defined as misplaced catheters and pneumothorax is quite high (27%). This is likely because the probe was not used during

TABLE 4.—Concordance Between Ultrasound and Chest Radiograph in Detecting Pneumothorax (n. Patient Examinations = 111; Concordance = 98%)

US	CXR	Positive	Negative
Positive		2	2
Negative		0	107

US, ultrasound examination; CXR, chest radiograph.

placement, and a single length (20 cm) catheter was placed from the right and the left sides. The rates of correlation with chest X-ray for determining these complications were quite high. From Table 4, it can be calculated that the negative predictive value was 98%, and positive predictive value was 50%. Although having a higher positive predictive value would be nice and may be seen when this study is repeated on a larger number of patients, the real issue for such a screening test is its negative predictive value. Given complications occurred so frequently for the reasons previously cited, a larger study is indeed needed where the ultrasound is used during placement and afterward. In addition, care to not place a 20 cm catheter to the hub or use of shorter central catheters from the right side of most patients should be considered as a means to further reduce misplacement from this side.

T. Dorman, MD

Differentiation of Pleural Effusions From Parenchymal Opacities: Accuracy of Bedside Chest Radiography

Kitazono MT, Lau CT, Parada AN, et al (Hosp of the Univ of Pennsylvania, Philadelphia)
AJR Am J Roentgenol 194:407-412, 2010

Objective.—The purpose of this study was to determine, with CT as the reference standard, the ability of radiologists to detect pleural effusions on bedside chest radiographs.

Materials and Methods.—Images of 200 hemithoraces in 100 ICU patients undergoing chest radiography and CT within 24 hours were reviewed. Four readers with varying levels of experience reviewed the chest radiographs and predicted the likelihood of the presence of an effusion or parenchymal opacity on independent 5-point scales. The results were compared with the CT findings.

Results.—All readers regardless of experience had similar accuracy in detecting pleural effusions. Among 117 pleural effusions, 66% were detected on chest radiographs (53%, 71%, and 92% of small, moderate, and large effusions) with 89% specificity. Similarly, 65% of all parenchymal opacities were detected on chest radiographs, also with 89% specificity. Most (93%) of the misdiagnosed pulmonary opacities were simply

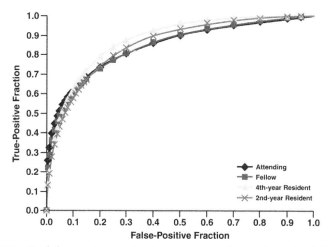

FIGURE 4.—Graph shows receiver operating characteristic curves for detection of pleural effusions of all sizes by readers with varying levels of experience. (Reprinted from Kitazono MT, Lau CT, Parada AN, et al. Differentiation of pleural effusions from parenchymal opacities: accuracy of bedside chest radiography. *AJR Am J Roentgenol.* 2010;194:407-412, with permission from the American Roentgen Ray Society.)

TABLE 2.—Reader Accuracy in Diagnosis of Pleural Effusion

Reader	Sensitivity (%)	Specificity (%)	Area Under ROC Curve
Attending	59 (69/117)	95 (79/83)	0.844
Fellow	62 (72/117)	90 (75/83)	0.843
Fourth-year resident	76 (89/117)	86 (71/83)	0.878
Second-year resident	66 (77/117)	93 (77/83)	0.855
Average	66 (309/468)[a]	89 (295/332)[a]	0.852

Note—Values in parentheses are raw numbers. ROC = receiver operating characteristic.
[a]Total number of effusions multiplied by four readers.

not seen. Meniscus, apical cap, lateral band, and subpulmonic opacity were highly specific findings but had low individual sensitivity for effusions. The finding of homogeneous opacity, including both layering and gradient opacities, was the most sensitive sign of effusion. Atelectasis can occasionally mimic the pleural veil sign of effusion, accounting for most false-positive findings.

Conclusion.—Radiologists interpreting bedside chest radiographs of ICU patients detect large pleural effusions 92% of the time and can exclude large effusions with high confidence. However, small and medium effusions often are misdiagnosed as parenchymal opacities (45%) or are not seen (55%). Pulmonary opacities often are missed (34%) but are rarely misdiagnosed as pleural effusions (7%).

▶ Diagnosis and management of pleural effusions start with recognizing their existence. This article evaluates the ability of a radiologist to identify a pleural effusion versus an infiltrate in the lower lobes using CT as the reference standard. Table 2 and Fig 4 show that all radiology readers had similar receiver operating characteristic (ROC) values for their ability to detect an effusion, and interestingly, the values are fairly homogenous despite a large variation in expertise. Unfortunately, the usefulness of this article in the critical care setting has several important limitations. First, a larger number of each type of radiology reader was needed to better characterize the sensitivity and specificity as these values represent only a single reviewer in this study. Importantly, most X-rays are reviewed and acted upon by the clinical intensive care unit (ICU) team long before a radiologist reviews the film, so this study would have greater applicability if the study participants included ICU physicians. Interpretation was commonly hurt by suboptimal bedside images, and clearly, this can be improved by standardization of body position, distance to the X-ray tube, and the kilovolts the film is taken at, while also trying to ensure that overlying equipment is minimized inside the film window. Finally, the real importance of detecting or missing a pleural effusion or lower lobe infiltrate is the impact on outcome and a future study should include such an assessment as detection of a small and clinically insignificant effusion is simply an unimportant outcome.

T. Dorman, MD

Femoral-Based Central Venous Oxygen Saturation Is Not a Reliable Substitute for Subclavian/Internal Jugular-Based Central Venous Oxygen Saturation in Patients Who Are Critically Ill
Davison DL, Chawla LS, Selassie L, et al (The George Washington Univ Med Ctr, DC)
Chest 138:76-83, 2010

Background.—Central venous oxygen saturation ($Scvo_2$) has been used as a surrogate marker for mixed venous oxygen saturation (Svo_2). Femoral venous oxygen saturation ($Sfvo_2$) is sometimes used as a substitute for $Scvo_2$. The purpose of this study is to test the hypothesis that these values can be used interchangeably in a population of patients who are critically ill.

Methods.—We conducted a survey to assess the frequency of femoral line insertion during the initial treatment of patients who are critically ill. $Scvo_2$ vs $Sfvo_2$ Study: Patients with femoral and nonfemoral central venous catheters (CVCs) were included in this prospective study. Two sets of paired blood samples were drawn simultaneously from the femoral and nonfemoral CVCs. Blood samples were analyzed for oxygen saturation and lactate.

Results.—One hundred and fifty physicians responded to the survey. More than one-third of the physicians insert a femoral line at least 10% of the time during the initial treatment of patients who were critically ill. $Scvo_2$ vs $Sfvo_2$ Study: Thirty-nine patients were enrolled. The mean $Scvo_2$ and $Sfvo_2$ were 73.1% ± 11.6% and 69.1% ± 12.9%, respectively

TABLE 2.—Baseline Demographics and Clinical Characteristics

Variable	Patients (N = 39)
Age, y	63 ± 17.9
Sex, male (female)	22 (17)
Mean arterial pressure, mm Hg	72 ± 12.7
SOFA scores	7.2 ± 4.17
APACHE II scores	18.0 ± 8.23
APACHE II predicted mortality, % average	32.8 ± 22.9
Actual mortality	12
Admitting diagnosis, No. of patients	
Pneumonia or respiratory failure	11
Cardiac arrest or ACS	6
Primary neurologic condition	6
Bacteremia (including endocarditis)	4
GI bleed	3
Surgical conditions	
Intraabdominal process	5
Postoperative valve repair	1
Other[a]	3
Sepsis, No. of patients (%)	11 (28.2)
Septic shock, No. of patients (%)	5 (12.8)

ACS = acute coronary syndrome; APACHE = Acute Physiology and Chronic Health Evaluation; SOFA = Sequential Organ Failure Assessment.

[a]Other diagnoses include acute renal failure, venous thrombosis/superior vena cava syndrome, and urosepsis.

($P = .002$), with a mean bias of 4.0% ± 11.2% (95% limits of agreement: −18.4% to 26.4%). The mean serum lactate from the nonfemoral and femoral CVCs was 2.84 ± 4.0 and 2.72 ± 3.2, respectively ($P = .15$).

Conclusions.—This study revealed a significant difference between paired samples of $Scvo_2$ and $Sfvo_2$. More than 50% of $Scvo_2$ and $Sfvo_2$ values diverged by > 5%. $Sfvo_2$ is not always a reliable substitute for $Scvo_2$ and should not routinely be used in protocols to help guide resuscitation (Table 2).

▶ Adequate resuscitation during any critical illness is important and linked to outcome. Several studies have shown that resuscitation titrated to a central venous oxygen saturation is an important approach for attenuation of mortality. Not all providers have accepted the results of these studies, especially given that the previous work using mixed venous oxygen saturation was not associated with improved mortality. Furthermore, a number of other clinically relevant differences between study groups have called some of these studies into doubt. With that said, many clinicians have avidly used this approach as a component of their early goal-directed therapy. These same physicians, at times, find themselves with a patient who meets the entry criteria they have established for use of an early goal-directed strategy, while having a femoral venous catheter and not a central venous catheter. Thus, if one assumes that indeed a venous saturation is important for resuscitation, then understanding if a femoral value correlates with a central value is clinically relevant. Unfortunately for those who have adopted this practice, this study demonstrates that oxygen saturation values obtained from a femoral catheter do not correlate with central values (Table 2 and Fig 4 in the original article). Consequently, use of the femoral site for management of early goal-directed therapy can be assumed to be supported by the previously published studies. One wonders if lactate clearance might prove adequate from the femoral site as a replacement for oxygen saturation.

T. Dorman, MD

How much of the intraaortic balloon volume is displaced toward the coronary circulation?

Kolyva C, Pantalos GM, Pepper JR, et al (Brunel Univ, Middlesex, UK; Univ of Louisville, KY; Royal Brompton Hosp, London, UK)

J Thorac Cardiovasc Surg 140:110-116, 2010

Objective.—During intraaortic balloon inflation, blood volume is displaced toward the heart (V_{tip}), traveling retrograde in the descending aorta, passing by the arch vessels, reaching the aortic root (V_{root}), and eventually perfusing the coronary circulation (V_{cor}). V_{cor} leads to coronary flow augmentation, one of the main benefits of the intraaortic balloon pump. The aim of this study was to assess V_{root} and V_{cor} in vivo and in vitro, respectively.

Methods.—During intraaortic balloon inflation, V_{root} was obtained by integrating over time the aortic root flow signals measured in 10 patients with intraaortic balloon assistance frequencies of 1:1 and 1:2. In a mock circulation system, flow measurements were recorded simultaneously upstream of the intraaortic balloon tip and at each of the arch and coronary branches of a silicone aorta during 1:1 and 1:2 intraaortic balloon support. Integration over time of the flow signals during inflation yielded V_{cor} and the distribution of V_{tip}.

Results.—In patients, V_{root} was 6.4% ± 4.8% of the intraaortic balloon volume during 1:1 assistance and 10.0% ± 5.0% during 1:2 assistance. In vitro and with an artificial heart simulating the native heart, V_{cor} was smaller, 3.7% and 3.8%, respectively. The distribution of V_{tip} in vitro varied, with less volume displaced toward the arch and coronary branches and more volume stored in the compliant aortic wall when the artificial heart was not operating.

Conclusion.—The blood volume displaced toward the coronary circulation as the result of intraaortic balloon inflation is a small percentage of the nominal intraaortic balloon volume. Although small, this percentage is still a significant fraction of baseline coronary flow (Fig 1).

▶ Use of an intra-aortic balloon (IAB) in patients who are unstable, secondary to severe coronary disease or a failing left ventricle, is common and has been shown to be quite effective. Inflation in diastole is known to lessen ischemia, while deflation in systole serves to afterload reduce the work for the ventricle. What is not known is the amount of blood displaced retrograde during inflation. Fig 1 in this article demonstrates the expected augmentation in diastolic

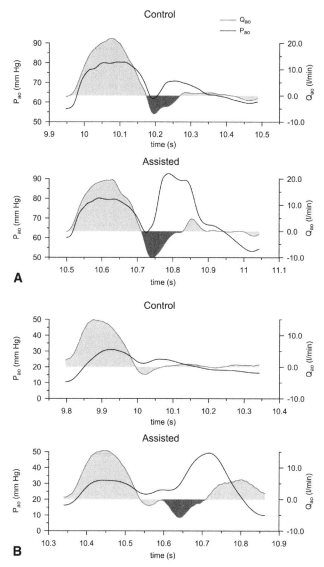

FIGURE 1.—Hemodynamic waveforms in vivo during 1:2 IABP support for a control (*top*) and an assisted (*bottom*) beat in 2 different patients (A, B). P_{ao}, aortic pressure (*solid black*); Q_{ao}, aortic flow (*filled grey*). In cases of correctly timed inflation (A), V_{root} was derived by subtracting the intrinsic backflow of the control beat from the backflow of the assisted beat (both areas shaded in *dark grey*). In cases of late inflation (B), V_{root} was derived directly from the assisted beat by integrating the area shaded in *dark grey*. (Reprinted from Kolyva C, Pantalos GM, Pepper JR, et al. How much of the intraaortic balloon volume is displaced toward the coronary circulation? *J Thorac Cardiovasc Surg.* 2010;140:110-116, with permission from The American Association for Thoracic Surgery.)

pressure by balloon inflation. The calculated retrograde flow corrected for IAB pump balloon volume was 6.4% during 1:1 and 10% during 1:2 support. These 2 values were not statistically different, although the study may have been underpowered to identify such a difference. More importantly though is that given 1:1 augments twice as frequently as 1:2, the total volume of blood moving in a retrograde fashion is actually higher as one would expect. The volumes represented by these percentage changes at first sounds quite low as they are in the 1 cc range. However, given that the calculated coronary flow is about 2.5 cc per cardiac cycle, these augmentation volumes are actually quite significant. Furthermore, these authors show in a model that most retrograde flow is lost secondary to aortic compliance, a fact that may or may not be true in case of atherosclerotic vessels. What also remains unclear from this work is whether the increase in coronary flow is secondary to the volume of retrograde displaced blood or the enhanced diastolic pressure or some combination of the 2.

T. Dorman, MD

Normative postpartum intraabdominal pressure: potential implications in the diagnosis of abdominal compartment syndrome
Abdel-Razeq SS, Campbell K, Funai EF, et al (Yale Univ School of Medicine, New Haven, CT)
Am J Obstet Gynecol 203:149.e1-149.e4, 2010

Objective.—We sought to establish normative values of intraabdominal pressure (IAP) in postpartum women with and without arterial hypertension.

Study Design.—Bladder pressure was measured via a Foley catheter 1 hour following completion of cesarean section in supine and semirecumbent positions in 21 patients.

Results.—Mean supine IAP (6.4 ± 5.2 mm Hg) was significantly lower than semirecumbent IAP (11.6 ± 7.2 mm Hg) ($P < .05$). Body mass index (BMI) was significantly correlated to IAP regardless of the gestational age (r^2 supine $= 0.46$, semirecumbent $= 0.37$; $P = .004$ for either). Increasing gravidity was associated with decreasing IAP. Patients with arterial hypertension had higher BMI, were delivered earlier, and had higher IAP than patients with normal arterial pressure, either in supine or semirecumbent position. However, these relationships were not significant when results were controlled for BMI.

Conclusion.—Postcesarean section IAP is higher than in the general surgical population. Patients with hypertensive disorders have IAPs approaching to intraabdominal hypertension range.

▶ These data from a single center remind us that patients must be in the supine position to effectively transduce bladder pressure using the height of a fluid column in the Foley catheter to evaluate intra-abdominal hypertension or determine criteria for abdominal compartment syndrome. Pregnancy is also an excellent model for elevated body mass index. Body mass index correlates with intra-abdominal pressure. These findings are not surprising, given work that has been done in other patient populations.[1]

The interesting observation in this small series of patients is that hypertensive disorders in pregnancy are associated with higher intra-abdominal pressures and appear to have an associated risk of abdominal compartment syndrome. The rationale provided by these authors is an increased likelihood for third space accumulation of fluid, presumably in the retroperitoneum and other intra-abdominal tissues during hypertensive disorders of pregnancy.[2]

While we need significant additional data to support this assertion, the authors point out that Centers for Disease Control and Prevention's statistics suggest that maternal mortality and the rate of cesarean section are reaching high levels in the United States. The authors question whether abdominal hypertension or abdominal compartment syndrome may cause some of the increasing morbidity seen in patients with hypertensive disorders of pregnancy. These data suggest that hospitalized patients with hypertensive disorders of pregnancy should be considered for routine measurement of intra-abdominal pressure.[3]

D. J. Dries, MSE, MD

References

1. Malbrain ML, Cheatham ML, Kirkpatrick A, et al. Results from the International Conference of Experts on Intra-abdominal Hypertension and Abdominal Compartment Syndrome. I. Definitions. *Intensive Care Med.* 2006;32:1722-1732.
2. Malbrain ML, Chiumello D, Pelosi P, et al. Incidence and prognosis of intraabdominal hypertension in a mixed population of critically ill patients: a multiple-center epidemiological study. *Crit Care Med.* 2005;33:315-322.
3. Malbrain ML, Chiumello D, Pelosi P, et al. Prevalence of intra-abdominal hypertension in critically ill patients: a multicentre epidemiological study. *Intensive Care Med.* 2004;30:822-829.

Passive leg raising is predictive of fluid responsiveness in spontaneously breathing patients with severe sepsis or acute pancreatitis
Préau S, Saulnier F, Dewavrin F, et al (Centre Hospitalier Jean Bernard, Valenciennes, France; Centre Hospitalier Universitaire de Lille, France)
Crit Care Med 38:819-825, 2010

Objective.—Rapid fluid loading is standard treatment for hypovolemia. Because volume expansion does not always improve hemodynamic status, predictive parameters of fluid responsiveness are needed. Passive leg raising is a reversible maneuver that mimics rapid volume expansion. Passive leg raising-induced changes in stroke volume and its surrogates are reliable predictive indices of volume expansion responsiveness for mechanically ventilated patients. We hypothesized that the hemodynamic response to passive leg raising indicates fluid responsiveness in nonintubated patients without mechanical ventilation.

Design.—Prospective study.

Setting.—Intensive care unit of a general hospital.

Patients.—We investigated consecutive nonintubated patients, without mechanical ventilation, considered for volume expansion.

Interventions.—We assessed hemodynamic status at baseline, after passive leg raising, and after volume expansion (500 mL 6% hydroxyethyl starch infusion over 30 mins).

Measurements and Main Results.—We measured stroke volume using transthoracic echocardiography, radial pulse pressure using an arterial catheter, and peak velocity of femoral artery flow using continuous Doppler. We calculated changes in stroke volume, pulse pressure, and velocity of femoral artery flow induced by passive leg raising (respectively, $\triangle$ stroke volume, $\triangle$ pulse pressure, and $\triangle$ velocity of femoral artery flow). Among 34 patients included in this study, 14 had a stroke volume increase of $\geq 15\%$ after volume expansion (responders). All patients included in the study had severe sepsis (n = 28; 82%) or acute pancreatitis (n = 6; 18%). The $\triangle$ stroke volume $\geq 10\%$ predicted fluid responsiveness with sensitivity of 86% and specificity of 90%. The $\triangle$ pulse pressure $\geq 9\%$ predicted fluid responsiveness with sensitivity of 79% and specificity of 85%. The $\triangle$ velocity of femoral artery flow $\geq 8\%$ predicted fluid responsiveness with sensitivity of 86% and specificity of 80%.

Conclusions.—Changes in stroke volume, radial pulse pressure, and peak velocity of femoral artery flow induced by passive leg raising are accurate and interchangeable indices for predicting fluid responsiveness in nonintubated patients with severe sepsis or acute pancreatitis.

▶ Assessment of volume status and potential need for volume resuscitation present many challenges at the bedside. Static measures such as central venous pressure and pulmonary artery occlusion pressure have limitations when used to predict fluid status. Many studies have suggested that dynamic measures, such as stroke volume (SV) or pulse pressure (PP), are more reliable. Passive leg raising (PLR) is a maneuver that mimics a bolus of fluid. In this study, the authors evaluated the ability of PLR to predict fluid responsiveness in a group of nonintubated patients with severe sepsis or acute pancreatitis. They performed several hemodynamic measurements before and after PLR, repeating them before and after volume expansion. The hemodynamic measurements included heart rate, blood pressure, SV by echocardiography, radial pulse pressure (PP) from arterial line, and peak velocity of femoral artery flow (VF) obtained via Doppler. The main finding of this article was that changes in SV, PP, and VF with PLR were good predictors of fluid responsiveness in nonintubated patients. Furthermore, the results from this study suggest that the different measurements are interchangeable. Finally, it is interesting to note that fluid responsiveness was found in only 41% of the study patients. This suggests that identifying patients who will benefit from continued volume expansion is important to avoid complications associated with volume overload and unnecessary intravenous fluid administration.

S. L. Zanotti-Cavazzoni, MD

Risk of Symptomatic DVT Associated With Peripherally Inserted Central Catheters

Evans RS, Sharp JH, Linford LH, et al (Intermountain Healthcare, Salt Lake City, UT; Med Ctr, Salt Lake City, UT; et al)
Chest 138:803-810, 2010

Background.—Previous studies undertaken to identify risk factors for peripherally inserted central catheter (PICC)-associated DVT have yielded conflicting results. PICC insertion teams and other health-care providers need to understand the risk factors so that they can develop methods to prevent DVT.

Methods.—A 1-year prospective observational study of PICC insertions was conducted at a 456-bed, level I trauma center and tertiary referral hospital affiliated with a medical school. All patients with one or more PICC insertions were included to identify the incidence and risk factors for symptomatic DVT associated with catheters inserted by a facility-certified PICC team using a consistent and replicated approach for vein selection and insertion.

Results.—A total of 2,014 PICCs were inserted during 1,879 distinct hospitalizations in 1,728 distinct patients for a total of 15,115 days of PICC placement. Most PICCs were placed in the right arm (76.9%) and basilic vein (74%) and were double-lumen 5F (75.3%). Of the 2,014 PICC insertions, 60 (3.0%) in 57 distinct patients developed DVT in the cannulated or adjacent veins. The best-performing predictive model for DVT (area under the curve, 0.83) was prior DVT (odds ratio [OR], 9.92; $P < .001$), use of double-lumen 5F (OR, 7.54; $P < .05$) or triple-lumen 6F (OR, 19.50; $P < .01$) PICCs, and prior surgery duration of > 1 h (OR, 1.66; $P = .10$).

Conclusions.—Prior DVT and surgery lasting > 1 h identify patients at increased risk for PICC-associated DVT. More importantly, increasing catheter size also is significantly associated with increased risk. Rates of PICC-associated DVT may be reduced by improved selection of patients and catheter size.

▶ The use of peripherally inserted central catheters (PICCs) has become a common tool in the management of patients who require long-term catheters. All procedures carry some risk, and PICCs are not different. Catheter-associated infections have been well studied and strategies developed to mitigate that risk have been studied and promulgated. A catheter in a vein alters flow in that vein and thus is associated with thrombosis of that vessel. When this involves larger veins, then such venous thrombosis also carries the risk of significant morbidity and mortality. Thus concern has been expressed related to the deep vein thrombosis (DVT) risk for PICCs. This single-institution study describes the rate and risk factors for PICC-related DVT in that institution. Fig 3 in the original article shows the most important findings of this study from the multivariate analysis. The highest risk predictor appears to be catheter size with a triple-lumen catheter having an odds ratio of up to almost 20 times baseline risk. The second highest risk factor was previous DVT, and the third and final identified risk was surgery of > 1 hour. As a single-institution study, it is impossible to know if these findings extrapolate to other institutions. The population studied may also have a significant impact on the findings, and of note is the low frequency of oncology patients in this study. Finally, although no one has ever determined that side of placement may impact thrombosis rate, most of these PICCs were placed on the right side via protocol.

T. Dorman, MD

Scar formation in the carotid sheath identified during carotid endarterectomy in patients with previous cardiac surgery: significance of history of intraoperative Swan-Ganz catheter insertion

Yoshida K, Ogasawara K, Kobayashi M, et al (Iwate Med Univ, Morioka, Japan)
J Neurosurg 113:885-889, 2010

Object.—Scar formation in the carotid sheath is often identified during carotid endarterectomy (CEA) in patients with previous cardiac surgery, and dissection of the carotid sheath and exposure of the carotid arteries in such patients are difficult. The purpose of the present study was to investigate factors related to scar formation identified during CEA in patients with previous cardiac surgery.

Methods.—Twenty-three patients with internal carotid artery stenosis ($\geq$ 70%) and previous cardiac surgery underwent CEA. A patient was prospectively defined as having scar formation during CEA when scissors were required throughout dissection of the carotid sheath and exposure of the carotid arteries.

Results.—Scar formation was identified during dissection of the carotid sheath in 7 patients (30.4%). In all 7 patients, the side of CEA was identical to the side on which the Swan-Ganz catheter was inserted during cardiac surgery, and the incidence of previous ipsilateral Swan-Ganz catheter insertion was significantly higher in patients with the scar formation (100%) than in those without (31.3%). Seven (58.3%) of 12 patients with a history of ipsilateral Swan-Ganz catheter insertion had scar formation. Two of the 7 patients with scar formation experienced complications after CEA, including one patient with hemiparesis due to artery-to-artery embolism during surgery, and another patient with transient vocal cord paralysis.

Conclusions.—A history of Swan-Ganz catheter insertion during previous cardiac surgery is associated with the presence of scar tissue in the ipsilateral carotid sheath and a higher risk of complications during CEA.

▶ Many complications of central venous access have been previously described and are well known to all health care providers. Strategies to successfully minimize these complications have been established. These strategies include multimodality programs designed to minimize central line–associated blood stream infections and the use of ultrasound to minimize mechanical complications. This article describes a potentially new complication of central venous access. The authors describe an association between previous placement of a central catheter, in this case, a pulmonary artery catheter (PAC) through a cordis and subsequently surgically identified scar formation in that ipsilateral carotid sheath. The study design does not permit causation to be determined, and thus, at best, the association should be considered preliminary at this time. Limitations include the nonrandomized nature of the study and, importantly, the subjective definition of scar formation. In addition, lack of findings associated with a carotid evaluation before the original cordis placement is not included. Finally, placement of central catheters of other sizes are not evaluated, and whether or not the sheath had multiple previous entries by double stick approaches is not described nor are patients who received a PAC for reasons other than cardiac surgery included. These limitations should not, however, remove all concerns, and clinicians will anxiously await additional studies, as impacting carotid flow would be considered a major complication that would indeed change practice.

T. Dorman, MD

4 Burns

Absence of pathological scarring in the donor site of the scalp in burns: An analysis of 295 cases

Farina JA Jr, Freitas FAS, Ungarelli LF, et al (Universidade de São Paulo, Brazil; et al)
Burns 36:883-890, 2010

Aim.—This study aims to describe the incidence of complications on scalp from which a thin split-skin graft was harvested (0.005–0.007 in.) of the donor site in children and adult burn victims.

Methods.—We reviewed the medical records of 295 burn patients admitted in the Burn Unit of the Clinical Hospital of the Faculty of Medicine of Ribeirão Preto, from January 1998 to December 2007, whose scalps were used as donor site for grafts. Skin-graft thickness varied from 0.005 in. to 0.007 in. The occurrence of pathological healing was evaluated clinically and the time of epithelisation by the main surgeon and a plastic surgeon or a staff nurse.

Results.—Of the 295 patients whose scalps were used as donor site, 274 were followed from 6 months to 10 years after the procedure (median 18.2 months). Twenty-one patients were lost to follow-up in the first 6 months. No hypertrophic scarring or keloids on the donor site was observed. Five patients (1.82%) presented with folliculitis and two of them were evaluated with small areas of alopecia (0.7%), treated with resection of these areas and primary suture. The average time of epithelisation of the donor site was 7 days.

Conclusion.—The harvest of thinner split graft from the scalp is a safe procedure.

▶ This is an excellent review of thin donor sites in the scalp. Over a 10-year period, the authors harvested skin from the scalp of 274 patients and had the patients available for follow-up for at least 6 months. There was no hypertrophic scarring (HTS) on the scalp, even in patients who developed HTS in donor sites on other body regions. The mean time to epithelialization was only 7 days. This study strongly supports my current bias and practice to use the scalp donor in pediatric patients as a hidden donor site. As the hair grows out, it covers any minor pigmentary changes, and using the sides of the scalp preferentially allows us to avoid the area of male pattern baldness when harvesting smaller donor sites. Additionally (and anecdotally), the scalp donor site is much less painful than other donor sites, and children seem to be unaware of a small bandage on their scalps. Use of a flexible semipermeable

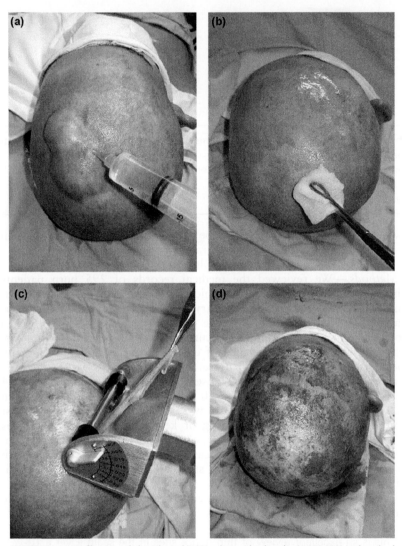

FIGURE 2.—(a) Infiltration of physiological 0.9% saline with adrenalin [1:500,000] in the subgaleal space. This was the second procedures to harvest the skin of scalp, after 12 days from the first one; (b) application of liquid Vaseline to facilitate sliding of the dermatome; (c) harvest of thin skin specimen, with a calibration of .005 in., using an electric dermatome; (d) scalp immediately after the harvest of the thin skin layers showing limited bleeding. (Reprinted from Farina JA Jr, Freitas FAS, Ungarelli LF, et al. Absence of pathological scarring in the donor site of the scalp in burns: an analysis of 295 cases. *Burns.* 2010;36:883-890, with permission from the International Society for Burn Injuries.)

dressing on the scalp donor site allows it to stay in place without bulky dressings, nicely adherent to the scalp during the first few days and then is gently pushed out with hair growth, thus requiring no painful dressing removal. Although I use plain saline to clyse the subcutaneous tissue prior to skin harvesting and topical epinephrine soaked laparotomy pads for hemostasis after harvesting (90 mg epinephrine/L normal saline), the technique shown by the authors in Fig 2 is otherwise very similar to that used at my institution.

Donor sites are one of the most problematic parts of burn care, from the pain, difficulty with bandages, donor site infections, itching during the healing process, and finally HTS. I would strongly encourage the more frequent use of scalp donor sites in adult patients to minimize the issues associated with a donor site elsewhere on the body.

B. A. Latenser, MD

Burn Rehabilitation and Research: Proceedings of a Consensus Summit
Richard R, Baryza MJ, Carr JA, et al (United States Army Inst of Surgical Res, Sam Houston, TX; Shriners Hosps for Children, Boston, MA; Westchester Burn Ctr, Valhalla, NY; et al)
J Burn Care Res 30:543-573, 2009

Burn rehabilitation is an essential component of successful patient care. In May 2008, a group of burn rehabilitation clinicians met to discuss the status and future needs of burn rehabilitation. Fifteen topic areas pertinent to clinical burn rehabilitation were addressed. Consensus positions and suggested future research directions regarding the physical aspects of burn rehabilitation are shared.

▶ Once the patient no longer requires the burn surgeons and nurses continuously at the bedside to survive the acute injury, there is no disagreement that burn rehabilitation is essential for optimal patient outcomes. And there the agreement ends. Practices in occupational and physical therapy vary widely between burn centers, and there is a paucity of data to direct practices in a scientific way. It is no longer acceptable to just survive a major burn injury. With overall mortality rates at 4%, outcomes must reflect the physical and psychological recuperation that occurs months to years post burn injury. Functioning at less than the highest level of wellness possible is not an appropriate target.

One of the main problems remains that there are no standards for therapist staffing needs for both in- and out-patient locations. There are no competencies for burn therapists, and new therapists may have had very little training in burn care. Again, competencies are dictated by the individual burn center, making it hard to standardize a knowledge base for therapists.

The literature that relates to burn therapy in general does not provide evidence-based guidance for many practices currently in place in burn centers. With few research-oriented burn therapists and few burn centers having the resources to have dedicated burn research therapists, the impediment remains. Organizing and participating in multicenter trials such as through the American Burn Association will be one way to provide scientific evidence for current practices.

There is agreement that burn patients need exercise, positioning, splinting, strengthening, and strategies to deal with pain, itch, and scars. Mr Richard and his conferees have put forth a well-defined program for moving forward with burn rehabilitation in a rigorous and scientific manner. For anyone working with burn patients, I recommend this in-depth analysis of burn rehabilitation and where we need to go.

B. A. Latenser, MD

Diagnosis and Grading of Inhalation Injury
Woodson LC (Shriners Hosp for Children, Galveston, TX)
J Burn Care Res 30:143-145, 2009

Background.—The risk of death or permanent pulmonary dysfunction after respiratory injury caused by inhaling smoke or other chemical irritants can be considerable. If cutaneous burns are also present, the patient will need more fluid for resuscitation and be at greater risk for pulmonary complications and death. The diagnosis of inhalation injury is an important but variable predictor of outcomes in these patients. Even with advances in understanding the pathophysiology of inhalation injury, few specific therapeutic options are available and treatment is generally supportive. Improved treatment of inhalation injuries has been hindered by the complexity of the clinical situation, the inflammatory responses triggered by inhalation injury, and lack of uniformity in the criteria used to diagnose inhalation injury and absence of a widely accepted and applied system for quantifying severity of injury.

Diagnosis.—The term *inhalation injury* covers a range of conditions that fall into the categories of thermal injury, which is restricted to the upper airway structures unless caused by a blast or steam; local chemical irritation affecting the entire respiratory tract; and systemic toxicity such as that caused when a toxin such as carbon monoxide is inhaled. The diagnosis is usually a subjective opinion based on the history, physical examination, and confirmatory diagnostic studies. Mechanism and duration of exposure as well as quality of the inhaled irritant are important elements in the history. The physical examination provides an estimate of the intensity of the exposure and yields evidence of exposure to extreme heat, soot deposits, and early signs of respiratory compromise. The clinical presentation can be extremely heterogeneous, making diagnostic criteria difficult to identify. Progressive respiratory failure does not always appear proportional to the smoke exposure suffered by the patient. Composition of the inhaled materials and/or differences in host response may alter the manifestations of injury. Sometimes the effects of exposure or signs of injury are delayed by a systemic inflammatory response to cutaneous burns or reperfusion injury. All of these make it difficult to define diagnostic criteria. In addition, clinical treatment decisions may be based on diagnostic criteria that differ from those used in scientific reports. Often burn center treatment decisions are based on the availability of resources and local practice, so they will vary between facilities. In contrast, criteria used for scientific reports are intended to identify patients with inhalation injury for the purpose of assessing a specific therapeutic intervention or making a prognosis.

Classification.—It is difficult to predict which patients will be vulnerable to resuscitation stresses, a higher rate of pulmonary complications, respiratory failure, and death. Reliable indicators of progressive respiratory failure in patients with smoke inhalation injury are lacking. Grading systems are needed to quantify the severity of inhalation injury. Most of those currently used rely on a combination of bronchoscopic findings and clinical findings, which can vary. However, the relationship between bronchoscopic findings and injury has been called into question, with proximal injury observed bronchoscopically often greater than the degree of peripheral parenchymyal injury and no correlation between bronchoscopic evidence and the development of ARDS or fluid resuscitation requirements.

Conclusions.—The criteria for diagnosing inhalation injury should be standardized to focus on modalities that are widely available and that do not require highly specialized skills. Criteria used for scientific reporting should clearly describe the injury and include sufficient data to compare the composition of inhaled irritants, the intensity of exposure, and measures of pulmonary dysfunction. Consensus in the diagnosis and quantification of inhalation injury may need to wait for the findings of a multicenter study to develop a predictive scoring system for patients with inhalation injury. The plan for such a study was outlined. It offers the potential benefits of providing burn centers with a way to predict outcomes after inhalation injury in children, standardize the diagnostic regimen for inhalation injury, and provide a foundation for future studies comparing therapeutic regimens to treat inhalation injury.

▶ Finally, someone has identified the weaknesses with current studies regarding inhalation injury (II): the main ones being lack of uniformity in diagnostic criteria, absence of a generally accepted system of quantifying the injury, and small numbers of patients with II at each burn center, thereby precluding single-center studies. The need for standard diagnostic criteria and quantification of severity has long been recognized but prospective multicenter studies have yet to be performed. A prospective, randomized, 2-phase study is recommended by the author.

II is a systemic injury, and even cutaneous burns without II may present as II or its sequelae, acute lung injury or adult respiratory distress syndrome, due to systemic inflammatory mediators, which further complicates the diagnostic picture. There are actually 3 types of II: upper airway, which may be due to thermal injury, chemical exposure, or a combination of the 2. This upper airway injury may be worsened by resuscitation, inflammatory mediators, loss of control of vascular permeability, paralyzed cilia, and/or denuded respiratory tract epithelium. Then there is the alveolar injury, wherein the type 2 pneumocytes are poisoned, surfactant is no longer produced, and alveoli are filled with mucus. Finally, the toxic inhaled gases such as carbon monoxide (CO) and cyanide, have known treatments. Although CO poisoning is treated with

100% oxygen to decrease the binding to hemoglobin, there are practitioners who insist that hyperbaric oxygen (HBO) should also be used. The data on HBO are unclear, and there are no randomized prospective studies showing improvement in patients without profound neurological deficits. The treatment for cyanide poisoning is worse than the toxicity itself, and yet, cyanide levels are known to be at least mildly elevated in all patients with II.

The recommendations for a 2-phase study put forth here are long overdue. Hopefully, II will move from the black box of unknowns to a disease where we can significantly improve the outcomes.

B. A. Latenser, MD

Glucose Variability is Associated With High Mortality After Severe Burn
Pidcoke HF, Wanek SM, Rohleder LS, et al (Univ of Texas Health Science Ctr, San Antonio; Brooke Army Med Ctr, San Antonio, TX)
J Trauma 67:990-995, 2009

Background.—Hyperglycemia is associated with increased mortality in the severely injured; intensive insulin protocols reduce mortality, improve wound healing, and decrease susceptibility to infection. High glucose variability creates challenges to glycemic control and may be a marker of poor outcome. We wondered whether glycemic variability alone might identify patients at higher risk of death.

Methods.—Burn patients admitted in 2005 with >20% total body surface area burned, ≥100 glucose measurements, and one hypo- and hyperglycemic event were included in the analysis; all were treated with intensive insulin (glycemic target: 80–110 mg/dL). Glycemic variability was the sum of percent excursions (defined as values <80 mg/dL or >110 mg/dL); variability above the mean was considered high.

Results.—Individual average variability in the 49 subjects was 50% ± 8% (range, 30–65%); the average number of glucose measurements per patient was 840 (range, 103–5314). Percent excursions in those with high (n = 26) compared with low (n = 23) variability scores was 56% ± 6% and 43% ± 5% ($p < 0.001$), respectively. No difference was found between groups in injury severity score, age, total body surface area burned, full thickness burns, gender, or inhalation injury. Both groups were similar for days of ventilator support, intensive care unit stay, and hospital stay. Mortality in the highly variable group was twice that of the less variable group (50% vs. 22%, $p = 0.041$).

Conclusions.—High glucose variability (>50% of values outside 80–110 mg/dL) is associated with increased mortality in the severely burned. Individuals with frequent excursions outside the glucose target range of 80 mg/dL to 110 mg/dL are at greater risk of death.

▶ We all read with interest the seminal article in 2001 by Van den Berghe et al[1] on maintaining euglycemia in a surgical intensive care unit population. They found reduced mortality, morbidity, duration of stay, and infection. Many facilities now use intensive insulin therapy to achieve tight glycemic control. Unfortunately, most studies investigating intensive insulin therapy heretofore have excluded patients with burns or had very small burn patient populations.

This study investigated only burn patients with large body surface area burns and an intensive insulin therapy protocol with target blood glucose 80 to 110 mg/dL. The group with the large glucose variability was the same as the low-variability group regarding injury severity, burn size, age, gender, inhalation injury, or pre-existing diabetes, and the same intensive insulin therapy protocol was used in both groups. Perhaps it is not the relative hyperglycemia or hypoglycemia, but the wide variability in glucose levels that is associated with poorer outcomes in the patient with burns. At the least, as these authors suggest, glucose variability should alert the clinician that more intensive monitoring is indicated.

Keep watch for future adequately powered studies investigating intensive insulin therapy in patients with burns as we seek to determine if it is the absolute glucose level, the lack of wide swings in glucose levels, the beneficial effects of exogenous insulin administration, or some combination of these factors that affect outcome in critically burned patients.

B. A. Latenser, MD

Reference

1. van den Berghe G, Wouters P, Weekers F, et al. Intensive insulin therapy in the critically ill patients. *N Engl J Med.* 2001;345:1359-1367.

Key Questions in Ventilator Management of the Burn-Injured Patient (First of Two Parts)
Dries DJ (Regions Hosp, St Paul, MN)
J Burn Care Res 30:128-138, 2009

Background.—In patients suffering thermal injury, preexisting patient condition, size of the cutaneous injury, and respiratory function, especially if compromised by smoke inhalation, will often indicate the likelihood of survival and attending complications. Respiratory failure occurring after burn trauma may be the result of a primary injury to the lung through the inhalation of toxic combustion products, but respiratory compromise can also occur without direct smoke inhalation. The effects of ventilation, oxygenation, and recruitment therapies on the outcome of respiratory injury were discussed.

Ventilation.—Current treatment for acute lung injury involves ventilator strategies that limit minute ventilation by using low tidal volumes. This produces a tendency to develop hypercapnia. Permissive hypercapnia is considered acceptable but, because of the potential for anti-inflammatory effects, is not routinely set as a goal for ventilator therapy. Significant morbidity and mortality accompany alveolar air leak during mechanical ventilation. Tomographic studies of patients with adult respiratory distress syndrome (ARDS) indicate there may be extensive collapse in dependent lung regions during mechanical ventilation in smaller nondependent lung areas. Hyperinflation of the nondependent areas may produce barotrauma, although some evidence indicates that alveolar wall necrosis with persistent collapse and inflammation in dependent lung zones also contributes. It is reasonable to maintain plateau airway pressure at less than 30 cm H_2O to keep all aerated lung regions at less than normal maximum volume. Unless there is significant airway resistance, peak inspiratory pressure can be maintained at less than 35 cm H_2O. There are cardiovascular advantages to performing less aggressive ventilation, such as avoiding elevation of pulmonary vascular resistance, increased pulmonary artery and right ventricular pressures, and compromised right ventricular performance. Hypercapnic acidosis also has protective effects, exerts anti-inflammatory effects, and reduces cytokine signaling.

Oxygenation.—The use of positive end-expiratory pressure (PEEP) remains a fundamental approach to elevating mean airway pressure and improving oxygenation. PEEP can be accompanied by adverse hemodynamic and anatomic effects, however. Setting PEEP at the highest level compatible with plateau pressure of 28 to 30 cm H_2O and tidal volume of 6 mL/kg predicted body weight is recommended. This approach should minimize injury to relatively normal lung where recruitment is not possible and injury caused by overdistention. For morbidly obese patients or persons with significant torso edema caused by thermal injury, higher pressure levels may be needed.

Recruitment.—Recruitment focuses on opening as many lung units as possible. The objective in managing lung injury is to apply sufficient pressure to keep the lung open without creating undue stress on tissues that remain closed or overdistending alveoli that are fully open during the tidal cycle. Recruitment or reopening of gas exchange units depends on the level and duration of transpulmonary pressure applied. The airway pressure needed to reopen an alveolus is considerably higher than the pressure needed to keep it from closing again, so once the small airways are open, they usually remain open. In recruitment, elevated pressure maneuvers are applied intermittently to avoid the extensive exposure of tissues to potentially damaging forces. Logically, PEEP would be applied after a recruitment maneuver to maintain airway and alveolar patency. However, the nature of recruitment maneuvers, the ideal number to perform, how to monitor recruitment, and safety issues remain controversial.

Conclusions.—The parameters used in caring for lung injury in burn injury patients and the physiologic rationales backing them are evolving. Simple ventilator prescriptions are still effective in a significant number of patients, but as more is learned about the physiology of ventilator management, approaches can be individualized and applications expanded.

▶ This article, along with the follow-on part 2 published in the next journal's issue,[1] provides a thorough overview of ventilator management focused on patients with burns. This part focuses on oxygenation and ventilation and should be recommended reading for those wanting to understand some of the unique issues associated with ventilator needs of the patients with inhalation injury and/or thermal burns. Dries makes several key points that the clinician not routinely providing burn critical care may not be aware:

1. Respiratory dysfunction with burn injury is a systemic process and may occur even in the absence of inhalation injury.

2. Hypercarbia in ventilated patients with burns should be tolerated if the goal is just to achieve a normal pH and pCO_2. High respiratory rates, tidal volumes, and pressures are inappropriate just to obtain a normal pH. A HCO_3 drip worsens the intracellular acidosis and provides no benefit to the patient. Hypercapnia may actually be protective, but the goal should not be to induce it.

3. Acute lung injury may just be a side effect of large volume resuscitation such as in burns or chemical pneumonitis. The recommendation for treating acute lung injury is to keep plateau pressures ≤30 to 35 mm Hg and positive end-expiratory pressure enough to maintain airway and alveolar patency. Lower tidal volumes and higher pCO_2 are frequent consequences of this strategy. Fancy pressure targets and ventilator modes are not beneficial with acute lung injury.

Part 2, published in the next issue,[1] is a good review on ventilator strategies relevant to burns as well as some consideration of the effect of fluids and certain medications. Some key points making burns different than other critical care patient populations include:

1. Although bronchoscopy within 24 hours of injury remains the gold standard of diagnosing inhalation injury, bronchoscopic findings do not predict severity of inhalation injury.

2. Even minor increases in pulmonary microvascular pressures (such as during burn resuscitation) will accentuate edema formation, and cutaneous burns + inhalation injury will require more resuscitation fluid.

I highly recommend this 2-part article as it provides insight into some recommendations and pitfalls in caring for critically burned patients.

B. A. Latenser, MD

Reference

1. Dries DJ. Key questions in ventilator management of the burn-injured patient (second of two parts). *J Burn Care Res.* 2009;30:211-220.

Outcome of acute kidney injury in severe burns: a systematic review and meta-analysis

Brusselaers N, Monstrey S, Colpaert K, et al (Ghent Univ, Belgium)
Intensive Care Med 36:915-925, 2010

Purpose.—The main objective of this review was to analyse the prevalence and outcome of acute kidney injury (AKI) in patients with severe burn injury. AKI is a common complication in patients with severe burn injury and one of the major causes of death (often combined with other organ dysfunctions). Several definitions of AKI have been used, but the RIFLE 'consensus' classification is nowadays considered the gold standard, enabling a more objective comparison of populations.

Methods.—We performed a systematic literature search (1960–2009), involving PubMed, the Web of Science, the search engine Google^{TM} and textbooks. Reference lists and the Science Citation Index search were also consulted. Attributable mortality was assessed by performing a metaanalysis.

Results.—This search yielded 57 articles and abstracts with relevant epidemiologic data of AKI in the burn population. Of these, 30 contained complete mortality data of the burn and control population, which revealed a 3- to 6-fold higher mortality for AKI patients in univariate analysis, depending on the applied definition. When defined by the RIFLE consensus classification, AKI occurred in one quarter of patients with severe burn injury (median mortality of 34.9%), and when defined by the need for renal replacement therapy (RRT), AKI occurred in 3% (median mortality of 80%). The prevalence of AKI slightly increased, but AKI-RRT decreased. However, the outcome in both groups improved.

Conclusion.—Despite the wide variation of the analysed burn populations and definitions of AKI, this review clearly showed that AKI remains prevalent and is associated with increased mortality in patients with severe burn injury.

▶ Acute kidney injury (AKI) is not something that burn care providers frequently have to address, especially when compared with nonburn critical care patients. One of the confounders is thinking about what constitutes AKI. Currently, the RIFLE consensus classification is the gold standard for a definition, but older publications may have only considered the need for dialysis when defining renal failure.

The decrease in mortality rates over time in patients with AKI is probably real, mirroring the total decrease in mortality rates in US burn centers. The 2010 National Burn Repository Report of Data from 2000-2009[1] puts the overall mortality for patients with burns at 4%, and for those with > 20% total body surface area burns, the mortality rate is 22.3%. For patients ≥60 years with inhalation injury (with or without any cutaneous burns), the mortality rate is 98.7%. Multisystem organ failure is listed as cause of death in 25% of cases, so isolating AKI as an independent predictor of outcome in this population is not really possible. As we refine our resuscitation techniques and monitoring tools and avoid abdominal compartment syndrome, the issue of AKI may become even less significant for severely burned patients.

B. A. Latenser, MD

Reference

1. American Burn Association. 2010 National Burn Repository: report of data from 2000-2009. Published 2010. Accessed November 11, 2010.

Perioperative use of cuffed endotracheal tubes is advantageous in young pediatric burn patients
Dorsey DP, Bowman SM, Klein MB, et al (Univ of Washington, Seattle; Univ of Arkansas for Med Sciences, Little Rock; et al)
Burns 36:856-860, 2010

Uncuffed endotracheal tubes traditionally have been preferred over cuffed endotracheal tubes in young pediatric patients. However, recent evidence in elective pediatric surgical populations suggests otherwise. Because young pediatric burn patients can pose unique airway and ventilation challenges, we reviewed adverse events associated with the perioperative use of cuffed and uncuffed endotracheal tubes. We retrospectively reviewed 327 cases of operating room endotracheal intubation for general anesthesia in burned children 0–10 years of age over a 10-year period. Clinical airway outcomes were compared using multivariable logistic regression, controlling for relevant patient and injury characteristics. Compared to those receiving cuffed tubes, children receiving uncuffed tubes were significantly more likely to demonstrate clinically significant loss of tidal volume (odds ratio 10.62, 95% confidence interval 2.2–50.5) and require immediate reintubation to change tube size/type (odds ratio 5.54, 95% confidence interval 2.1–13.6). No significant differences were noted for rates of post-extubation stridor. Our data suggest that operating room use of uncuffed endotracheal tubes in such patients is associated with increased rates of tidal volume loss and reintubation. Due to the frequent challenge of airway management in this population, strategies should emphasize cuffed endotracheal tube use that is associated with lower rates of airway manipulation.

▶ Although this is a retrospective study covering 10 years, all operating room records for pediatric patients were reviewed, focusing on records where it was clear whether a cuffed or uncuffed tube was used. The uncuffed tube was significantly more likely to have a clinically significant air leak with difficulty in maintaining ventilation, leading to a fairly emergent tube change.

Endotracheal tube changes in small patients with burns can be a pretty scary process, as they are more likely to have problems with the small cross-sectional diameter of their airway, now compromised by edema early and scar contractures later. With inhalation injury, resuscitation, or prior excision and grafting, this can truly be the airway from your worst nightmare. The risks of repeated laryngoscopy and reintubation are more problematic in burned children. Patients with burns in general are at higher risk for postextubation stridor. In addition, health care providers in the operating room should not be exposed to inhalational agents as they leak around an uncuffed tube or during a tube change.

Pediatric patients with burns should be cared for by experienced pediatric anesthesiologists with specific burn experience. This study is compelling and implementation of cuffed endotracheal tubes for all pediatric patients with burns is recommended. Another sacred cow bites the dust.

B. A. Latenser, MD

The Efficacy of Hair and Urine Toxicology Screening on the Detection of Child Abuse by Burning

Hayek SN, Wibbenmeyer LA, Kealey LDH, et al (American Univ of Beirut, Lebanon; Univ of Iowa Carver College of Medicine)
J Burn Care Res 30:587-592, 2009

Abuse by burning is estimated to occur in 1 to 25% of children admitted with burn injuries annually. Hair and urine toxicology for illicit drug exposure may provide additional confirmatory evidence for abuse. To determine the impact of hair and urine toxicology on the identification of child abuse, we performed a retrospective chart review of all pediatric patients admitted to our burn unit. The medical records of 263 children aged 0 to 16 years of age who were admitted to our burn unit from January 2002 to December 2007 were reviewed. Sixty-five children had suspected abuse. Of those with suspected abuse, 33 were confirmed by the Department of Health and Human Services and comprised the study group. Each of the 33 cases was randomly matched to three pediatric (0–16 years of age) control patients (99). The average annual incidence of abuse in pediatric burn patients was 13.7 ± 8.4% of total annual pediatric admissions (range, 0–25.6%). Age younger than 5 years, hot tap water cause, bilateral, and posterior location of injury were significantly associated with nonaccidental burn injury on multivariate analysis. Thirteen (39.4%) abused children had positive ancillary tests. These included four (16%) skeletal surveys positive for fractures and 10 (45%) hair samples positive for drugs of abuse (one patient had a fracture and a positive hair screen). In three (9.1%) patients who were not initially suspected of abuse but later confirmed, positive hair test for illicit drugs was the only indicator of abuse. Nonaccidental injury can be difficult to confirm. Although inconsistent injury history and burn injury pattern remain central to the diagnosis of abuse by burning, hair and urine toxicology offers a further means to facilitate confirmation of abuse.

▶ Child abuse is a universal problem and has been implicated in up to one-fourth of children admitted with burn injuries. Although health care providers may be astute at recognizing child abuse, many injuries still go undetected. Methods to increase recognition of child abuse have been successful, but the concern for unrecognized intentional burn injuries remain. This study investigated hair and urine toxicology and found that 9% of children not suspected of being abused by any other screening criteria had hair samples positive for illicit drugs. Although this is a retrospective study, and a routine protocol for child abuse was not followed in the early part of the study, the fact remains that 9% of children not suspected of abuse by any other screening criteria had illegal drugs in their systems. Based upon these findings, a routine system of child abuse investigation is now standard protocol in our burn center. Protecting children and helping families is a part of our mandate, and although expensive, the cost of detecting even 1 abused child is less than the future psychological costs of providing physical and psychological care for the child who has been abused.

The policy for child abuse investigation of burn injuries at my institution is included below. If you do not have such a policy, please feel free to adapt ours for your institution. Web links are provided to view all policies and forms.[1]

Burn Center: Child Abuse and Neglect Workup (ages 0-14 years)

Determine if injury is suspicious:

- Obtain thorough history of event from everyone present. Attempt to interview them independently. Conflicting stories raise suspicion of intentional injury.
- Determine if the injury story matches the developmental age of the child (ie, a 12-month old will not be able to turn the hot water on).
- Recreate the injury as best as you can and confirm with the person present at the injury that you are correct in your recreation.
- Take a thorough history of the child. All pertinent history should be obtained on the children. History is expanded in children to include immunization history, emergency room visits/hospitalizations, developmental progress, emergency room visits/hospitalizations in other siblings, as well as ages of other siblings, primary care giver and other caregivers, and caregivers present in the house.
- Examine the child for the burn pattern looking at the injury pattern.
  - ▶ Suspicious injuries often have straight lines (immersion lines), no splash marks, and occur on posterior surfaces (dorsum of hand, posterior torso) or are bilateral lower leg burns.
  - ▶ Look for other signs of injuries (bruises, welts, abrasions, scars, and alopecia). Suspicious injuries may have patterns of objects (ie, coat hangers, grill marks) and occur on covered parts of the body (torso, back, abdomen, and inner thighs).
  - ▶ Uniform injury is also suspicious. Burn injuries are usually a mixture of many different depths depending on the exposure time.
  - ▶ Finally, determine if the injury pattern matches the story that the caregiver gave you.
- An emergency room social worker is available 24×7. Their services should be obtained during off hours on all pediatric burn patients who have suspicious

injuries or are aged < 1 year or are younger than 5 years with a tap water scald or have had their injury reported to the Department of Human Services (DHS).

- A social services consult should also be obtained on every clinic patient with a suspicious injury before they are discharged from the clinic.
- Social services should be notified at any time when DHS arrives on the nursing unit to interview families and/or to assess pediatric patients.
- Have a pediatric huddle (during day time hours) either at admission or soon after. Team members required are attending MD, primary nurse, and social worker.

Perform a diagnostic workup:

- A diagnostic workup should be performed on all children younger than or equal to 5 years with admission with a tap water burn injury.
- A diagnostic workup should be performed on all children younger than or equal to 1 year.
- Workup is dependent on age and physical examination.
- Please see the University of Iowa Health Care (UIHC) link for full detailed examination. Please see the link http://forms.uihc.uiowa.edu/pdf/abuseforms/index.htm for burn specific workup.
- Consult #9760 (Dr Oral or covering pediatrician) in all suspected cases of abuse or when in doubt that the case is the result of abuse.

Suspected abuse diagnostic workup for children 0 to 12 months:

- All UIHC mandatory reporters must make a verbal report of suspected child or dependent adult abuse to the Iowa DHS (1-800-362-2178) within 24 hours of such a determination. Within 48 hours of this determination a written report, B-22a UIHC Suspected Child and Dependent Adult Abuse Reporting Form (found as a template in electronic medical record) must be filed with DHS. http://forms.uihc.uiowa.edu/pdf/abuseforms/5.iv-diagchildabuse.pdf.
- Retinal examination on all children aged < 6 months or if shaken baby syndrome is presumed or if intracranial trauma is presumed.
- Head CT on all children < 6 months and in all children with neurologic findings or positive retinal hemorrhages.
- Skeletal survey on all children who are aged < 12 months.
- Hair and urine toxicology testing.
- Coagulation profile if bruising or bleeding is found.
- Sexual abuse workup if suspected (consult #9760—Dr Oral or covering pediatrician).
- Genetic workup if multiple fractures are found (consult #9760—Dr Oral or covering pediatrician).
- Digital photography of burns and other injuries (upload to Evidence Photographers International Council [EPIC] as soon as possible or forward to Dr Oral or covering pediatrician via e-mail).
- Pediatric huddle during day hours (attending MD, primary nurse, and social worker).

Suspected abuse diagnostic workup for children 1 to 2 years:

- All UIHC mandatory reporters must make a verbal report of suspected child or dependent adult abuse to the Iowa DHS (1-800-362-2178) within 24 hours of such a determination. Within 48 hours of this determination, a written report, B-22a UIHC Suspected Child and Dependent Adult Abuse Reporting Form (found as a template in electronic medical record) must be filed with DHS. http://forms.uihc.uiowa.edu/pdf/abuseforms/5.iv-diagchildabuse.pdf.
- Retinal examination on all children aged 1 to 2 years with rib fractures or metaphyseal fractures or spiral fractures or with neurologic findings.
- Head CT on all children aged 1 to 2 years with neurologic findings or positive retinal hemorrhages.
- Skeletal survey on all children 1 to 2 years of age or as directed by physical examination.
- Hair and urine toxicology testing.
- Coagulation profile if bruising or bleeding is found.
- Sexual abuse workup if suspected (consult #9760—Dr Oral or covering pediatrician).
- Genetic workup if multiple fractures are found (consult #9760—Dr Oral or covering pediatrician).
- Digital photography of burns and other injuries (upload to EPIC as soon as possible or forward to Dr Oral or covering pediatrician via e-mail).
- Pediatric huddle during day hours (attending MD, primary nurse, and social worker).

Suspected abuse diagnostic workup for children 2 to 5 years:

- All UIHC mandatory reporters must make a verbal report of suspected child or dependent adult abuse to the Iowa DHS (1-800-362-2178) within 24 hours of such a determination. Within 48 hours of this determination a written report, B-22a UIHC Suspected Child and Dependent Adult Abuse Reporting Form (found as a template in electronic medical record) must be filed with DHS. http://forms.uihc.uiowa.edu/pdf/abuseforms/5.iv-diagchildabuse.pdf.
- Retinal examination on all children aged 2 to 5 years with neurological findings.
- Head CT on all children aged 2 to 5 years with neurologic findings or positive retinal hemorrhages.
- Skeletal survey on all children aged 2 to 5 years as directed by physical examination.
- Hair and urine toxicology testing.
- Coagulation profile if bruising or bleeding is found.
- Sexual abuse workup if suspected (consult #9760—Dr Oral or covering pediatrician).
- Genetic workup if multiple fractures are found (consult #9760—Dr Oral or covering pediatrician).
- Digital photography of burns and other injuries (upload to EPIC as soon as possible or forward to Dr Oral or covering pediatrician via e-mail).

- Pediatric huddle during day hours (attending MD, primary nurse, and social worker).

Please refer to Policies and Procedures for Suspected Child and Dependant Adult Abuse policy PC-SOC-05.16 for definitions of types of abuse and mandatory reporting requirements.

Burn Treatment Center multidisciplinary team meeting led by Dr Barbara Latenser, Director, with consults from UIHC pediatric abuse specialists and social services.

B. A. Latenser, MD

Reference

1. PC-SOC-05.16 Policies and Procedures for Suspected Child and Dependant Adult Abuse. Child Protection Clinical Guidelines page. http://forms.uihc.uiowa.edu/pdf/abuseforms/index.htm. Page 4. Accessed October 15, 2010.

The year in burns 2008

Wolf SE (Univ of Texas Health Science Ctr – San Antonio and the United States Army Inst of Surgical Res, Floyd Curl)
Burns 35:1057-1070, 2009

For 2008, approximately 1200 original burn research articles were published in scientific journals using the English language. This article reviews those with the most impact on burn treatment according to the Editor of one of the major journals (Burns). As in the previous year's review, articles were divided into the following topic areas: epidemiology, wound characterisation, critical care physiology, inhalation injury, infection, metabolism and nutrition, psychological considerations, pain management, rehabilitation, and burn reconstruction. Each selected article is mentioned briefly with editorial comment.

▶ As editor of the journal *Burns*, Dr Wolf has again provided us with his annual overview of 92 of the most impactful English language articles relating to burns. He summarizes a few key articles in each of his categories such as burn epidemiology, wound treatment, critical care, inhalation injury, infection, nutrition, pain and psychosocial considerations, rehabilitation, and burn reconstruction. Although cursory, the citations allow further in-depth focus for those interested in a complete article on a particular topic. Admittedly, the articles are chosen by an individual, leading to inevitable bias, and in the future, some peer-reviewed publications omitted from this review will prove to be landmark articles. However, for the busy clinician, it is impossible to read every burn-related article as it is published. At the annual American Burn Association meeting, the session entitled, "The Year in Review" is always a standing room only session. I recommend this 10 000 foot view of current thinking in burn research as well as giving a glimpse of what is most likely on the horizon.

B. A. Latenser, MD

5 Infectious Disease

Miscellaneous

Antibiotic Therapy and Treatment Failure in Patients Hospitalized for Acute Exacerbations of Chronic Obstructive Pulmonary Disease

Rothberg MB, Pekow PS, Lahti M, et al (Baystate Med Ctr, Springfield, MA; Univ of Massachusetts School of Public Health, Amherst)
JAMA 303:2035-2042, 2010

Context.—Guidelines recommend antibiotic therapy for acute exacerbations of chronic obstructive pulmonary disease (COPD), but the evidence is based on small, heterogeneous trials, few of which include hospitalized patients.

Objective.—To compare the outcomes of patients treated with antibiotics in the first 2 hospital days with those treated later or not at all.

Design, Setting, and Patients.—Retrospective cohort of patients aged 40 years or older who were hospitalized from January 1, 2006, through December 31, 2007, for acute exacerbations of COPD at 413 acute care facilities throughout the United States.

Main Outcome Measures.—A composite measure of treatment failure, defined as the initiation of mechanical ventilation after the second hospital day, inpatient mortality, or readmission for acute exacerbations of COPD within 30 days of discharge; length of stay, and hospital costs.

Results.—Of 84 621 patients, 79% received at least 2 consecutive days of antibiotic treatment. Treated patients were less likely than nontreated patients to receive mechanical ventilation after the second hospital day (1.07%; 95% confidence interval [CI], 1.06%-1.08% vs 1.80%; 95% CI, 1.78%-1.82%), had lower rates of inpatient mortality (1.04%; 95% CI, 1.03%-1.05% vs 1.59%; 95% CI, 1.57%-1.61%), and had lower rates of readmission for acute exacerbations of COPD (7.91%; 95% CI, 7.89%-7.94% vs 8.79%; 95% CI, 8.74%-8.83%). Patients treated with antibiotic agents had a higher rate of readmissions for *Clostridium difficile* (0.19%; 95% CI, 0.187%-0.193%) than those who were not treated (0.09%; 95% CI, 0.086%- 0.094%). After multivariable adjustment, including the propensity for antibiotic treatment, the risk of treatment failure was lower in antibiotic-treated patients (odds ratio, 0.87; 95% CI, 0.82-0.92). A grouped treatment approach and hierarchical modeling to account for potential confounding of hospital effects yielded similar results. Analysis stratified by risk of treatment failure found similar magnitudes of benefit across all subgroups.

Conclusion.—Early antibiotic administration was associated with improved outcomes among patients hospitalized for acute exacerbations of COPD regardless of the risk of treatment failure.

▶ The role of empiric antibiotic therapy in the absence of overt bacterial infection during exacerbations of chronic obstructive pulmonary disease (COPD) has been debated. Based on a very small number of trials, current recommendations call for antibiotic treatment of hospitalized patients with acute COPD exacerbations associated with purulent or increased sputum or shortness of breath, despite the fact that the trigger for exacerbation in over half of these cases is likely viral infection.[1] The authors of this study demonstrate in a large cohort (almost 85 000 cases identified from International Classification of Diseases coding) from a national database comprised of small to medium sized nonteaching hospitals that early antimicrobial therapy was associated with improved clinical outcome, including intensive care unit admission and mortality. These results held even after various adjustments for severity of illness and potential disparities in the 2 populations that were taken into account. The only notable risk associated with antimicrobial therapy was, predictably, a high risk of readmissions for *Clostridium difficile* infection. Of course, the study is a retrospective analysis with all the attendant issues of confounding/nonrandom allocation. Nonetheless, these data suggest that current recommendations for antibiotic therapy of COPD exacerbations are appropriate and should be routinely implemented particularly in severe cases of illness.

A. Kumar, MD

Reference

1. Snow V, Lascher S, Mottur-Pilson C. Evidence based for management of acute exacerbations of chronic obstructive pulmonary disease. *Ann Intern Med.* 2001; 134:595-599.

Can Preemptive Cytomegalovirus Monitoring Be As Effective As Universal Prophylaxis When Implemented As the Standard of Care in Patients at Moderate Risk?
McGillicuddy JW, Weimert NA, Taber DJ, et al (Med Univ of South Carolina, Charleston)
Transplantation 89:1218-1223, 2010

Background.—Cytomegalovirus (CMV) is a significant cause of morbidity, mortality, and cost in solid organ transplant recipients. This study was conducted to measure both the clinical efficacy and the pharmacoeconomic impact of implementing, as standard of care, an abbreviated preemptive monitoring strategy compared with universal prophylaxis in a large teaching hospital.

Methods.—This prospective observational study included only recipients at moderate risk for CMV infection, specifically recipients who were CMV seropositive before transplant. Recipients transplanted between February 2006 and December 2006 received prophylactic valganciclovir for 90 days after transplant, and those transplanted between January 2007 and December 2007 were enrolled in a preemptive monitoring strategy that included no anti-CMV prophylaxis but instead used serial CMV polymerase chain reactions in weeks 4, 6, 8, 10, 12, 16, 20, and 24 to monitor the development of CMV DNAemia. Costs were analyzed from a societal perspective.

Results.—A total of 130 patients were included in this study. Baseline and transplant demographics are well matched between groups. CMV syndrome occurred in three patients in each group, and one patient in the preemptive group developed CMV disease. Thirty-seven percent of patients in the preemptive group developed CMV DNAemia, 68% of these patients received antiviral therapy. Personnel and laboratory monitoring costs were significantly higher in the preemptive group, whereas medication cost was significantly higher in the prophylaxis group.

Conclusions.—Although outcomes and the overall cost of (1) universal prophylaxis and (2) preemptive monitoring are similar, universal prophylaxis places the cost burden on the patient whereas preemptive monitoring shifts the cost burden to the healthcare system (Tables 2 and 4).

▶ Cytomegalovirus (CMV) disease remains an important complication in patients with transplant. Consequently, effective management strategies are important, but given the potential impact of the disease, preventive strategies are more important. Secondary to these concerns, many centers prophylactically treat all transplant patients, whereas some treat all those calculated to be at higher risk. This article evaluates a strategy that would further limit the use of prophylaxis to a subset of patients who demonstrate viral replication by polymerase chain reaction. Importantly, all patients at high risk received prophylaxis,

TABLE 2.—Overall CMV, Patient, and Allograft Outcomes

	Universal (n = 71)	Preemptive Group (n = 59)	P
CMV syndrome (%)	4	5	0.67
CMV disease (%)	0	2	0.45
Median days to CMV (d)	181	63	0.10
Mean total WBC count (10^3 cells/mm^3)			
1 (mo)	8.3 ± 4.3	9.6 ± 3.7	0.06
3 (mo)	6.6 ± 4.3	7.2 ± 3.1	0.40
6 (mo)	7.2 ± 3.1	6.9 ± 2.7	0.60
Borderline acute rejection (%)	15	14	1.00
Acute rejection (%)	10	5	0.34
1 yr graft loss[a] (%)	4	0	0.25
1 yr death (%)	4	0	0.25

CMV, cytomegalovirus; WBC, white blood cells.
[a]Death censored.

TABLE 4.—Mean Universal Vs. Preemptive Cost Per Patient

	Universal	Preemptive	P
Total (mean ± SD)	$6674 ± 4173	$3955 ± 5428	0.001
Valganciclovir (mean ± SD)	$5870 ± 3221	$1542 ± 3832	0.001
CMV-PCR[a]	$129 ± 285	$1939 ± 706	0.001
Provider time	$62 ± 135	$612 ± 287	0.001

CMV, cytomegalovirus; PCR, polymerase chain reaction.
[a]Includes provider time.

and all patients received prophylaxis for the first 90 days after transplant. Table 2 shows that no statistical differences could be identified between the 2 strategies, while Table 4 shows this was accomplished at a lower cost. Before one changes the practice at their center, it should be notified that the study is very underpowered and thus a lack of difference between the groups may or may not be found if a higher number of patients were studied. This sort of study needs to be powered based upon the expectant rate of outcomes, which in this case, as can be seen in Table 2, are quite low necessitating a much larger study, especially given the percentage of patients with either CMV syndrome or disease was higher in the prophylactic group.

T. Dorman, MD

CD64 Index Provides Simple and Predictive Testing for Detection and Monitoring of Sepsis and Bacterial Infection in Hospital Patients

Icardi M, Erickson Y, Kilborn S, et al (Iowa City Veterans Hosp)
J Clin Microbiol 47:3914-3919, 2009

The rapid diagnosis and management of bacterial infection are heavily dependent upon clinical assessment. Blood culture may take up to 2 days for results and may be suspect. Surface neutrophil CD64 expression has been shown to be upregulated in cases of bacterial infection. Recently, a standardized kit for the CD64 index was used in neonatal intensive care units, showing high sensitivity and specificity for bacterial infections. Our study was designed to confirm and extend these results to adult hospital patients and to determine the impact of this testing on a clinical laboratory's finances and staffing. CD64 indices were performed with peripheral blood drawn in tandem with blood cultures from 109 patients over a 2-month period. We found that a CD64 index of ≤1.19 was predictive of "no growth" blood culture results. An index of >1.19 was predictive of an ultimate clinical and/or culture diagnosis of infection with a sensitivity and specificity of 94.6% and 88.7%, respectively. Positive and negative predictive values were 89.8% and 94%, respectively. The CD64 index was easily performed using our flow cytometer and staff, producing minimal alteration in clinical workflow. A 7-day-a-week testing schedule will result in some additional expense but will be more than offset by the expected cost savings. The CD64 index is a useful and inexpensive test for improving the diagnosis and management of hospital patients with bacterial infection. It can be readily performed by clinical laboratories and could result in considerable savings for the institution.

▶ Identifying infected patients accurately is extremely important for effective management. This allows early initiation of broad-spectrum coverage and ensures a better outcome. At the same time, overuse of antibiotics creates environmental pressure for the development of resistance. Thus there is always a tension between overuse and underuse of antibacterial coverage. This article looks at the use of CD64 index as a means to better identify an infected patient and finds a positive predictive value (PPV) of 89.8% and a negative predictive value (NPV) of 94%. These values make the possibility that CD64 index may play a role in antibiotic decision making in the future. Unfortunately, these predictive values also demonstrate why CD64 index is not an ideal independent tool. As a screening tool the PPV needs to be very high, and the 11% this test is off from 100% means millions of patients may go under treated and thus be harmed. Furthermore, the NPV is too low as even small percentages off mean millions at risk given the frequency of infected patients. Fig 2 in the original article shows this cross over of values. CD64 may, however, contribute to the assessment of an infected patient. Note in Fig 4 in the original article how the value falls after successful treatment and increases again with a new intercurrent process. It would be interesting to see a study where this value is used to help make the decision to stop antibiotics' faster initiation and thus help protect potentially infected patients, while limiting antibiotic exposure. For instance a study where this was used in conjunction with procalcitonin for stopping rules might prove quite fruitful. Finally, the comparison to WBC is not very useful. Although WBC is a frequent consideration, it is well known that WBC increases may lag and that with overwhelming infection of bone marrow suppressants that it may fall in the face of infectious process.

T. Dorman, MD

Early Removal of Central Venous Catheter in Patients with Candidemia Does Not Improve Outcome: Analysis of 842 Patients from 2 Randomized Clinical Trials

Nucci M, Anaissie E, Betts RF, et al (Hospital Universitário Clementino Fraga Filho, Rio de Janeiro, Brazil; Univ of Arkansas for Med Sciences, Little Rock; Univ of Rochester, NY; et al)
Clin Infect Dis 51:295-303, 2010

Background.—Patients with candidemia frequently have a central venous catheter (CVC) in place, and its early removal is considered the standard of care.

Methods.—We performed a subgroup analysis of 2 phase III, multicenter, double-blind, randomized, controlled trials of candidemia to examine the effects of early CVC removal (within 24 or 48 h after treatment initiation) on the outcomes of 842 patients with candidemia. Inclusion criteria were candidemia, age >16 years, CVC at diagnosis, and receipt of ≥1 dose of the study drug. Six outcomes were evaluated: treatment success, rates of persistent and recurrent candidemia, time to mycological eradication, and survival at 28 and 42 days. Univariate and multivariate analyses were performed, controlling for potential confounders.

Results.—In univariate analysis, early CVC removal did not improve time to mycological eradication or rates of persistent or recurrent candidemia but was associated with better treatment success and survival. These benefits were lost in multivariate analysis, which failed to show any beneficial effect of early CVC removal on all 6 outcomes and identified Acute Physiology and Chronic Health Evaluation II score, older age, and persistent neutropenia as the most significant variables. Our findings were consistent across all outcomes and time points (removal within 24 or 48 h and survival at 28 and 42 days). The median time to eradication of candidemia was similar between the 2 study groups.

Conclusions.—In this cohort of 842 adults with candidemia followed up prospectively, early CVC removal was not associated with any clinical benefit. These findings suggest an evidence-based re-evaluation of current treatment recommendations (Tables 3 and 5).

▶ The correct approach to management of central access in a patient with candidemia is simply not known. Many experts have advocated for removal of all access for as long as can be clinically tolerated, given the propensity of *Candida* to attach to access devices. Whether or not this is truly required and/or beneficial remains unknown. This article seems to show little benefit to early removal of central catheters when assessed by multivariate analysis (Table 5). However, when one looks at the univariate data in Table 3, it appears that there may be an association or possibly that the association may have been missed in an underpowered study. Importantly, this study was a retrospective

TABLE 3.—Univariate Analysis of 5 Predefined Outcomes Among 842 Patients with Candidemia According to Time of Removal of the Central Venous Catheter (CVC) (within 24 or 48 h After Treatment Initiatin)

Outcome	CVC Removed within 24 h			CVC Removed within 48 h		
	Yes ($n = 318$)	No ($n = 524$)	P	Yes ($n = 354$)	No ($n = 488$)	P
Overall treatment success	237 (74.5)	360 (68.7)	.07	266 (75.1)	331 (67.8)	.02
Persistent candidemia[a]	30/292 (10.3)	66/493 (13.4)	.20	34/328 (10.4)	62/457 (13.6)	.18
Recurrent candidemia	18 (5.7)	42 (8.0)	.21	22 (6.2)	38 (7.8)	.42
Survival at 28 days	244 (76.7)	369 (70.4)	.046	274 (77.4)	339 (69.4)	.01
Survival at 42 days	228 (71.6)	341 (65.0)	.046	256 (72.3)	313 (64.1)	.01

Note. Data are no. (%) of patients, unless indicated otherwise.
[a]Data were missing for 57 patients.

TABLE 5.—Multivariate Analysis of the Effect of Early Removal of the Central Venous Catheter (CVC) on Treatment Success and Survival At 28 and 42 Days After Treatment Initiation in 842 Patients with Candidemia

Variable	Treatment Success OR (95% CI)	P	Survival at 28 Days OR (95% CI)	P	Survival at 42 Days OR (95% CI)	P
CVC removal within 24 h after treatment initiation						
CVC removal	NT	NT	1.15 (0.79–1.67)	.45	1.19 (0.84–1.67)	.33
Persistent neutropaenia	NT	NT	0.36 (0.15–0.88)	.03	0.38 (0.16–0.90)	.03
Higher APACHE II score	NT	NT	0.90^a (0.88–0.93)	<.001	0.91^a (0.89–0.93)	<.001
Liver failure	NT	NT	0.23 (0.07–0.72)	.01	NT	NT
Surgery	NT	NT	1.46 (0.87–2.47)	.16	1.97 (1.23–3.18)	.005
Older age	NT	NT	0.98^a (0.97–0.99)	.02	0.98^a (0.97–0.99)	.02
CVC removal within 48 h after treatment initiation						
CVC removal	1.20 (0.86–1.69)	.26	1.23 (0.85–1.75)	.27	1.25 (0.88–1.75)	.20
Receipt of corticosteroids	0.64 (0.44–0.94)	.02	0.77 (0.51–1.16)	.21	0.70 (0.47–1.02)	.06
Persistent neutropaenia	0.42 (0.18–0.98)	.04	0.36 (0.15–0.89)	.03	0.38 (0.16–0.90)	.03
Higher APACHE II score	0.93^a (0.91–0.96)	<.001	0.90^a (0.88–0.93)	<.001	0.91^a (0.89–0.93)	<.001
Liver failure	NT	NT	0.22 (0.07–0.72)	.01	NT	NT
Surgery	1.25 (0.80–1.95)	.33	1.46 (0.86–2.46)	.16	1.96 (1.22–3.17)	.006
Older age	0.99^a (0.98–1.01)	.31	0.98^a (0.97–0.99)	.02	0.98^a (0.97–0.99)	.02

Note. Analysis of time to mycological eradication, success rate, and rates of persistent and recurrent candidemia was not performed because of the lack of significant effect of CVC removal on these outcomes by univariate analysis (Figure 1 and Table 2 in the original article). APACHE, Acute Physiology and Chronic Health Evaluation; CI, confidence interval; NT, not tested because this variable was not significant by univariate analysis; OR, odds ratio.
^{a}The OR is the incremental increased risk for each additional point in the scale.

subgroup analysis of a non a priori intervention, and thus any association or lack thereof requires prospective analysis before fully impacting clinical decision making. Furthermore, it is important to remember that these candidemic patients had no evidence of the catheter being infected, as these were not known to be catheter-related infections, a fact that may influence the outcome. Finally, for those that are removing all catheters in such patients, it must be remembered that older data regarding complications of line placement may not be applicable in this era of ultrasound-guided catheter placement.

T. Dorman, MD

Fever and Leukocytosis in Critically Ill Trauma Patients: It Is Not the Blood

Claridge JA, Golob JF Jr, Fadlalla AMA, et al (Case Western Reserve Univ School of Medicine, Cleveland, OH; Cleveland State Univ, OH)
Am Surg 75:405-410, 2009

The diagnosis of bacteremia in critically ill patients is classically based on fever and/or leukocytosis. The objectives of this study were to determine 1) if our intensive care unit obtains blood cultures based on fever and/or leukocytosis over the initial 14 days of hospitalization after trauma; and 2) the efficacy of this diagnostic workup. An 18-month retrospective cohort analysis was performed on consecutively admitted trauma patients. Data collected included demographics, injuries, and the first 14 days maximal daily temperature, leukocyte count, and results of blood and catheter tip cultures. Fever was defined as a maximum daily temperature of 38.5°C or greater and leukocytosis as a leukocyte count $12,000/mm^3$ or greater of blood. Five hundred ten patients were evaluated for a total of 3,839 patient-days. The mean age and injury severity score were 49 ± 1 years and 19 ± 1, respectively. Four hundred twenty-five blood culture episodes were obtained and 25 (6%) bacteremias were identified in 23 patients (5%). A significant association was found between obtaining blood cultures in patients with fever (relative risk [RR], 7.7), leukocytosis (RR, 1.3), and fever + leukocytosis (RR, 3.2). However, no significant association was found between these clinical signs and the diagnosis of bacteremia. In fact, fever alone was inversely associated with bacteremia. Our intensive care unit follows the common "fever workup" practice and obtains blood cultures based on the presence of fever and leukocytosis. However, fever and leukocytosis were not associated with bacteremia, suggesting inefficiency and that other factors are more important after trauma (Fig 1, Table 5).

▶ The authors appropriately relate early fever and leukocytosis to inflammation related to the blunt mechanism of trauma that affects most patients studied. Examination of the data tables effectively characterizes the patients who are likely to have positive blood cultures. These individuals have longer stay in the intensive care unit (ICU) and greater reliance on central venous catheters.[1,2] Injury severity is also greater, and these patients spend more time on mechanical ventilation. In fact, at our institution, catheter-related bloodstream infection, typically, is not seen until the end of the second week of a critical care unit stay with a central venous catheter. Thus, catheter-related bacteremia should be unlikely in the patients studied here.

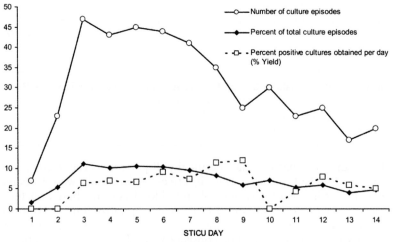

FIGURE 1.—Blood culture episodes by day. (Courtesy of Claridge JA, Golob JF Jr, Fadlalla AMA, et al. Fever and leukocytosis in critically ill trauma patients: it is not the blood. *Am Surg*. 2009;75:405-410.)

TABLE 5.—Outcome Comparison of Patients with and without Bacteremia*

	Patients with Bacteremia (n = 23)	Nonbacteremic Patients (n = 487)	P Value
Surgical and trauma intensive care unit length of stay (days)	21.6 ± 2.8	9.8 ± 0.5	<0.001
Hospital length of stay (days)	26.1 ± 4.3	12.6 ± 0.5	<0.001
Ventilator-days	9.0 ± 1.3	5.2 ± 0.2	<0.001
Central line-days	5.9 ± 1.3	1.9 ± 0.2	<0.001
Antibiotic-days	6.9 ± 1.1	2.1 ± 0.2	<0.001
Mortality	22%	6%	0.016

*Values expressed as means ± SE of the mean.

It is interesting to speculate whether the authors can provide additional insight into the etiology of early bacteremia after injury. Based on data provided in the article, in the first 2 weeks after injury, it is best to consider bacteremia in patients where clinical signs of respiratory infection are also present. Patients with evidence of lower respiratory infection are good candidates for blood and sputum cultures during the initial 2 weeks after injury. The authors must be complimented on a low rate of catheter-related bloodstream infection.

D. J. Dries, MSE, MD

References

1. McGee DC, Gould MK. Preventing complications of central venous catheterization. N Engl J Med. 2003;348:1123-1133.
2. Kusminsky RE. Complications of central venous catheterization. J Am Coll Surg. 2007;204:681-696.

Impact of the Implementation of a Sepsis Protocol for the Management of Fluid-Refractory Septic Shock: A Single-Center, Before-and-After Study

Gurnani PK, Patel GP, Crank CW, et al (Rush Univ Med Ctr, Chicago, IL)
Clin Ther 32:1285-1293, 2010

Background.—Evidence-based guidelines have been published for the acute management of severe sepsis and septic shock. Key goals of institution-driven protocols include timely fluid resuscitation and antibiotic selection, as well as source control.

Objective.—This study assessed the impact of a sepsis protocol on the timeliness of antibiotic administration, the adequacy of fluid resuscitation, and 28-day mortality in patients with fluid-refractory septic shock.

Methods.—This was a single-center, before-and-after study (18 months before July 2007 and 18 months after) with prospective data collection evaluating the outcomes of a sepsis protocol in adult patients with fluid-refractory septic shock. All patients received a fluid challenge and antibiotics; those who did not were excluded from this analysis. Preprotocol findings led to the development of the sepsis protocol, which emphasized fluid resuscitation, timely administration of antibiotic therapy, and collection of specimens for culture at the onset of septic shock. In the pre- and postprotocol phases of the study, data were collected prospectively and analyzed for demographic characteristics; Acute Physiology and Chronic Health Evaluation (APACHE) II score; appropriateness of fluid resuscitation; antibiotic use; number of vasopressor, ventilator, and intensive care unit (ICU) days; and 28-day mortality. Outcomes were measured prospectively at any time during the patient's hospital admission. The primary end points were the time to administration of antimicrobial therapy and the appropriateness of fluid resuscitation before and after implementation of the sepsis protocol.

Results.—A total of 118 patients were included in the analysis: 64 and 54 in the pre- and postprotocol groups, respectively. Patients in the preprotocol group were primarily women (53% [34/64]) and had a mean (SD) age of 61 (15.5) years and a mean APACHE II score of 28 (6.0). Patients in the postprotocol group were primarily men (54% [29/54]) and had a mean age of 52 (18.0) years and a mean APACHE II score of 27 (6.4). Implementation of the sepsis protocol resulted in a greater percentage of patients receiving timely antibiotic therapy (ie, within 4.5 hours of refractory shock; 85% [46/54] vs 56% [36/64]; $P = 0.001$) and adequate fluid resuscitation (72% [39/54] vs 31% [20/64]; $P < 0.001$) compared with the preprotocol group. Post hoc analysis found significant decreases in the number of vasopressor days (mean [SD], 3.8 [2.7] to 1.4 [1.5]; $P < 0.001$), ventilator days (9.1 [12.2] to 2.7 [4.0]; $P < 0.001$), and ICU days (12.3 [12.6] to 4.9 [3.9]; $P < 0.001$) in the postprotocol group. In-hospital mortality was not significantly different between the groups (survival 46% [28/61] before vs 54% [33/61] after the protocol). Multivariate analysis for predictors of in-hospital mortality identified an interval between shock and empiric antibiotic administration of >4.5 hours (odds ratio [OR] = 5.54; 95% CI, 1.91–16.07; $P < 0.002$), vasopressor duration in days (OR = 1.27; 95% CI, 1.01–1.59; $P = 0.037$), APACHE II score (OR = 1.14; 95% CI, 1.05–1.24; $P = 0.003$), and type of infection (community vs nosocomial, OR = 0.18; 95% CI, 0.05–0.61; $P = 0.006$) as significant predictors. The 28-day mortality decreased from 61% (39/64) to 33% (18/54) after implementation of the protocol ($P = 0.004$).

Conclusion.—Implementation of a sepsis protocol emphasizing early administration of antibiotic therapy and adequate fluid resuscitation was associated with improved clinical outcomes and lower 28-day mortality in patients with fluid-refractory septic shock at this institution.

▶ An extensive literature has developed on the importance of early antimicrobial therapy of septic shock. Data have consistently shown that delays in antimicrobial therapy are associated with increased inflammatory markers,[1] risk of renal failure[2] and acute lung injury,[3] as well as mortality[4] in serious infections and septic shock. This before-and-after study by Gurnani of 118 patients with septic shock within a single institution extends this observation by showing that the implementation of a sepsis protocol can shorten time to anti-microbial therapy yielding significant improvement in duration of pressor therapy and ventilator support, intensive care unit length of stay, and 28-day survival. Interestingly, the authors do not report an association of outcome with fluid resuscitation. To date, no randomized controlled studies of the impact of accelerated antimicrobial therapy of critical infection have been performed. In the absence of such studies, before-and-after studies such as the one by Gurnani and colleagues are the best evidence that will be available. Based on such studies, protocol-driven therapy (including efforts to speed antimicrobial delivery) of life-threatening infections is necessary for optimal outcomes.

A. Kumar, MD

References

1. Calbo E, Alsina M, Rodriguez-Carballeira M, Lite J, Garau J. The impact of time on the systemic inflammatory response in pneumococcal pneumonia. *Eur Respir J.* 2010;35:614-618.
2. Bagshaw SM, Lapinsky S, Dial S, et al. Acute kidney injury in septic shock: clinical outcomes and impact of duration of hypotension prior to initiation of antimicrobial therapy. *Intensive Care Med.* 2009;35:871-881.
3. Iscimen R, Cartin-Ceba R, Yilmaz M, et al. Risk factors for the development of acute lung injury in patients with septic shock: an observational cohort study. *Crit Care Med.* 2008;36:1518-1522.
4. Kumar A, Roberts D, Wood KE, et al. Duration of hypotension before initiation of effective antimicrobial therapy is the critical determinant of survival in human septic shock. *Crit Care Med.* 2006;34:1589-1596.

Late Admission to the ICU in Patients With Community-Acquired Pneumonia Is Associated With Higher Mortality
Restrepo MI, Mortensen EM, Rello J, et al (South Texas Veterans Health Care System, San Antonio; Hosp Universitario de Tarragona Joan XXIII, Spain; et al)
Chest 137:552-557, 2010

Background.—Limited data are available on the impact of time to ICU admission and outcomes for patients with severe community acquired pneumonia (CAP). Our objective was to examine the association of time to ICU admission and 30-day mortality in patients with severe CAP.

Methods.—A retrospective cohort study of 161 ICU subjects with CAP (by *International Classification of Diseases, 9th edition,* codes) was conducted over a 3-year period at two tertiary teaching hospitals. Timing of the ICU admission was dichotomized into early ICU admission (EICUA, direct admission or within 24 h) and late ICU admission (LICUA, ≥ day 2). A multivariable analysis using Cox proportional hazard model was created with the primary outcome of 30-day mortality (dependent measure) and the American Thoracic Society (ATS) severity adjustment criteria and time to ICU admission as the independent measures.

Results.—Eighty-eight percent (n = 142) were EICUA patients compared with 12% (n = 19) LICUA patients. Groups were similar with

TABLE 2.—Etiologic Diagnosis With an Identifiable Pathogen Causing Disease in CAP of Patients With EICUA vs LICUA

Microorganisms	EICUA (n = 57)	LICUA (n = 8)
Streptococcus pneumoniae	21 (36.8)	2 (25.0)
Staphylococcus aureus	12 (21.1)	4 (50.0)
Methicillin-resistant *S aureus*	2 (5.8)	0
Pseudomonas aeruginosa	8 (14.0)	0
Haemophilus influenzae	3 (5.3)	0
Escherichia coli	1 (1.8)	0
Klebsiella pneumoniae	2 (3.5)	1 (12.5)
Proteus mirabilis	1 (1.8)	1 (12.5)
Other[a]	3 (5.3)	0
Polymicrobial	6 (10.5)	0

Values are given as N (%). No comparisons showed statistical significant differences among the groups. Percentages have been rounded and may not sum 100.
[a]Other consists of *Aspergillus* spp, *Haemophilus parainfluenzae*, and *Enterococcus* spp.

respect to age, gender, comorbidities, clinical parameters, CAP-related process of care measures, and need for mechanical ventilation. LICUA patients had lower rates of ATS severity criteria at presentation (26.3% vs 53.5%; $P = .03$). LICUA patients (47.4%) had a higher 30-day mortality compared with EICUA (23.2%) patients ($P = .02$), which remained after adjusting in the multivariable analysis (hazard ratio 2.6; 95% CI, 1.2-5.5; $P = .02$).

Conclusion.—Patients with severe CAP with a late ICU admission have increased 30-day mortality after adjustment for illness severity. Further research should evaluate the risk factors associated and their impact on clinical outcomes in patients admitted late to the ICU (Table 2).

▶ Patients with community-acquired pneumonia (CAP) are typically assessed for severity and then started on guideline-based antibiotic treatment as soon as feasible.[1] The assessment of severity assists the clinician in determining the site of care, that is, which patients can be managed as an outpatient and which patients have severe CAP and require care in the intensive care unit (ICU).[1] Past studies have demonstrated higher mortality rates for patients with CAP who are admitted to the ICU versus the general floor.[2] Recent data have also demonstrated increased mortality associated with higher bacterial loads.[3] This retrospective 3-year study of 2 academic institutions evaluated the survival difference between those patients admitted initially or early on to the ICU for severe CAP in comparison with patients with delayed or late admission to the ICU for management of severe CAP. The late ICU patients tended to have a higher number of *Staphylococcus aureus* infections and had a significantly higher mortality rate. The higher mortality rate may reflect that these patients who required late transfer to the ICU for care did not respond to the initial antibiotic therapy or possibly had other factors that would adversely effect mortality. Late transfer to the ICU for management of CAP is a marker for poor outcome. While we cannot always predict in advance which patients will not appropriately respond to directed therapy of their CAP, these data do support early identification of patients with severe CAP and caring for them in the ICU to obtain the best possible outcome.

R. A. Balk, MD

References

1. Mandell LA, Wunderink RG, Anzueto A, et al. Infectious Disease Society of America; American Thoracic Society. Infectious Disease Society of America/American Thoracic Society Consensus guidelines on the management of community-acquired pneumonia in adults. *Clin Infect Dis.* 2007;44:S27-S72.
2. Restrepo MI, Mortensen EM, Velez JA, Frei C, Anzueto A. A comparative study of community-acquired pneumonia patients admitted to the ward and the ICU. *Chest.* 2008;133:610-617.
3. Rello J, Lisboa T, Lujan M, et al. DNA-Neumococo Study Group. Severity of pneumococcal pneumonia associated with genomic bacterial load. *Chest.* 2009; 136:832-840.

Management of the Catheter in Documented Catheter-Related Coagulase-Negative Staphylococcal Bacteremia: Remove or Retain?

Raad I, Kassar R, Ghannam D, et al (The Univ of Texas MD Anderson Cancer Ctr, Houston; Kadlec Med Ctr, Richland, WA)
Clin Infect Dis 49:1187-1194, 2009

Background.—Studies and guidelines recommending the retention of the central venous catheter (CVC) in patients with coagulase-negative staphylococcal bacteremia were based on loose definitions of bacteremia and/or did not evaluate the risk of recurrence. In this study, we used strict definitions of coagulase-negative staphylococcal bacteremia to determine the impact of CVC retention on response to and recurrence of infection.

Methods.—During the period from July 2005 through December 2007, we retrospectively evaluated 188 patients with coagulase-negative staphylococcal bacteremia. Bacteremia was defined using the strict Centers for Disease Control and Prevention criteria of 2 positive blood culture results. Catheter-related bacteremia was confirmed by differential quantitative blood cultures ($\geq$3:1) or time to positivity (>2 h).

Results.—Resolution of infection within 48 h after commencement of antimicrobial therapy was not influenced by CVC removal or exchange versus retention and occurred in 175 patients (93%). Multiple logistic regression analysis showed that infection was 7.0 times (95% confidence interval [CI], 1.5–32.6 times) more likely to fail to resolve in patients with an intensive care unit stay prior to infection ($P=.013$) and 3.8 times (95% CI, 1.1–13.3 times) more likely to fail to resolve in patients who had other concurrent sites of infection ($P=.041$). Duration of therapy did not affect recurrence. Multiple logistic regression analysis revealed that patients with catheter retention were 6.6 times (95% CI, 1.8–23.9 times) more likely to have a recurrence than were those whose catheter was removed or exchanged ($P=.004$).

Conclusions.—CVC retention does not have an impact on the resolution of coagulase-negative staphylococcal bacteremia but is a significant risk factor of recurrence.

▶ The management of catheter-related coagulase-negative staphylococcal bacteremia, one of the most common infections seen in the intensive care unit, has been controversial. In the past, many have recommended routine removal of such catheters, but the most recent Infectious Diseases Society of America guidelines do not support routine removal.[1] However, the basis of this recommendation was primarily on studies that examined resolution of acute infectious manifestations with and without line removal.[2,3] This retrospective single-center study re-examines the issue from another angle. It supports the idea that careful antibiotic therapy for appropriately chosen patients suffices in terms of resolution of clinical infection but adds to the controversy by showing that catheter retention was strongly associated with recurrence, particularly for tunneled catheters. The isolated organism for all recurrences tested was the same organism as the original infection. These data do not suggest that current recommendations are inappropriate but should be taken as a warning to monitor cured catheter infections closely for recurrence. Under the circumstance of recurrent clinical or microbiologic infection, catheter removal may be the only prudent option.

A. Kumar, MD

References

1. Mermel LA, Farr BM, Sheretz RJ, et al. Guidelines for the management of intravascular catheter-related infections. *Clin Infect Dis.* 2001;32:1249-1272.
2. Rijnders BJ, Peetermans WE, Verwaest C, Wilmer A, Van Wijngaerden E. Watchful waiting versus immediate catheter removal in ICU patients with suspected catheter-related infection: a randomized trial. *Intensive Care Med.* 2004;30: 1073-1080.
3. Capdevila JA, Segarra A, Planes AM, et al. Successful treatment of haemodialysius catheter-related sepsis without catheter removal. *Nephrol Dial Transplant.* 1993; 8:231-234.

Use of procalcitonin to reduce patients' exposure to antibiotics in intensive care units (PRORATA trial): a multicentre randomised controlled trial
Bouadma L, for the PRORATA trial group (Université Paris 7–Denis-Diderot, France; et al)
Lancet 375:463-474, 2010

Background.—Reduced duration of antibiotic treatment might contain the emergence of multidrug-resistant bacteria in intensive care units. We aimed to establish the effectiveness of an algorithm based on the biomarker procalcitonin to reduce antibiotic exposure in this setting.

Methods.—In this multicentre, prospective, parallel-group, open-label trial, we used an independent, computer-generated randomisation sequence to randomly assign patients in a 1:1 ratio to procalcitonin (n=311 patients) or control (n=319) groups; investigators were masked to assignment before, but not after, randomisation. For the procalcitonin group, antibiotics were started or stopped based on predefined cut-off ranges of procalcitonin concentrations; the control group received antibiotics according to present guidelines. Drug selection and the final decision to start or stop antibiotics were at the discretion of the physician. Patients were expected to stay in the intensive care unit for more than 3 days, had suspected bacterial infections, and were aged 18 years or older. Primary endpoints were mortality at days 28 and 60 (non-inferiority analysis), and number of days without antibiotics by day 28 (superiority analysis). Analyses were by intention to treat. The margin of non-inferiority was 10%. This trial is registered with ClinicalTrials.gov, number NCT00472667.

Findings.—Nine patients were excluded from the study; 307 patients in the procalcitonin group and 314 in the control group were included in analyses. Mortality of patients in the procalcitonin group seemed to be non-inferior to those in the control group at day 28 (21·2% [65/307] *vs* 20·4% [64/314]; absolute difference 0·8%, 90% CI −4·6 to 6·2) and day 60 (30·0% [92/307] *vs* 26·1% [82/314]; 3·8%, −2·1 to 9·7). Patients in the procalcitonin group had significantly more days without antibiotics than did those in the control group (14·3 days [SD 9·1] *vs* 11·6 days [SD 8·2]; absolute difference 2·7 days, 95% CI 1·4 to 4·1, p<0·0001).

Interpretation.—A procalcitonin-guided strategy to treat suspected bacterial infections in non-surgical patients in intensive care units could

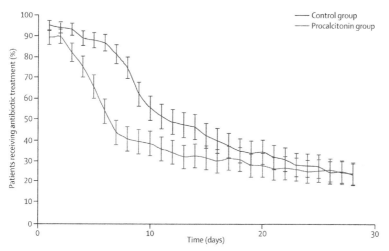

FIGURE 4.—Patients receiving antibiotics for days 1–28. Significantly fewer patients assigned to the procalcitonin group received antibiotics than did those assigned to the control group (p<0·0001, generalised linear model test for repeated measures). (Reprinted from Bouadma L, for the PRORATA trial group. Use of procalcitonin to reduce patients' exposure to antibiotics in intensive care units (PRORATA trial): a multicentre randomised controlled trial. *Lancet.* 2010;375:463-474, with permission from Elsevier.)

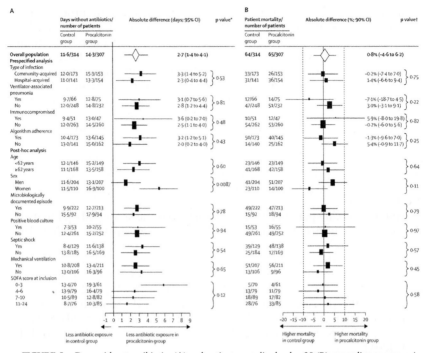

FIGURE 5.—Days without antibiotics (A) and patient mortality by day 28 (B), according to prespecified and post-hoc baseline characteristics. Dotted vertical lines in B show clinical non-inferiority margins that were calculated a priori. SOFA=sequential organ-failure assessment. *p values show the interaction between the subgroup and days without antibiotics. †p values show the interaction between the subgroup and patient mortality. (Reprinted from Bouadma L, for the PRORATA trial group. Use of procalcitonin to reduce patients' exposure to antibiotics in intensive care units (PRORATA trial): a multicentre randomised controlled trial. *Lancet.* 2010;375:463-474, with permission from Elsevier.)

reduce antibiotic exposure and selective pressure with no apparent adverse outcomes (Figs 4 and 5, Table 2).

▶ Treating patients with documented infection or suspected of being infected is a commonplace occurrence in ICUs. Published data show that delays in treatment lead to worse outcomes. Thus, clinicians tend to start treatment for a host of reasons if infection is even on the possible differential. Then, because the rules for stopping coverage are quite vague and clinicians are also concerned about stopping even when cultures are negative, overuse of antibiotics continues. Thus, too frequent initiation and prolonged unjustified use contribute potentially to the overuse of antibiotics that could be causing a progression of resistance in organisms. This study evaluated an algorithm using procalcitonin levels for both the initiation and stopping of coverage. This was compared with a more standard approach for which the clinicians received a simple reminder of general guidelines. Fig 4 shows the main outcomes consistent with the procalcitonin arm patients receiving less total coverage. In addition, Fig 5 shows that there were fewer days of coverage in

TABLE 2.—Main Outcome Variables

	Procalcitonin Group (n=307)	Control Group (n=314)	Between-Group Absolute Difference	p Value
Primary endpoints				
28-day mortality*	65 (21·2%)	64 (20·4%)	0·8% (−4·6 to 6·2)	NA
60-day mortality*	92 (30·0%)	82 (26·1%)	3·8% (−2·1 to 9·7)	NA
Number of days without antibiotics	14·3 (9·1)	11·6 (8·2)	2·7 (1·4 to 4·1)	<0·0001
Secondary endpoints (days 1–28)				
Relapse	20 (6·5%)	16 (5·1%)	1·4% (−2·3 to 5·1)	0·45
Superinfection	106 (34·5%)	97 (30·9%)	3·6% (−3·8 to 11·0)	0·29
Number of days without mechanical ventilation	16·2 (11·1)	16·9 (10·9)	−0·7 (−2·4 to 1·1)	0·47
SOFA score				
Day 1	7·5 (4·4)	7·2 (4·4)	0·3 (−0·4 to 1·0)	0·39
Day 7	4·1 (4·2)	4·0 (4·2)	0·1 (−0·6 to 0·8)	0·73
Day 14	2·8 (3·5)	2·8 (3·6)	0 (−0·6 to 0·7)	0·87
Day 21	2·1 (3·3)	1·9 (3·1)	0·2 (−0·4 to 0·8)	0·52
Day 28	1·5 (3·0)	0·9 (2·4)	0·6 (0·0 to 1·1)	0·0370
Length of stay in ICU from inclusion (days)	15·9 (16·1)	14·4 (14·1)	1·5 (−0·9 to 3·9)	0·23
Length of stay in hospital from inclusion (days)	26·1 (19·3)	26·4 (18·3)	−0·3 (−3·2 to 2·7)	0·87
Multidrug-resistant bacteria[†]	55 (17·9%)	52 (16·6%)	1·3% (−4·6 to 7·2)	0·67
Days of antibiotic exposure per 1000 inpatient days	653	812	−159 (−185 to −131)	<0·0001
Duration of first episode of antibiotic treatment (number [%]; days [SD])				
Overall population	307 (100%); 6·1 (6·0)	314 (100%); 9·9 (7·1)	−3·8 (−4·8 to −2·7)	<0·0001
Community-acquired pneumonia	79 (26%); 5·5 (4·0)	101 (32%); 10·5 (6·4)	−5·0 (−6·6 to −3·4)	<0·0001
Ventilator-associated pneumonia	75 (24%); 7·3 (5·3)	66 (21%); 9·4 (5·7)	−2·1 (−4·0 to −0·3)	0·0210
Intra-abdominal infection	14 (5%); 8·1 (7·7)	20 (6%); 10·8 (6·7)	−2·7 (−7·7 to 2·4)	0·29
Urinary tract infection	24 (8%), 7·4 (6·3)	18 (6%), 14·5 (9·3)	−7·1 (−11·9 to −2·2)	0·0053
Infection with positive blood culture	55 (18%), 9·8 (7·7)	53 (17%), 12·8 (8·1)	−3·0 (−6·0 to 0·1)	0·06

Data are number (%), difference (95% CI), or mean (SD), unless otherwise indicated. NA = not applicable. SOFA = sequential organ-failure assessment. ICU = intensive care unit.
*Difference (90% CI).

essentially all subgroups evaluated. This sounds great at first review but needs to be weighed against several concerns. First, there were a large number of treatment violations in both arms. Second, the procalcitonin arm had a recommended hard stop based on level, whereas the more standard group had the general treatment duration of the distributed materials. Fig 5 also shows that the fewer days of coverage did not translate into a mortality benefit. Furthermore, Table 2 shows some concerning trends in the data, with the procalcitonin arm having higher relapse rates, higher rates of superinfection, longer stays in the ICU and hospital, and a higher rate of multidrug-resistant organisms. Further study is clearly needed.

T. Dorman, MD

Use of procalcitonin to reduce patients' exposure to antibiotics in intensive care units (PRORATA trial): a multicentre randomised controlled trial

Bouadma L, for the PRORATA trial group (Université Paris 7–Denis-Diderot, France; et al)
Lancet 375:463-474, 2010

Background.—Reduced duration of antibiotic treatment might contain the emergence of multidrug-resistant bacteria in intensive care units. We aimed to establish the effectiveness of an algorithm based on the biomarker procalcitonin to reduce antibiotic exposure in this setting.

Methods.—In this multicentre, prospective, parallel-group, open-label trial, we used an independent, computer generated randomisation sequence to randomly assign patients in a 1:1 ratio to procalcitonin (n=311 patients) or control (n=319) groups; investigators were masked to assignment before, but not after, randomisation. For the procalcitonin group, antibiotics were started or stopped based on predefined cut-off ranges of procalcitonin concentrations; the control group received antibiotics according to present guidelines. Drug selection and the final decision to start or stop antibiotics were at the discretion of the physician. Patients were expected to stay in the intensive care unit for more than 3 days, had suspected bacterial infections, and were aged 18 years or older. Primary endpoints were mortality at days 28 and 60 (non-inferiority analysis), and number of days without antibiotics by day 28 (superiority analysis). Analyses were by intention to treat. The margin of non-inferiority was 10%. This trial is registered with ClinicalTrials.gov, number NCT00472667.

Findings.—Nine patients were excluded from the study; 307 patients in the procalcitonin group and 314 in the control group were included in analyses. Mortality of patients in the procalcitonin group seemed to be non-inferior to those in the control group at day 28 (21·2% [65/307] *vs* 20·4% [64/314]; absolute difference 0·8%, 90% CI −4·6 to 6·2) and day 60 (30·0% [92/307] *vs* 26·1% [82/314]; 3·8%, −2·1 to 9·7). Patients in the procalcitonin group had significantly more days without antibiotics than did those in the control group (14·3 days [SD 9·1] *vs* 11·6 days [SD 8·2]; absolute difference 2·7 days, 95% CI 1·4 to 4·1, p<0·0001).

Interpretation.—A procalcitonin-guided strategy to treat suspected bacterial infections in non-surgical patients in intensive care units could reduce antibiotic exposure and selective pressure with no apparent adverse outcomes.

▶ Antimicrobial resistance has become a huge factor in the management of intensive care unit (ICU) patients. Every succeeding year seems to usher in

new resistant isolates of common nosocomial pathogens, which then dissemi-
nate to ICUs across the world. For example, enteric isolates carrying the
New Delhi metallo beta lactamase resistance to all antibiotics except colistin
and tigecycline have recently been described in patients in ICUs in England,
Canada, and the United States. For the most part, the response to resistance
problems has been the development of even more powerful antibiotics.
However, science may be reaching the limits of its ability to counter microbial
evolution in this manner because the very driving force behind this evolution
to resistant pathogens is the worldwide indiscriminate overuse of potent
antimicrobials.

A more rationale approach to the problem is to focus on reduction of inappropriate use of potent antimicrobials, particularly in the ICU, where much of
this misuse occurs. The authors of this study performed a complex but important study of the use of the infection biomarker, procalcitonin, as a tool to
reduce the initial and continued use of antimicrobial therapy in the critically
ill, including a significant fraction with septic shock.

Plasma concentrations of procalcitonin, an intermediate to calcitonin, have
been shown to be specifically elevated in the presence of serious infection.[1]
The use of this biomarker appears to limit antimicrobial use in some clinical
situations[2-4] but had not been tested extensively in a general ICU population.
That has changed.

In this randomized study, the authors tested the use of procalcitonin in
a general ICU population to determine whether its use could reduce antimicrobial consumption while not adversely affecting outcome. In the experimental
group, an algorithm recommended starting, continuation, or discontinuation
of antimicrobials based on blood procalcitonin levels that were drawn
throughout the course of suspected infection, but physicians were free to
make the final decision. The control group consisted of patients treated under
standard guidelines and clinical judgment.

The experimental group did have about 3 days less antimicrobial use than did
the control group without a significant difference in mortality over 28 days even
though physicians followed the procalcitonin level–assigned recommendations
only about half the time. This may create some serious confounding in terms of
outcomes. Nonetheless, this result does suggest a significant clinical potential
for this approach. One worrying element in the findings is the trend toward
increased mortality (about 4%) later in the hospital stay (day 29-60). Although
the authors suggest this appeared to be unrelated to infection issues, the possibility of increased mortality is of concern.

Although perhaps not entirely read for broad adoption, it is clear that there
are clinical scenarios where procalcitonin may be useful, and further research
is to be encouraged.

A. Kumar, MD

References

1. Suprin E, Camus C, Gacouin A, et al. Procalcitonin: a valuable indicator of infection in a medical ICU? *Intensive Care Med.* 2000;26:1232-1238.

2. Boussekey N, Leroy O, Georges H, Devos P, d'Escrivan T, Guery B. Diagnostic and prognostic values of admission procalcitonin levels in community-acquired pneumonia in an intensive care unit. *Infection.* 2005;33:257-263.
3. Christ-Crain M, Jaccard-Stolz D, Bingisser R, et al. Effect of procalcitonin-guided treatment on antibiotic use and outcome in lower respiratory tract infections: cluster-randomised, single-blinded intervention trial. *Lancet.* 2004;363:600-607.
4. Clec'h C, Ferriere F, Karoubi P, et al. Diagnostic and prognostic value of procalcitonin in patients with septic shock. *Crit Care Med.* 2004;32:1166-1169.

Nosocomial/Ventilator-Acquired Pneumonia

A multifaceted program to prevent ventilator-associated pneumonia: Impact on compliance with preventive measures

Bouadma L, Mourvillier B, Deiler V, et al (Université Paris 7-Denis Diderot, France)
Crit Care Med 38:789-796, 2010

Objective.—To determine the effect of a 2-yr multifaceted program aimed at preventing ventilator-acquired pneumonia on compliance with eight targeted preventive measures.

Design.—Pre- and postintervention observational study.

Setting.—A 20-bed medical intensive care unit in a teaching hospital.

Patients.—A total of 1649 ventilator-days were observed.

Interventions.—The program involved all healthcare workers and included a multidisciplinary task force, an educational session, direct observations with performance feedback, technical improvements, and reminders. It focused on eight targeted measures based on well-recognized published guidelines, easily and precisely defined acts, and directly concerned healthcare workers' bedside behavior. Compliance assessment consisted of five 4-wk periods (before the intervention and 1 month, 6 months, 12 months, and 24 months thereafter).

Measurements and Main Results.—Hand-hygiene and glove-and-gown use compliances were initially high (68% and 80%) and remained stable over time. Compliance with all other preventive measures was initially low and increased steadily over time (before 2-yr level, $p < .0001$): backrest elevation (5% to 58%) and tracheal cuff pressure Maintenance (40% to 89%), which improved after simple technical equipment implementation; orogastric tube use (52% to 96%); gastric overdistension avoidance (20% to 68%); good oral hygiene (47% to 90%); and nonessential tracheal suction elimination (41% to 92%). To assess overall performance of the last six preventive measures, using ventilator-days as the unit of analysis, a composite score for preventive measures applied (range, 0–6) was developed. The median (interquartile range) composite scores for the five successive assessments were 2 (1–3), 4 (3–5), 4 (4–5), 5 (4–6), and 5 (4–6) points; they increased significantly over time ($p < .0001$). Ventilator-acquired pneumonia prevalence rate decreased by 51% after intervention ($p < .0001$).

Conclusions.—Our active, long-lasting program for preventing ventilator-acquired pneumonia successfully increased compliance with preventive

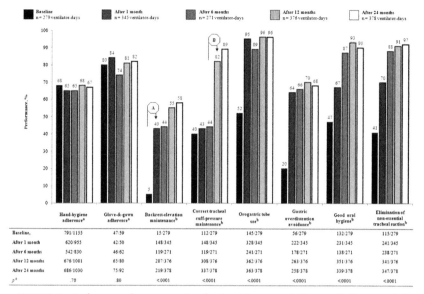

	Baseline,	After 1 month	After 6 months	Correct tracheal cuff-pressure maintenance[b]	Orogastric tube use[b]	Gastric overdistention avoidance[b]	Good oral hygiene[b]	Elimination of non-essential tracheal suction[b]
Baseline,	791/1155	47/59	15/279	112/279	145/279	56/279	132/279	115/279
After 1 month	620/955	42/50	148/345	148/345	328/345	222/345	231/345	241/345
After 6 months	542/830	46/62	119/271	119/271	241/271	178/271	138/271	238/271
After 12 months	676/1001	65/80	207/376	308/376	362/376	263/376	351/376	341/376
After 24 months	686/1030	75/92	219/378	337/378	363/378	258/378	339/378	347/378
p^c	.70	.80	<.0001	<.0001	<.0001	<.0001	<.0001	<.0001

FIGURE 2.—Performance changes over time for the eight process indicators. Performance during each 4-wk-long assessment was defined for each process indicator (Table 1) and is represented as a percentage. A and B show the times the technical improvements were implemented. Values are: [a]number of observed episodes/number of opportunities; [b]number of ventilator-days with strict recommendation adherence, as defined in Table 1 for each item; [c]determined with Cochran-Armitage tests for change over time. Only hand hygiene and glove-and-gown use compliances, which were initially high (68% and 80%), did not improve significantly. (Reprinted from Bouadma L, Mourvillier B, Deiler V, et al. A multifaceted program to prevent ventilator-associated pneumonia: impact on compliance with preventive measures. Crit Care Med. 2010;38:789-796, with permission from the Society of Critical Care Medicine and Lippincott Williams & Wilkins.)

measures directly dependent on healthcare workers' bedside performance. The multidimensional framework was critical for this marked, progressive, and sustained change (Fig 2).

▶ Ventilator-associated pneumonia (VAP) is a common complication in patients who are on ventilatory support. As we all target our clinical efforts to reduce or eliminate hospital-acquired infections and other complications in hospitalized patients, it is helpful to find techniques that work, both in the short-term and the long-term follow-up. These investigators evaluated the use of 8 common targets demonstrated in previous studies and/or guidelines to decrease the development of VAP. The investigators used a combination of education and follow-up reminders to ensure that adherence to the preventive targets did not wane over time. The success rate over the 2-year follow-up time of the various component targets in this effort is displayed in Fig 2. Use of the targeted preventive measures did successfully reduce the development of VAP in this academic medical intensive care unit.

The real value of this effort will be in the ability of the health care workers in this unit to maintain these practices and continue to reduce or eliminate the complication of VAP in the mechanically ventilated population. Unfortunately, human nature typically results in returning to past habits and constant reminders and surveillance are likely necessary to maintain this benefit.

R. A. Balk, MD

Adherence to Ventilator-Associated Pneumonia Bundle and Incidence of Ventilator-Associated Pneumonia in the Surgical Intensive Care Unit

Bird D, Zambuto A, O'Donnell C, et al (Boston Med Ctr, MA)
Arch Surg 145:465-470, 2010

Objective.—To examine the impact of adherence to a ventilator-associated pneumonia (VAP) bundle on the incidence of VAP in our surgical intensive care units (SICUs).

Design.—Prospectively collected data were retrospectively examined from our Infection Control Committee surveillance database of SICU patients over a 38-month period. Cost of VAP was estimated at $30 000 per patient stay.

Setting.—Two SICUs at a tertiary care academic level I trauma center.

Patients.—Ventilated patients admitted to a SICU.

Intervention.—The Institute for Healthcare Improvement VAP bundle was instituted at the beginning of the study and included head-of-bed elevation, extubation assessment, sedation break, peptic ulcer prophylaxis, and deep vein thrombosis prophylaxis. A daily checklist was considered compliant if all 5 items were performed for each patient.

Main Outcome Measures.—Patients were assessed for VAP. Staff were assessed for compliance with the VAP bundle.

Results.—Prior to initiation of the bundle, VAP was seen at a rate of 10.2 cases/1000 ventilator days. Compliance with the VAP bundle increased over the study period from 53% and 63% to 91% and 81% in each respective SICU. The rate of VAP decreased to 3.4 cases/1000 ventilator days. A cost savings of $1.08 million was estimated.

TABLE 1.—Ventilator-Associated Pneumonia Bundle Compliance

	Mean Compliance, % (95% CI)					
	2007		2008		2009	
Bundle Item	SICU	TICU	SICU	TICU	SICU	TICU
DVT prophylaxis	83 (77-88)	78 (73-84)	96 (94-98)	98 (97-99)	96 (91-100)	100 (100)
HOB elevation	77 (73-82)	65 (57-72)	84 (80-89)	90 (86-93)	85 (77-94)	99 (98-100)
Peptic ulcer prophylaxis	98 (96-99)	99 (98-100)	99 (98-100)	98 (97-99)	100 (99-100)	100 (99-100)
Sedation break	98 (97-99)	97 (96-99)	97 (96-98)	99 (98-100)	95 (89-100)	98 (95-100)
Assessment for extubation	96 (94-98)	92 (87-97)	97 (95-98)	97 (96-99)	99 (98-100)	94 (88-99)
Total bundle compliance	63 (57-69)	53 (46-60)	78 (73-83)	85 (82-89)	81 (72-90)	91 (85-97)

Abbreviations: CI, confidence interval; DVT, deep vein thrombosis; HOB, head-of-bed; SICU, surgical intensive care unit; TICU, trauma intensive care unit.

Conclusions.—Initiation of the VAP bundle is associated with a significantly reduced incidence of VAP in patients in the SICU and with cost savings. Initiation of a VAP bundle protocol is an effective method for VAP reduction when compliance is maintained (Table 1).

▶ To overcome the forgetfulness of human nature and to improve compliance with strategies to reduce the development of ventilator-associated pneumonia (VAP), most of our intensive care units have resorted to the use of bundles of care.[1] Studies have demonstrated the success of using a VAP prevention bundle to improve care and decrease the development of VAP. Here is another testimonial to the success of bundles.

R. A. Balk, MD

Reference

1. Resar R, Pronovost P, Haraden C, Simmonds T, Rainey T, Nolan T. Using a bundle approach to improve ventilator care processes and reduce ventilator-associated pneumonia. *Jt Comm J Qual Patient Saf.* 2005;31:243-248.

Does De-Escalation of Antibiotic Therapy for Ventilator-Associated Pneumonia Affect the Likelihood of Recurrent Pneumonia or Mortality in Critically Ill Surgical Patients?
Eachempati SR, Hydo LJ, Shou J, et al (Weill Cornell Med College, NY)
J Trauma 66:1343-1348, 2009

Background.—Ventilator-associated pneumonia (VAP) is a leading cause of mortality in critically ill patients. Although previous studies have shown that de-escalation therapy (DT) of antibiotics may decrease costs and the development of resistant pathogens, minimal data have shown its effect in surgical patients or in any patients with septic shock. We hypothesized that DT for VAP was not associated, with an increased rate of recurrent pneumonia (RP) or mortality in a high acuity cohort of critically ill surgical patients.

Methods.—All surgical intensive care unit (SICU) patients from January 2005 to May 2007 with VAP diagnosed by quantitative bronchoalveolar lavage with a positive threshold of 10,000 CFU/mL were identified. Data collected included age, gender, Acute Physiologic and Chronic Health Evaluation Score III (A3), type of bacterial or other pathogen, antibiotics used for initial and final therapy, mortality, RP, and appropriateness of initial therapy (AIT). Patients were designated as receiving AIT, DT, or escalation of antibiotic therapy based on microbiology for their VAP.

Results.—One hundred thirty-eight of 1,596 SICU patients developed VAP during the study period (8.7%). For VAP patients, the mean Acute Physiologic and Chronic Health Evaluation III score was 82.7 points with a mean age of 63.8 years. The RP rate was 30% and did not differ between patients receiving DT (27.3%) and those who did not receive DT (35.1%). Overall mortality was 37% (55% predicted by A3 norms) and did not differ between those receiving DT (33.8%) or not (42.1%). The most common pathogens for primary VAP were methicillin-resistant *Staphylococcus aureus* (14%), *Escherichia coli* (11%), and *Pseudomonas aeruginosa* (9%) whereas *P. aeruginosa* was the most common pathogen in RP. The AIT for all VAP was 93%. De-escalation of therapy occurred in 55% of patients with AIT whereas 8% of VAP patients required escalation of antibiotic therapy. The most commonly used initial antibiotic choice was vancomycin/piperacillin-tazobactam (16%) and the final choice was piperacillin-tazobactam (20%). Logistic regression demonstrated no specific parameter correlated with development of RP. Higher A3 (Odds ratio, 1.03; 95% confidence interval, 1.01–1.05) was associated with mortality whereas lack of RP (odds ratio, 0.31; 95% confidence interval, 0.12–0.80), and AIT reduced mortality (odds ratio, 0.024; 95% confidence interval, 0.007–0.221). Age, gender, individual pathogen, individual antibiotic regimen, and the use of DT had no effect on mortality.

Conclusion.—De-escalation therapy did not lead to RP or increased mortality in critically ill surgical patients with VAP. De-escalation therapy was also shown to be safe in patients with septic shock. Because of its acknowledged benefits and lack of demonstrable risks, de-escalation therapy should be used whenever possible in critically ill patients with VAP.

▶ In this era of ever-expanding resistance patterns common microorganisms, it is important to practice good antibiotic stewardship to decrease pressure on microorganisms to develop resistance mechanisms and prolong the efficacy of our current antibiotic regimens. Antibiotic stewardship includes de-escalating therapy when there is clinical improvement and when it is possible to administer more targeted antibiotic therapy based on culture and sensitivity results. In the intensive care patient with ventilator-associated pneumonia, there are often multiple factors at play that can have substantial impact on outcome. When the patient continues to be critically ill, it is often difficult to reduce antibiotic treatment for fear of recurrence or lack of success, even when good antibiotic stewardship would tell us that it is time to de-escalate therapy. These authors evaluated the use of de-escalation and antibiotic stewardship in their surgical intensive care unit (ICU) in a large academic medical center. Importantly, they were able to de-escalate antibiotic management in 55% of the patients and noted the same rate of mortality in those who received de-escalation of antibiotics and in those patients who did not receive de-escalation. They concluded that this practice is safe to use in a critically ill population of patients in the ICU and with septic shock.

I support these authors for their commitment to demonstrate the safety of de-escalation therapy in critically ill patients. The next step should be to evaluate whether or not good antibiotic stewardship with de-escalation of antibiotics, truly does result in an improved antibiogram in the ICU and reduces the development of resistance in organisms.

R. A. Balk, MD

Early Bacteremia After Solid Organ Transplantation

Linares L, García-Goez JF, Cervera C, et al (Barcelona-IDIBAPS-Univ of Barcelona, Spain)
Transplant Proc 41:2262-2264, 2009

Objective.—Bloodstream infections (BSI) are a major cause of morbidity and mortality after solid organ transplantation. Our aim was to analyze early BSI after solid organ transplantation.

Materials and Methods.—A prospective cohort study included patients undergoing a kidney, simultaneous kidney-pancreas (SPK), or orthotopic liver transplantation (OLT) from 2003–2007. We prospectively collected demographic variables, underlying chronic diseases, transplantation procedures, and posttransplant complications. Recorded cases of BSI were defined as significant according to CDC criteria. Early BSIs were considered to be those appearing within 30 days posttransplantation.

Results.—During the study period, we performed 902 transplantations: 474 renal, 340 liver, and 88 pancreas. Seventy episodes of early BSI were diagnosed in 67 patients (7.4%). The incidences of BSI according to the type of transplantation were: 4.8% in renal, 4.5% in SPK, and 12% in OLT ($P < .001$). Sixty-three percent of the bacteria isolated were gram-negative, the most frequent being *Escherichia coli*, of which 18 (54%) were extended-spectrum beta-lactamase-producing (ESBL), and *Pseudomonas aeruginosa*, of which 18 (31%) were multidrug-resistant. The most frequent gram-positive bacteria were coagulase-negative staphylococci (20%). The urinary tract was a frequent source of BSI (27%), followed by a catheter (18%). Two patients (3%) died, both liver recipients, but neither death was related to the BSI.

Conclusions.—In our setting, the incidence of early BSI among solid organ transplant recipients was high, especially liver recipients, but with low associated mortality. The most frequent sources of infection were urinary tract and catheter. Gram-negative BSI showed a high rate of multidrug resistance.

▶ In this series, infectious complications after liver transplantation are more common than those following pancreatic and renal replacement. Clearly, replacement of the liver is a larger surgical procedure and may be associated with additional blood product use, which increases infectious complications.[1-3] In general, infectious complications after liver transplantation are relatively common. In the first month after transplantation, infections are, typically, related to surgical complications, comorbid conditions, or initial graft function. Risk factors, more likely to be seen in the setting of hepatic transplantation include prolonged operation, large volume blood transfusion, and reoperation for bleeding or bile leakage.

We are told little about these transplant patients to gain additional insight into the risk of infection. However, it is important to note that multidrug resistant organisms are quite common. I was impressed at a near 50% incidence of extended-spectrum beta-lactamase-producing organisms. Although CDC criteria are used to identify infections, I am concerned that we are told little about general aspects of care among these patient groups. For example, coagulase-negative staphylococci were isolated in 50% of catheter-related bloodstream infections among liver transplant recipients. We are not told whether these staphylococci are methicillin resistant. In our critical care population, a high incidence of methicillin resistance is seen. Are these bacteria pathogens or contaminants?

Finally, I would like to know more about catheter management and culture procedures in these patients. Additional outcome data with transplant patients from this group could shed additional light on risk factors for bacteremia.

D. J. Dries, MSE, MD

References

1. Sihler KC, Napolitano LM. Complications of massive transfusion. *Chest.* 2010; 137:209-220.
2. McGilvray ID, Greig PD. Critical care of the liver transplant patient: an update. *Curr Opin Crit Care.* 2002;8:178-182.
3. Bernard AC, Davenport DL, Chang PK, Vaughan TB, Zwischenberger JB. Intraoperative transfusion of 1 U to 2 U packed red blood cells is associated with increased 30-day mortality, surgical-site infection, pneumonia, and sepsis in general surgery patients. *J Am Coll Surg.* 2009;208:931-939.

Enteric absorption and pharmacokinetics of oseltamivir in critically ill patients with pandemic (H1N1) influenza

Ariano RE, Sitar DS, Zelenitsky SA, et al (St Boniface General Hosp, Winnipeg, Manitoba, Canada; Univ of Manitoba, Winnipeg, Canada; et al)
CMAJ 182:357-363, 2010

Background.—Whether the enteric absorption of the neuraminidase inhibitor oseltamivir is impaired in critically ill patients is unknown. We documented the pharmacokinetic profile of oseltamivir in patients admitted to intensive care units (ICUs) with suspected or confirmed pandemic (H1N1) influenza.

Methods.—We included 41 patients 18 years of age and older with suspected or confirmed pandemic (H1N1) influenza who were admitted for ventilatory support to nine ICUs in three cities in Canada and Spain. Using tandem mass spectrometry, we assessed plasma levels of oseltamivir free base and its active metabolite carboxylate at baseline (before gastric administration of the drug) and at 2, 4, 6, 9 and 12 hours after the fourth or later dose.

Results.—Among the 36 patients who did not require dialysis, the median concentration of oseltamivir free base was 10.4 (interquartile range [IQR] 4.8–14.9) µg/L; the median concentration of the carboxylate metabolite was 404 (IQR 257–900) µg/L. The volume of distribution of the carboxylate metabolite did not increase with increasing body weight ($R^2 = 0.00$, $p = 0.87$). The rate of elimination of oseltamivir carboxylate was modestly correlated with estimations of creatinine clearance ($R^2 = 0.27$, $p < 0.001$). Drug clearance in the five patients who required continuous renal replacement therapy was about one-sixth that in the 36 patients with relatively normal renal function.

Interpretation.—Oseltamivir was well absorbed enterically in critically ill patients admitted to the ICU with suspected or confirmed pandemic (H1N1) influenza. The dosage of 75 mg twice daily achieved plasma levels that were comparable to those in ambulatory patients and were far in excess of concentrations required to maximally inhibit neuraminidase activity of the virus. Adjustment of the dosage in patients with renal dysfunction requiring continuous renal replacement therapy is appropriate; adjustment for obesity does not appear to be necessary.

▶ Current guidelines from the World Health Organization recommend that all patients with pandemic (H1N1) influenza be treated with oseltamivir. They have also recommended that in cases of progressive or severe disease, a higher dose (150 mg twice a day) be considered. However, little data exist regarding the pharmacokinetics of oseltamivir, especially in a critically ill patient. In this elegant study, the authors evaluated the pharmacokinetics and enteric absorption of oseltamivir in a group of critically ill patients with pandemic (H1N1) influenza. Patients were treated with oral oseltamivir 75 mg or 150 mg twice daily. Blood samples were obtained at baseline and at preidentified time points after achievement of a steady state. The findings of the study are significant because they provide the much needed pharmacokinetic information on a drug that is used to treat a novel form of influenza in critically ill patients. It also provides some very clinically useful information for intensivists dealing with patients with H1N1. The authors report excellent enteric absorption of oseltamivir. In this study, the average plasma concentration of oseltamivir was well over the 50 percent maximal inhibitory concentration reported for influenza (H1N1) virus. Furthermore, there was no relationship between increase in weight of patients and plasma levels achieved. These 2 findings suggest that perhaps there is no need to use the high-dose regime (150 mg twice daily) in an obese or a critically ill patient. A limitation pointed out by the authors was that there were no data obtained on lung levels of the drug. Finally, they also evaluated patients undergoing renal replacement therapy. The findings of this study suggest that dose adjustment for patients on renal replacement is appropriate because they achieve much higher levels than patients who have normal renal function. This is an important contribution to our understanding of the pharmacokinetics of oseltamivir in critically ill patients. The findings of this study should be taken into account when prescribing this drug in the intensive care unit.

S. L. Zanotti-Cavazzoni, MD

How Many Lumens Should Be Cultured in the Conservative Diagnosis of Catheter-Related Bloodstream Infections?

Guembe M, Rodríguez-Créixems M, Sánchez-Carrillo C, et al (Universidad Complutense, Madrid, Spain)
Clin Infect Dis 50:1575-1579, 2010

Background.—Recent practice guidelines for the diagnosis of catheter-related bloodstream infection (CRBSI) describe as an "unresolved issue" the number of lumens from which blood culture specimens should be drawn to make a conservative diagnosis of CRBSI. Our objective was to determine how many CRBSI episodes would be missed if not all catheter lumens were sampled.

Methods.—We performed a retrospective study (1 January 2003– 31 May 2009) in patients with microbiologically proven CRBSI in which all available catheter lumens (those that did not contain clots) were used to draw blood culture samples. We calculated the number of episodes that would have been missed in double- and triple-lumen catheters if the culture of samples obtained from ≥1 lumens had been eliminated.

Results.—We studied 171 episodes of proven CRBSI in 154 patients. Overall, if 1 lumen-associated culture had been eliminated for both double-lumen and triple-lumen catheters, we would have missed 27.2% and 15.8% of episodes of CRBSI, respectively. If we had eliminated 2 cultures for triple-lumen catheters, 37.3% of episodes would have been missed.

Conclusions.—Samples for blood culture should be obtained through all catheter lumens to establish a diagnosis of CRBSI (Table 4).

▶ Knowing how to best address central access in a patient suspected of being infected is of utmost importance to clinicians. Years ago, it was believed to be best to change the site of access every 3 days. Then the literature demonstrated that rewiring and culturing the catheter was a better approach in most patients as it led to fewer mechanical complications. Recently, there has been a growing number of advocates for culturing these percutaneous catheters through

TABLE 4.—Number and Percentage of Missed Episodes

Variable	Double-Lumen Catheters ($n = 112$)	Triple-Lumen Catheters ($n = 59$)
When eliminating 1 lumen		
No. (%) of episodes	81.4 (72.8)	49.7 (84.2)
95% CI, %	65.2–81.3	74.6–93.2
P	<.001	.001
When eliminating 2 lumens		
No. (%) of episodes	...	37 (62.7)
95% CI, %		49.2–74.6
P		<.001

NOTE. CI, confidence interval.

a lumen and looking at differential time to positivity as compared with peripherally obtained blood cultures. What has not been clear from that body of literature is how many lumens must be cultured from a multilumen catheter to confidently rule out a catheter-related infection. This article demonstrates through retrospective analysis that a statistically and clinically significant number of infections would have been missed (Table 4). Thus, it would seem unacceptable to culture only some of the lumens of a multilumen catheter. Although this has not been shown to be true prospectively, it would be prudent to adopt such a practice until more data can inform our decision making. Of course, one could choose to simply rewire catheters and avoid this situation completely.

T. Dorman, MD

Procalcitonin for reduced antibiotic exposure in ventilator-associated pneumonia: a randomised study

Stolz D, Smyrnios N, Eggimann P, et al (Univ Hosp, Basel, Switzerland; Univ Hosp, Lausanne, Switzerland; UMass Memorial Med Ctr, Worcester, MA; et al)
Eur Respir J 34:1364-1375, 2009

In patients with ventilator-associated pneumonia (VAP), guidelines recommend antibiotic therapy adjustment according to microbiology results after 72 h. Circulating procalcitonin levels may provide evidence that facilitates the reduction of antibiotic therapy.

In a multicentre, randomised, controlled trial, 101 patients with VAP were assigned to an antibiotic discontinuation strategy according to guidelines (control group) or to serum procalcitonin concentrations (procalcitonin group) with an antibiotic regimen selected by the treating physician. The primary end-point was antibiotic-free days alive assessed 28 days after VAP onset and analysed on an intent-to-treat basis.

Procalcitonin determination significantly increased the number of antibiotic free-days alive 28 days after VAP onset (13 (2–21) days *versus* 9.5 (1.5–17) days). This translated into a reduction in the overall duration of antibiotic therapy of 27% in the procalcitonin group (p = 0.038). After adjustment for age, microbiology and centre effect, the rate of antibiotic discontinuation on day 28 remained higher in the procalcitonin group compared with patients treated according to guidelines (hazard rate 1.6, 95% CI 1.02–2.71). The number of mechanical ventilation-free days alive, intensive care unit-free days alive, length of hospital stay and mortality rate on day 28 for the two groups were similar.

Serum procalcitonin reduces antibiotic therapy exposure in patients with ventilator associated pneumonia (Figs 2 and 3, Table 4).

▶ Initiating early broad-spectrum antibiotic coverage for a patient with a potential infectious process is important to help ensure a better outcome. The ongoing use of antibiotics after negative cultures exposes the patient and the

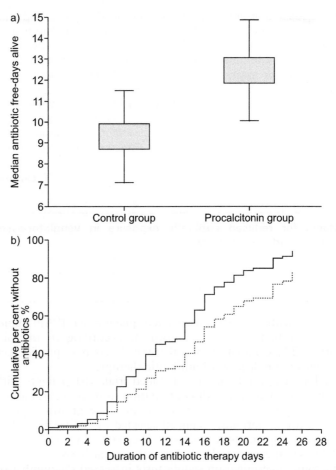

FIGURE 2.—a) Median number of antibiotic-free days alive in patients in the control and the procalcitonin group at 28 days after onset of ventilator-associated pneumonia. p = 0.049. b) Cumulative frequency distribution curve for the time to discontinuation of antibiotics in patients in the control (······) and the procalcitonin (——) group on day 28. Adjusted by age, respiratory tract culture results and centre effect. p = 0.043. (Reprinted from Stolz D, Smyrnios N, Eggimann P, et al. Procalcitonin for reduced antibiotic exposure in ventilator-associated pneumonia: a randomised study. *Eur Respir J.* 2009;34:1364-1375, with permission from ERS Journals Ltd.)

environment needlessly to antibiotic pressures that generate resistant organisms. Strategies that help limit this misuse of coverage are important. Fig 2 shows that the strategy used in this article of monitoring procalcitonin concentrations to help guide decision making indeed led to fewer days of antibiotic coverage. Fig 3 shows how all patients were equally exposed at the outset and how there was a trend to declining therapy in both groups, but how the procalcitonin strategy led to a greater decrease in subsequent antibiotic use. Unfortunately, even in the procalcitonin group, the primary physician had the final decision to decrease therapy or not and, thus, the results are biased

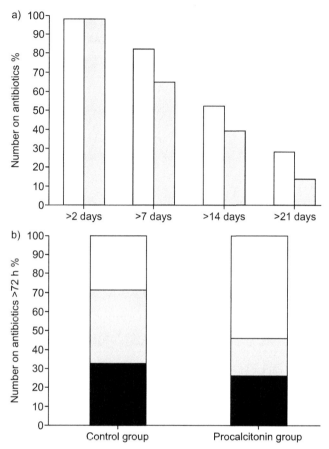

FIGURE 3.—a) Duration of antibiotic therapy. Percentage of patients in control (□) and procalcitonin (□) group on antibiotics beyond 2, 7, 14 and 21 days. b) Antibiotic reduction profile. Percentage of patients in control group and procalcitonin group on monotherapy and combination therapy with one (□), two (□) or three or more (■) antibiotics after 72 h. $p = 0.008$. (Reprinted from Stolz D, Smyrnios N, Eggimann P, et al. Procalcitonin for reduced antibiotic exposure in ventilator-associated pneumonia: a randomised study. *Eur Respir J*. 2009;34:1364-1375, with permission from ERS Journals Ltd.)

because of the manner in which the study group may have had even greater degrees of decreased usage. In fact, this lack of compliance with guidance demonstrates the cultural barrier to change commonly seen in health care and, thus, alerts future researchers in this domain to address this barrier in advance stages of their study. In addition, Table 4 shows that although the primary outcome of less antibiotic use was achieved, this did not translate into meaningful clinical benefit. This study was not powered to find that benefit, so a type 2 error may exist. These results do, however, justify a larger study of this strategy to test for changes in clinical outcome.

T. Dorman, MD

TABLE 4.—Secondary Study Outcomes in Patients with Ventilator-Associated Pneumonia (VAP) According to the Treatment Algorithm

	Control Group[#]	Procalcitonin Group[¶]	p-Value
MV-free days alive, days 1–28			
All patients	19 (8.5–22.5)	21 (2–24)	0.455
Nonfermenting GNB	15 (7–20)	12 (0.3–23)	0.867
MRSA	15 (0–22)	14 (6–21)	1
Other bacteria	19 (1.8–24.8)	22 (15.5–24.5)	0.284
No bacteria	21.5 (18.8–23.3)	23 (3.5–27)	0.563
ICU-free days alive, days 1–28			
All patients	8.5 (0–18)	10 (0–18)	0.526
Nonfermenting GNB	0 (0–11)	4 (0–13.5)	0.683
MRSA	15 (2–17)	9 (1.5–15)	0.548
Other bacteria	7.5 (1–17.8)	14 (7.5–20)	0.139
No bacteria	18 (1.5–20)	10 (1.–19.5)	0.554
Length of hospital stay days			
All patients	26 (16.8–22.3)	26 (7–21)	0.153
Nonfermenting GNB	34 (26–46)	31 (13–35.5)	0.130
MRSA	28 (17–41)	26 (23.5–37.5)	1.0
Other bacteria	24 (16.5–32.5)	21.5 (14–28)	0.442
No bacteria	28.5 (16–38)	29 (9.5–33)	0.343
VAP-related clinical deterioration days 1–28[+]	7 (14)	5 (10)	0.759
Discharge home days 1–28	3 (6)	5 (10)	0.479
Discharge to another institution days 1–28	32 (64)	35 (69)	0.509
Death from all causes days 1–28	12 (24)	8 (16)	0.327
In-hospital mortality	14 (28)	10 (20)	0.322

Data are presented as median (interquartile range) and n (%), unless otherwise stated. MV: mechanical ventilation; GNB: Gram-negative bacilli; MRSA: methicillin-resistant *Staphylococcus aureus*; ICU: intensive care unit.
[#]n = 50.
[¶]n = 51.
[+]Defined as an increase in clinical pulmonary infection score more than two points.

6 Postoperative Management

Cardiovascular Surgery

Analysis of the Impact of Early Surgery on In-Hospital Mortality of Native Valve Endocarditis: Use of Propensity Score and Instrumental Variable Methods to Adjust for Treatment-Selection Bias
Lalani T, for the International Collaboration on Endocarditis–Prospective Cohort Study (ICE-PCS) Investigators (Duke Univ Med Ctr, Durham, NC; et al)
Circulation 121:1005-1013, 2010

Background.—The impact of early surgery on mortality in patients with native valve endocarditis (NVE) is unresolved. This study sought to evaluate valve surgery compared with medical therapy for NVE and to identify characteristics of patients who are most likely to benefit from early surgery.
Methods and Results.—Using a prospective, multinational cohort of patients with definite NVE, the effect of early surgery on in-hospital mortality was assessed by propensity-based matching adjustment for survivor bias and by instrumental variable analysis. Patients were stratified by propensity quintile, paravalvular complications, valve perforation, systemic embolization, stroke, *Staphylococcus aureus* infection, and congestive heart failure. Of the 1552 patients with NVE, 720 (46%) underwent early surgery and 832 (54%) were treated with medical therapy. Compared with medical therapy, early surgery was associated with a significant reduction in mortality in the overall cohort (12.1% [87/720] versus 20.7% [172/832]) and after propensity-based matching and adjustment for survivor bias (absolute risk reduction [ARR] −5.9%, P<0.001). With a combined instrument, the instrumental-variable–adjusted ARR in mortality associated with early surgery was −11.2% (P<0.001). In subgroup analysis, surgery was found to confer a survival benefit compared with medical therapy among patients with a higher propensity for surgery (ARR−10.9% for quintiles 4 and 5, P=0.002) and those with paravalvular complications (ARR −17.3%, P<0.001), systemic embolization (ARR −12.9%, P=0.002), *S aureus*

NVE (ARR −20.1%, *P*<0.001), and stroke (ARR−13%, *P*=0.02) but not those with valve perforation or congestive heart failure.

Conclusions.—Early surgery for NVE is associated with an in-hospital mortality benefit compared with medical therapy alone.

▶ Native valve endocarditis (NVE) is associated with a significant mortality risk, estimated at 15% to 30%. Consensus guidelines advocate early surgery if it is associated with complications,[1] but these are based largely on limited data, which have been retrospective in nature and have included small sample sizes. In this article, Lalani and colleagues used a subset of patients from a prospective cohort of patients with definite NVE to evaluate whether early surgery impacted in-hospital mortality. This prospective cohort is part of the larger cohort of the International Collaboration on Endocarditis-Prospective Cohort Study. The entire cohort includes 2760 patients with definitive endocarditis as defined by the modified Duke criteria.[2] One thousand five hundred fifty-two met the inclusion criteria for this report. It is important to note that they excluded patients with prosthetic valves, nonnative valve infective endocarditis (ie, pacemaker), in-hospital death, and patients with intravenous (IV) drug use. Patients with IV drug use constituted 44% of their entire patient population. The authors report that early surgical intervention for NVE is associated with lower in-hospital mortality (Table 2). Early intervention was defined as replacement or repair of the valve during the index hospitalization.

While this study has limitations associated with all observational studies—an important one of which is the risk of unmeasured confounders introduced by the lack of randomization, that is, care providers use an array of data to guide the decision of whether or not to operate early, and these variables are not captured in the database and are thus unmeasured—the authors have taken steps to minimize these. The strengths of this study are that a prospective cohort

TABLE 2.—Unadjusted and Adjusted ARRs and Odds Ratios for Mortality Associated with Early Surgery and Medical Therapy

Risk-Adjustment Method for In-Hospital Mortality	ARR, %*	P	Odds Ratio	95% Confidence Interval
Unadjusted	−8.6	<0.001	0.53	0.40–0.70
Logistic regression[†]	−5.9	<0.001	0.56	0.38–0.82
Propensity matched, survivor-bias adjusted[‡]	−5.9	<0.001	0.55	0.31–0.96
Instrumental-variable adjusted[§]	−11.2	<0.001	0.44	0.33–0.59

*A negative value represents the percent difference in mortality between patients undergoing early surgery and medical therapy, in favor of early surgery.

[†]Logistic regression of mortality against 27 measured covariates and 5 interaction terms (see Table II in the online-only Data Supplement).

[‡]Patients matched on the basis of the propensity for surgery (see Table I in the online-only Data Supplement for propensity-score model) and follow-up times such that each patient in the medical therapy group survived at least as long as the time to surgery in the surgically treated patient. Logistic regression was performed with clustered standard errors, to account for matching with replacement, and interaction terms.

[§]Using the combined instrument, 22 measured covariates, and 5 interaction terms as the independent variables and mortality and early surgery as the dependent variable. Independent variable analysis was performed with the bivariate probit (biprobit) method.

was used in addition to advanced statistical modeling to attempt to account for measured and unmeasured confounding factors. The authors used multiple methods to account for these, including propensity matching, based on the likelihood that a patient would undergo surgery adjusted for survival time and instrumental variable methods. Propensity score matching has become a well-accepted methodology for adjusting for factors that, in this case, contributed to the decision to operate early. Frequently, well-performed multivariable logistic regressions result in similar qualitative findings compared with propensity matching techniques, which is the case in this study (Table 2).

What is very unique in this article is the use of instrumental variable methods. Instrumental variables are described as those variables that impact the decision to operate but are not associated with mortality. By teasing these out and adjusting for these, the authors argue that they are accounting to a great extent for those unmeasured, and unknown, biases or confounders, and the results more accurately reflect the true impact of surgery. This methodology is a well-established technique.[3] Table 2 reflects the quantitative differences in the absolute risk reduction found using the different methodologies. All of the methodologies used resulted in consistent qualitative findings (ie, all showed a risk reduction with surgery). While there may be some disagreement about the exact variables used in the final analysis,[4] the consistency of the findings is certainly suggestive that early surgery is truly protective in this patient population. It is important to note that this patient population does not include patients who are IV drug users, a significant proportion of individuals in the parent cohort, and that there was a lack of stratification of the severity of heart failure or its response to initial medical treatment,[4] making it challenging to generalize these findings. Furthermore, this cohort is cared for by a group of providers who have experience with early surgery, and this also may limit generalizability to centers with a different level of experience.

This article is an important contribution to the literature in its incorporation of advanced statistical modeling to gain greater insight into the management of NVE. However, no matter what statistical modeling is used, this remains an observational trial, and questions remain unanswered. The authors identify 2 potentially very important prospective randomized trials evaluating the use of surgery in patients with NVE that are underway, of which we anxiously await the results.

E. A. Martinez, MD, MHS

References

1. Bonow RO, Carabello BA, Kanu C, et al. ACC/AHA 2006 guidelines for the management of patients with valvular heart disease: a report of the American College of Cardiology/American Heart Association Task Force on Practice Guidelines (writing committee to revise the 1998 Guidelines for the Management of Patients With Valvular Heart Disease): developed in collaboration with the Society of Cardiovascular Anesthesiologists: endorsed by the Society for Cardiovascular Angiography and Interventions and the Society of Thoracic Surgeons. *Circulation.* 2006;114:e84-e231.
2. Li JS, Sexton DJ, Mick N, et al. Proposed modifications to the Duke criteria for the diagnosis of infective endocarditis. *Clin Infect Dis.* 2000;30:633-638.

3. Newhouse JP, McClellan M. Econometrics in outcomes research: the use of instrumental variables. *Annu Rev Public Health.* 1998;19:17-34. 10.1146/annurev.publhealth.19.1.17.
4. Farzaneh-Far R, Bolger AF. Surgical timing in infectious endocarditis: wrestling with the unrandomized. *Circulation.* 2010;121:960-962.

Effect of the Perioperative Blood Transfusion and Blood Conservation in Cardiac Surgery Clinical Practice Guidelines of the Society of Thoracic Surgeons and the Society of Cardiovascular Anesthesiologists upon Clinical Practices

Likosky DS, FitzGerald DC, Groom RC, et al (Dartmouth-Hitchcock Med Ctr Dartmouth College, Lebanon, NH; Harvard Med School, Boston, MA; Maine Med Ctr, Portland; et al)
Anesth Analg 111:316-323, 2010

Background.—The 2007 Society of Thoracic Surgeons and the Society of Cardiovascular Anesthesiologists Clinical Practice Guideline for Perioperative Blood Transfusion and Blood Conservation in Cardiac Surgery was recently promulgated and has received much attention. Using a survey of cardiac anesthesiologists and perfusionists' clinical practice, we aimed to assess the current practices of perfusion, anesthesia, and surgery, as recommended by the Guidelines, and to also determine the role the Guidelines had in changing these practices.

Methods.—Nontrainee members of the Society of Cardiovascular Anesthesiologists, the American Academy of Cardiovascular Perfusion, the Canadian Society of Clinical Perfusion, and the American Society of Extra-Corporeal Technology were surveyed using a standardized survey instrument that examined clinical practices and responses to the Guidelines.

Results.—A total of 1402 surveys from 1061 institutions principally in the United States (677 institutions) and Canada (34 institutions) were returned, a 32% response rate. There was wide distribution of the Guidelines with 78% of anesthesiologists and 67% of perfusionists reporting having read all, part, or a summary of the Guidelines. However, only 20% of respondents reported that an institutional discussion had taken place as a result of the Guidelines, and only 14% of respondents reported that an institutional monitoring group had been formed. There was wide variability in current preoperative testing, perfusion, surgical, and pharmacological practices reported by respondents. Twenty-six percent of respondents reported 1 or more practice changes in response to the Guidelines. The changes made were reported to be highly (9%) or somewhat (31%) effective in reducing overall transfusion rates. Only 4 of 38 Guideline recommendations were reported by >5% of respondents to have been changed in response to the Guidelines.

Conclusions.—Wide variation in clinical practices of cardiac surgery was reported. Little change in clinical practices was attributed to the

Society of Thoracic Surgeons/Society of Cardiovascular Anesthesiologists Guidelines.

▶ With the introduction of the Institute of Medicine's report, "To Err is Human," the problem of medical errors became widely publicized and evident to practitioners. What is frequently forgotten is that errors include the lack of the delivery of evidence-based care. For example, McGlynn and colleagues demonstrated that less than 55% of patients received recommended practices for a number of chronic care conditions.[1] This article by Likosky and colleagues takes a very important look at the incorporation of evidence-based guidelines into clinical practice for cardiac surgical patients and how perioperative cardiac surgery providers are performing with these new guidelines. Not surprisingly, they found wide variation in adoption of these guidelines. They cite many of the common reasons or barriers as to why this occurs.[2] One of the most common barriers is lack of knowledge about the guidelines. This important issue was identified in the survey by Likosky, who found that over 20% of the respondents reported that they had not read the guidelines, and only 20% reported that they had an institutional discussion about the guidelines. Thus, in this study Likosky and colleagues identify an important gap in the quality of care for cardiac surgery patients and discuss what barriers may be playing a role in the lack of incorporation of these into practice.

An important area of study in medicine is the identification of barriers to the implementation of guidelines.[2] Barriers to implementation are local and must be systematically identified and addressed if we are to improve adherence. This can be challenging. Gurses and colleagues present a novel tool to facilitate the local identification and elimination of barriers.[3]

E. A. Martinez, MD, MHS

References

1. McGlynn EA, Asch SM, Adams J, et al. The quality of health care delivered to adults in the United States. *N Engl J Med.* 2003;348:2635-2645.
2. Cabana MD, Rand CS, Powe NR, et al. Why don't physicians follow clinical practice guidelines? A framework for improvement. *JAMA.* 1999;282:1458-1465.
3. Gurses AP, Murphy DJ, Martinez EA, Berenholtz SM, Pronovost PJ. A practical tool to identify and eliminate barriers to compliance with evidence-based guidelines. *Jt Comm J Qual Patient Saf.* 2009;35:526-532.

Frail Patients Are at Increased Risk for Mortality and Prolonged Institutional Care After Cardiac Surgery
Lee DH, Buth KJ, Martin B-J, et al (Dalhousie Univ, Halifax, Nova Scotia, Canada)
Circulation 121:973-978, 2010

Background.—Frailty is an emerging concept in medicine yet to be explored as a risk factor in cardiac surgery. Where elderly patients are increasingly referred for cardiac surgery, the prevalence of a frail group among these is also on the rise. We assessed frailty as a risk factor for adverse outcomes after cardiac surgery.

Methods and Results.—Functional measures of frailty and clinical data were collected prospectively for all cardiac surgery patients at a single center. Frailty was defined as any impairment in activities of daily living (Katz index), ambulation, or a documented history of dementia. Of 3826 patients, 157 (4.1%) were frail. Frail patients were older, were more likely to be female, and had risk factors for adverse surgical outcomes. By logistic regression, frailty was an independent predictor of in-hospital mortality (odds ratio 1.8, 95% CI 1.1 to 3.0), as well as institutional discharge (odds ratio 6.3, 95% CI 4.2 to 9.4). Frailty was an independent predictor of reduced midterm survival (hazard ratio 1.5, 95% CI 1.1 to 2.2).

Conclusions.—Frailty is a risk for postoperative complications and an independent predictor of in-hospital mortality, institutional discharge, and reduced midterm survival. Frailty screening improves risk assessment in cardiac surgery patients and may identify a subgroup of patients who may benefit from innovative processes of care.

▶ This observational study was designed to explore the association of frailty and outcomes following cardiac surgery. The authors included all cardiac surgical procedures and defined frailty as any impairment in activities of daily living (using the Katz[1] index), ambulation, or a documented history of dementia. Frailty, as they describe, is an emerging concept and risk factor. Frailty, in general, is a marker of biological age and in theory is independent of age. It has previously been shown to be associated with falls, hospitalizations, institutionalization, and mortality. This report is the first look at this marker and its association with multiple outcomes following cardiac surgery. The authors found a significant association between frailty and the outcomes of interest. Using logistic regression and adjusting for important variables that were shown to be associated with these outcomes, for those patients designated as frail, the risk of in-hospital mortality was increased by 80%; the risk of institutional discharge was increased by 6 times; and midterm survival was decreased by 50% compared with those who did not meet the frailty criteria. These findings were independent of age, and there was no interaction with age identified (using an interaction term in the analysis).

While this article clearly demonstrates a consistent association between frailty and outcomes, the limitations are important to note. First, the definition of frailty varies in the literature. The authors have certainly identified important clinical parameters, but to further the study of frailty, a definition that can be used across patient populations will be necessary for us to begin to be able to understand the broader impact of frailty on health outcomes. Second, the authors did not include other important clinical parameters that may reflect the aging or frail population, for example the pulse pressure difference, which has been shown to be associated with worse outcomes in the cardiovascular patient population. Nonetheless, as the authors point out, these findings are important for discussing risks with our patients and for designing potential interventions targeted to improve outcomes in this subset of patients.

E. A. Martinez, MD, MHS

Reference

1. Katz S, Ford AB, Moskowitz RW, Jackson BA, Jaffe MW. Studies of illness in the aged. the index of Adl: a standardized measure of biological and psychosocial function. *JAMA*. 1963;185:914-919.

Hemofiltration During Cardiopulmonary Bypass Does Not Decrease the Incidence of Atrial Fibrillation After Cardiac Surgery
Mauermann WJ, Nuttall GA, Cook DJ, et al (Mayo Clinic, Rochester, MN)
Anesth Analg 110:329-334, 2010

Background.—Atrial fibrillation (AF) occurs in 20%–50% of patients after cardiac surgery and is associated with increased morbidity and mortality. Corticosteroids are reported to decrease the incidence of postoperative AF, presumably by attenuating inflammation caused by surgery and cardiopulmonary bypass (CPB). We hypothesized that hemofiltration during CPB, which may attenuate inflammation, might decrease the incidence of AF after cardiac surgery.

Methods.—This was a retrospective review of patients previously enrolled in a double-blind, placebo-controlled trial evaluating the effects of perioperative steroid therapy and hemofiltration during CPB on duration of postoperative mechanical ventilation. In that study, 192 patients undergoing cardiac surgery were randomized to 1 of 3 groups: controls (placebo), hemofiltration during CPB, or perioperative steroid therapy. Patient records were reviewed to determine the incidence of new onset AF defined as any electrocardiogram evidence of AF or AF diagnosed by the patients' clinicians.

Results.—Of the 192 enrolled patients, 3 were excluded for protocol violations and 4 were excluded for history of chronic AF. Data from 185 patients from the original study were available for review. Sixty patients (32%) had new onset AF after cardiac surgery. There was no difference among groups in the incidence of AF (control group, 21%; steroid group, 41%; hemofiltration group, 36%; $P = 0.057$ among groups). The only risk factor for the development of AF was age (mean age of patients with AF, 65.4 ± 10.1 yr vs patients without AF, 61.4 ± 11.5 yr; $P = 0.024$). When age, procedure type, and presence or absence of chronic obstructive pulmonary disease were controlled for in multivariate analysis, the difference among study groups remained nonsignificant ($P = 0.108$).

Conclusions.—Perioperative corticosteroids or the use of hemofiltration during CPB did not decrease the incidence of AF after cardiac surgery. Further studies evaluating the efficacy and safety of perioperative corticosteroids for prevention of postoperative AF are warranted before their routine use can be recommended.

▶ Atrial fibrillation (AF) remains a common complication following cardiac surgery.[1] Patients who develop postoperative AF have been shown to have increased morbidity and mortality. Many factors have been implicated in the genesis of AF. Perioperative inflammation has been increasingly implicated, and the interventions evaluated in these 2 articles target this mechanism.[2,3]

Mauermann and colleagues performed a post hoc analysis of patients who were previously enrolled in a double-blinded randomized controlled trial evaluating the impact of perioperative steroids or intraoperative hemofiltration on postoperative pulmonary complications. They retrospectively reviewed the records for episodes of AF, as this was not collected as part of the prospective trial. The groups were similar at baseline, and they report the incidence of AF to be 30%, which is consistent with the literature. When they adjusted for age, procedure type (valve vs no valve), and chronic obstructive pulmonary disease, there was no difference in the incidence of postoperative AF among the 3 groups (control, steroids, and hemofiltration). These independent variables were predetermined based on the literature. Only age was associated with AF in the univariate analysis. Two of the key limitations to this study are that they retrospectively identified AF and they did not measure inflammatory markers. For the first limitation, the diagnosis of AF in this study relied heavily on surveillance and documentation, and both of these may introduce an important bias. For example, the identification of the outcome of interest depended on the bedside provider's identification and documentation. There may have been self-limited episodes of AF that did not require intervention, regardless of their duration, and may not have been captured. However, it is likely that this would not have resulted in a systematic bias, but instead random bias, and therefore would be distributed equally between the 3 groups, so the results would likely not change. With regard to the second limitation, the authors have not demonstrated the adequacy of the interventions to actually suppress inflammation.

In another article, Heidarsdottir and colleagues[3] used a much stronger study design as they prospectively identified episodes of AF. They evaluated a novel intervention: treatment with n-3 polyunsaturated fatty acids (n-3 PUFAs), an anti-inflammatory agent, for the prevention of AF using a randomized controlled blinded design. While they report in the abstract that there were no differences at baseline, they show in the article that the patient groups differed in length of bypass time: those in the placebo group have a median length of 100.5 minutes compared with 83 minutes in the intervention group ($P = .047$). They too did not find a difference in incidence of AF. Importantly, they did track C-reactive protein levels, a reasonable marker of inflammation, but they were unable to demonstrate a difference in the concentration of the peak postoperative C-reactive protein levels between the 2 groups with the dose of n-3-PUFA used.

These articles highlight that while we have identified a potential target for intervention—inflammation—we still do not have a magic bullet. We may either not have the correct pharmacologic intervention or we do not understand the appropriate dose. In addition, they highlight that we may need to continue to look for other targets for reducing the incidence of postoperative AF. Given the lack of breakthroughs in treatment, current therapy should still include the use of perioperative beta blockers. The most recent guidelines[4] suggest that the best interventions are prophylactic beta blockers (and amiodarone in patients who do not tolerate beta blockers) and biatrial pacing out for 3 days postoperatively.

E. A. Martinez, MD, MHS

References

1. Hogue CW Jr, Creswell LL, Gutterman DD, Fleisher LA. Epidemiology, mechanisms, and risks: American College of Chest Physicians guidelines for the prevention and management of postoperative atrial fibrillation after cardiac surgery. *Chest.* 2005;128:9S-16S.
2. Mauermann WJ, Nuttall GA, Cook DJ, Hanson AC, Schroeder DR, Oliver WC. Hemofiltration during cardiopulmonary bypass does not decrease the incidence of atrial fibrillation after cardiac surgery. *Anesth Analg.* 2010;110:329-334.
3. Heidarsdottir R, Arnar DO, Skuladottir GV, et al. Does treatment with n-3 polyunsaturated fatty acids prevent atrial fibrillation after open heart surgery? *Europace.* 2010;12:356-363.
4. McKeown PP, Gutterman D. Executive summary: American College of Chest Physicians guidelines for the prevention and management of postoperative atrial fibrillation after cardiac surgery. *Chest.* 2005;128:1S-5S.

No Major Differences in 30-Day Outcomes in High-Risk Patients Randomized to Off-Pump Versus On-Pump Coronary Bypass Surgery: The Best Bypass Surgery Trial

Møller CH, Perko MJ, Lund JT, et al (Copenhagen Univ Hosp, Denmark)
Circulation 121:498-504, 2010

Background.—Off-pump coronary artery bypass grafting compared with coronary revascularization with cardiopulmonary bypass seems safe and results in about the same outcome in low-risk patients. Observational studies indicate that off-pump surgery may provide more benefit in high-risk patients. Our objective was to compare 30-day outcomes in high-risk patients randomized to coronary artery bypass grafting without or with cardiopulmonary bypass.

Methods and Results.—We randomly assigned 341 patients with a Euro-SCORE ≥5 and 3-vessel coronary disease to undergo coronary artery bypass grafting without or with cardiopulmonary bypass. Patients were followed through the Danish National Patient Registry. The primary outcome was a composite of adverse cardiac and cerebrovascular events (ie, all-cause mortality, acute myocardial infarction, cardiac arrest with successful resuscitation, low cardiac output syndrome/cardiogenic shock, stroke, and coronary reintervention). An independent adjudication committee blinded to treatment allocation assessed the outcomes. Baseline characteristics were well balanced between groups. The mean number of grafts per patient did not differ significantly between groups (3.22 in off-pump group and 3.34 in on-pump group; $P=0.11$). Fewer grafts were performed to the lateral part of the left ventricle territory during off-pump surgery (0.97 versus 1.14 after on-pump surgery; $P=0.01$). No significant differences in the composite primary outcome (15% versus 17%; $P=0.48$) or the individual components were found at 30-day follow-up.

Conclusions.—Both off- and on-pump coronary artery bypass grafting can be performed in high-risk patients with low short-term complications.

Clinical Trial Registration.—clinicaltrials.gov. Identifier: NCT00120991.

▶ With the introduction of off-pump coronary artery bypass (OPCAB) surgery, there was the expectation that there would be broad improvements in outcomes, such as decreased stroke with the avoidance of an aortic cross clamp and decreased postoperative pulmonary complications with the avoidance of cardiopulmonary bypass. Since that time, there have been numerous studies to compare outcomes. A recent meta-analysis, which included randomized controlled trials (RCTs), suggested that there was no difference in outcomes, except for possibly a reduced risk of postoperative atrial fibrillation.[1] Some of the criticisms of the RCTs to date are that they only included lower risk patients. Some of the observational studies, however, have included high-risk patients and did show benefit from OPCAB. Two recent RCTs have been added to the literature. In the first, Moller and colleagues report findings from a single-center study that evaluated the short-term (30-day) outcomes in a group of high-risk patients (EuroSCORE ≥5; approximately 50% of patients had an ejection fraction [EF] ≤50%) from Denmark, who were randomized to OPCAB versus on-pump CAB. They used a composite outcome at 30 days postoperation and showed no significant difference in this outcome (all-cause mortality, acute myocardial infarction [MI], cardiac arrest with successful resuscitation, low cardiac output syndrome/cardiogenic shock, stroke, and coronary reintervention) or any of the individual component outcomes between the 2 groups. This held true for both the intention-to-treat analysis and when a sensitivity analysis was done (a total of 14 treatment crossovers occurred). There were no reported differences between the groups at baseline and no patients were lost to follow-up—an important advantage when national longitudinal databases are available. One of the findings of this trial and others was that there were fewer grafts to the lateral wall of the left ventricle.

Another study by Hueb[2] reported on the long-term outcomes of the MASS III Trial. This was also a single-center RCT that included patients who may have been at a lower risk (excluded patients with left ventricular EF < 40%; mean EF approximately 69%) than those in the Moller trial. The strength of this trial is that patients were followed out to 5 years. The authors report that there were no differences in the primary composite end point (death, MI, further revascularization, or stroke) at 5 years. They did, however, identify some significant differences in some intermediate outcomes. There was a statistically significant decrease in duration of surgery, intensive care unit and hospital length of stay, time to extubation, incidence of atrial fibrillation, and blood requirements in the OPCAB group. However, these did not seem to have any impact on all-cause mortality or the composite end point.

The limitations of both of these trials are that they are single-center studies with a subset of surgeons who are likely experienced with OPCAB and that the lack of risk or benefit with OPCAB on long-term outcomes may not be evident because of surgeon experience. While the expected broad benefits of OPCAB do not seem to be realized, these studies are important in that they show that there does not appear to be an increase in risk with this technique, at least in the hands of experienced surgeons. The question remains how generalizable these findings are to one's patient population and skill level.

E. A. Martinez, MD, MHS

References

1. Møller CH, Penninga L, Wetterslev J, Steinbruchel DA, Gluud C. Clinical outcomes in randomized trials of off-vs. on-pump coronary artery bypass surgery: systematic review with meta-analyses and trial sequential analyses. *Eur Heart J.* 2008;29:2601-2616.
2. Hueb W, Lopes NH, Pereira AC, et al. Five-year follow-up of a randomized comparison between off-pump and on-pump stable multivessel coronary artery bypass grafting. The MASS III Trial. *Circulation.* 2010;122:S48-S52.

Postoperative and Long-Term Outcome of Patients With Chronic Obstructive Pulmonary Disease Undergoing Coronary Artery Bypass Grafting

Angouras DC, Anagnostopoulos CE, Chamogeorgakis TP, et al (Attikon Univ Hosp, Athens, Greece; Columbia Univ, NY)
Ann Thorac Surg 89:1112-1118, 2010

Background.—Chronic obstructive pulmonary disease (COPD) has been conventionally associated with increased operative mortality and morbidity after coronary artery bypass grafting. Some studies, however, challenge this association. Moreover, the effect of COPD on long-term survival after coronary artery bypass grafting has not been adequately assessed. Thus, in this clinical setting, both early and late outcome require further examination.

Methods.—We studied 3,760 consecutive patients who underwent isolated coronary artery bypass grafting between 1992 and 2002. The propensity for COPD was determined by logistic regression analysis, and each patient with COPD was matched with 3 patients without COPD. Matched groups were compared for early outcome and long-term survival (mean follow-up, 7.6 years). Long-term survival data were obtained from the National Death Index.

Results.—There were 550 patients (14.6%) with COPD. Multivariate analysis showed that patients with COPD were older and sicker. However, propensity-matched groups did not differ in terms of hospital mortality or major morbidity, although COPD was associated with a slightly longer hospital stay. In contrast, COPD patients had increased long-term mortality, with a hazard ratio of 1.28 (95% confidence intervals, 1.11 to 1.47; $p = 0.001$). Freedom from all-cause mortality at 7 years after CABG was 65% and 72% in matched patients with and without COPD, respectively ($p = 0.008$). In patients with COPD, the hazard estimate was consistently increased up to 9 years postoperatively.

Conclusions.—Chronic obstructive pulmonary disease, although not an independent predictor of increased early mortality and morbidity in this series, is a continuing detrimental risk factor for long-term survival.

▶ The presence of chronic obstructive pulmonary disease (COPD) is typically accepted as a risk factor for increased morbidity and mortality following cardiac surgery and is incorporated into both the Society of Thoracic Surgeons and the EuroSCORE risk models for operative mortality. These investigators performed an observational prospective study evaluating the association between COPD and outcomes following coronary artery bypass grafting (CABG) surgery, given that there still are conflicting data supporting the use of COPD as an independent predictor for worse outcomes. In this article, they have demonstrated that patients with COPD were older and sicker and that they had a slightly longer hospital length of stay and a 30% increased long-term mortality risk, even when adjusted for baseline characteristics (propensity-matched groups).

The strengths of this study are that they followed patients out to a mean follow-up of 7.6 years, they used data that were collected prospectively, and used propensity score matching, a well-accepted statistical technique for accounting for unmeasured confounders. However, the limitations need to be considered. First, this study is by its nature observational, so is marked by the limitations inherent to this design. Importantly, however, they have attempted to account for this using propensity score matching. We will always be limited to observational data when assessing the impact of COPD on outcomes. Second, the definition of COPD that was used for this, while allowing for a reproducible definition, did not allow for discerning mild versus severe COPD. Clumping all patients with COPD into 1 group may have had significant impact on the outcome of interest and may have resulted in missing true differences in some of the other outcomes of interest. Third, the authors appropriately elected to censor those patients for whom they could not ascertain their death status at hospital discharge. However, they did not perform a sensitivity analysis to evaluate the impact of these patients on the outcomes of interest. If these patients do not have a social security number and therefore cannot be tracked, they may be very different than the overall cohort (unmeasured confounders), for example, if they included a group of undocumented aliens whose long-term risks may be increased. Fourth, they did not look for temporal trends, and this study spanned a 10-year period. During this time, the management of these patients may have changed and the risk of dying may have changed over this time course. Fifth, they utilized the social security index to define mortality, and the cause of death is not known. The natural history of the disease of COPD is that these patients are at increased risk of morbidity and mortality. Perhaps a more interesting question is how their mortality risk is modified by the intervention. To better understand this association between CABG and the natural history of COPD, we might compare this patient population to patients with COPD who do not have coronary artery disease (CAD) and those with COPD and CAD but who are medically managed or underwent percutaneous procedures. The addition of a comparison group would give the reader important insight into these issues because the real questions are what might be done for these patients in the perioperative and follow-up periods to modify their long-term mortality risk and whether these interventions are any different than for those who did not undergo CABG.

E. A. Martinez, MD, MHS

Predicting Hospital Mortality and Analysis of Long-Term Survival After Major Noncardiac Complications in Cardiac Surgery Patients
Rahmanian PB, Adams DH, Castillo JG, et al (Univ Hosp Cologne, Germany; Mount Sinai School of Medicine, NY)
Ann Thorac Surg 90:1221-1229, 2010

Background.—This study was designed to investigate the incidence of and early and midterm outcomes after major complications in cardiac surgery patients. We determined independent predictors of operative mortality to create a model for prediction of outcome. A particular focus was the fate of patients after the occurrence of these complications.

Methods.—Prospectively collected data of 6,641 patients (mean age, 64 ± 14 years; n = 2,499 female [38%]) undergoing cardiac surgery between January 1998 and December 2006 were retrospectively analyzed. Outcome measures were six index complications: respiratory failure, sepsis, dialysis-dependent renal failure, mediastinitis, gastrointestinal complication, and stroke; and their impact on operative mortality, hospital length of stay, and midterm survival using multivariate regression models. The discriminatory power was evaluated by calculating the area under the receiver operating characteristic curves (C statistic).

Results.—A total of 1,354 complications were observed in 826 (12.4%) patients: respiratory failure (n = 634; 9.5%), sepsis (n = 202; 3%), stroke (n = 163; 2.5%), dialysis-dependent renal failure (n = 145; 2.2%), mediastinitis (n = 111; 1.7%), and gastrointestinal complication (n = 99; 1.5%). Overall operative mortality was 20% and correlated with the number of complications (single, 12.0%; n = 58 of 485; double, 25.5%; n = 52 of 204; ≥ 3, 40.1%; n = 55 of 137). Ten preoperative and five postoperative predictors of operative mortality were identified and included in the logistic model, which accurately predicted outcome (C statistic, 0.866). One-year survival was less than 50% in patients with three or more complications and a length of stay greater than 60 days.

Conclusions.—With a worsening in the risk profile of patients undergoing cardiac surgery, an increasing number of patients develop major complications leading to increased length of stay and mortality, which is correlated to the number and severity of these complications. Our

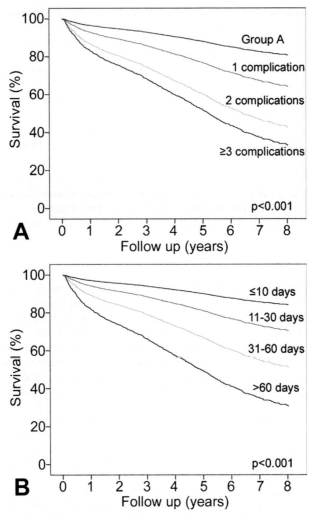

FIGURE 3.—Adjusted long-term survival according to the number of postoperative index complications (A) and to the length of hospitalization (B). Adjusted for age, sex, ejection fraction, diabetes, peripheral vascular disease, and type of procedure. (Reprinted from Rahmanian PB, Adams DH, Castillo JG, et al. Predicting hospital mortality and analysis of long-term survival after major noncardiac complications in cardiac surgery patients. *Ann Thorac Surg*. 2010;90:1221-1229, with permission from The Society of Thoracic Surgeons.)

predictive model based on preoperative and postoperative variables allowed us to determine with accuracy the operative mortality in critically ill patients after cardiac surgery. One-year survival after multiple complications and prolonged length of stay remains marginal (Fig 3, Table 4).

▶ As interventional cardiologists and radiologists expand their repertoire and increase their expertise with minimally invasive percutaneous procedures to

TABLE 4.—Predictors of In-Hospital Mortality in Multivariate Analysis

Variable	Coefficient B	OR	95% CI	p Value
Preoperative variables				
Female sex	0.5	1.7	(1.3–2.3)	<0.001
Age >70 y	0.4	1.4	(1.1–1.9)	0.016
Ejection fraction <0.30	0.6	1.8	(1.3–2.5)	<0.001
Peripheral vascular disease	0.7	2.0	(1.4–2.8)	<0.001
Creatinine >2.5 no dialysis	0.9	2.4	(1.3–4.4)	0.006
Acute MI	1.1	2.9	(1.3–6.4)	0.009
Hemodynamic instability	0.8	2.2	(1.2–3.9)	0.007
Emergent procedures	0.6	1.8	(1.1–3.1)	0.032
Reoperation	0.4	1.5	(1.1–2.1)	0.019
Other than CABG	0.5	1.6	(1.2–2.3)	0.006
Postoperative morbidities				
Respiratory failure	0.9	2.5	(1.7–3.6)	<0.001
Sepsis	0.5	1.6	(1.0–2.6)	0.042
Stroke	1.2	3.4	(2.1–5.4)	<0.001
Renal failure (dialysis)	2.1	8.2	(5.2–12.9)	<0.001
GIC	1.2	3.2	(1.8–5.6)	<0.001
Intercept (a)	−5.0			

CABG = coronary artery bypass grafting; CI = confidence interval; GIC = gastrointestinal complication; MI = myocardial infarction; OR = odds ratio.

correct vascular and valvular abnormalities, the cardiovascular surgeon is left operating on those individuals who have too difficult an abnormality or other clinical attributes that deem them to be of high risk for the less invasive procedure. The fallout from this practice is a significant increase in morbidity and mortality associated with cardiovascular procedures performed on this higher risk profile population of patients. This retrospective review of over 6600 cardiovascular surgery patients evaluated the impact of 6 common complications on important outcome parameters, including operative mortality and hospital length of stay. Table 4 lists the preoperative and postoperative conditions identified in multivariate analysis as predictive of in-hospital mortality. Fig 3 illustrates the significant impact the presence of single and multiple complications has on mortality. While sepsis was the most common complication found in these individuals, those who developed renal failure requiring dialysis had the highest odds ratio for increased mortality.

These data illustrate how important it is to continually evaluate the outcome data for the procedures we perform to understand the dramatic impact changes in technology and patient selection have on these variables.

R. A. Balk, MD

Predicting Hospital Mortality and Analysis of Long-Term Survival After Major Noncardiac Complications in Cardiac Surgery Patients

Rahmanian PB, Adams DH, Castillo JG, et al (Univ Hosp Cologne, Germany; Mount Sinai School of Medicine, NY)

Ann Thorac Surg 90:1221-1229, 2010

Background.—This study was designed to investigate the incidence of and early and midterm outcomes after major complications in cardiac surgery patients. We determined independent predictors of operative mortality to create a model for prediction of outcome. A particular focus was the fate of patients after the occurrence of these complications.

Methods.—Prospectively collected data of 6,641 patients (mean age, 64 ± 14 years; n = 2,499 female [38%]) undergoing cardiac surgery between January 1998 and December 2006 were retrospectively analyzed. Outcome measures were six index complications: respiratory failure, sepsis, dialysis-dependent renal failure, mediastinitis, gastrointestinal complication, and stroke; and their impact on operative mortality, hospital length of stay, and midterm survival using multivariate regression models. The discriminatory power was evaluated by calculating the area under the receiver operating characteristic curves (C statistic).

Results.—A total of 1,354 complications were observed in 826 (12.4%) patients: respiratory failure (n = 634; 9.5%), sepsis (n = 202; 3%), stroke (n = 163; 2.5%), dialysis-dependent renal failure (n = 145; 2.2%), mediastinitis (n = 111; 1.7%), and gastrointestinal complication (n = 99; 1.5%). Overall operative mortality was 20% and correlated with the number of complications (single, 12.0%; n = 58 of 485; double, 25.5%; n = 52 of 204; ≥3, 40.1%; n = 55 of 137). Ten preoperative and five postoperative predictors of operative mortality were identified and included in the logistic model, which accurately predicted outcome (C statistic, 0.866). One-year survival was less than 50% in patients with three or more complications and a length of stay greater than 60 days.

Conclusions.—With a worsening in the risk profile of patients undergoing cardiac surgery, an increasing number of patients develop major complications leading to increased length of stay and mortality, which is correlated to the number and severity of these complications. Our predictive model based on preoperative and postoperative variables allowed us to determine with accuracy the operative mortality in critically ill patients after cardiac surgery. One-year survival after multiple complications and prolonged length of stay remains marginal.

▶ Multiple reasons have led to a growing cardiac surgery population of older patients with multiple preoperative comorbid conditions. This not only entails them having multiple pre-existing comorbidities but also requiring more complex procedures than isolated coronary artery bypass grafting. The study in consideration aimed at formulating a model using pre- and postoperative variables and accurately predicting the operative mortality in critically ill patients undergoing cardiac surgery depending on these variables. The study identified a large and heterogeneous group of patients, all of whom underwent a variety of procedures. It also identified the 15 independent predictors of in-hospital mortality, including preoperative ejection fraction, history of congestive heart failure, hemodynamic parameters at the time of admission, and the emergent nature of the procedure. The most common postoperative complications were respiratory failure, stroke, and dialysis-dependent renal failure. The 1-year survival was associated with the number of complications. In patients with 3 or more postoperative complications, 1-year survival was only 50%. The in-hospital length of stay (LOS), especially the intensive care unit LOS, correlated directly with the decline in survival in the first 6 months after discharge. This well-designed study sheds some light into some of the determinants of prognosis in the changing population of patients undergoing cardiac surgery.

S. L. Zanotti-Cavazzoni, MD

Preoperative C-reactive Protein Predicts Long-term Mortality and Hospital Length of Stay after Primary, Nonemergent Coronary Artery Bypass Grafting
Perry TE, for the CABG Genomics Investigators (Harvard Med School, Boston, MA; et al)
Anesthesiology 112:607-613, 2010

Background.—Preoperative C-reactive protein (CRP) levels more than 10 mg/l have been shown to be associated with increased morbidity and mortality after cardiac surgery. We examine the value of preoperative CRP levels less than 10 mg/l for predicting long-term, all-cause mortality and hospital length of stay in surgical patients undergoing primary, non-emergent coronary artery bypass graft-only surgery.

Methods.—We examined the association between preoperative CRP levels stratified into four categories (< 1, $1–3$, $3–10$, and > 10 mg/l), and 7-yr all-cause mortality and hospital length of stay in 914 prospectively enrolled primary, nonemergent coronary artery bypass graft-only surgical patients using a proportional hazards regression model.

Results.—Eighty-seven patients (9.5%) died during a mean follow-up period of 4.8 ± 1.5 yr. After proportional hazards adjustment, the 3–10 and > 10 mg/l preoperative CRP groups were associated with long-term, all-cause mortality (hazards ratios [95% CI]: 2.50 [1.22–5.16], $P = 0.01$ and 2.66 [1.21–5.80], $P = 0.02$, respectively) and extended hospital length of stay (1.32 [1.07–1.63], $P < 0.001$ and 1.27 [1.02–1.62], $P = 0.001$, respectively).

Conclusion.—We demonstrate that preoperative CRP levels as low as 3 mg/l are associated with increased long-term mortality and extended hospital length of stay in relatively lower-acuity patients undergoing primary, nonemergent coronary artery bypass graft-only surgery. These important findings may allow for more objective risk stratification of patients who present for uncomplicated surgical coronary revascularization.

▶ C-reactive protein (CRP) is a marker for systemic inflammation and may also be a mediator of inflammation. It is a well-known marker for cardiovascular risk in nonsurgical patients. There are also data regarding cardiac surgery showing that levels > 10 mg/L are associated with increased postoperative morbidity and mortality. However, a level of 10 mg/dL is in the very high range, and many of these studies were done in higher-acuity patients who are generally accepted as in the highest risk category for postoperative morbidity and mortality. This is in comparison to a level of > 3 mg/L, which is generally the cutoff for high in the medical population and has been shown to be associated with a marked increase in risk of cardiovascular events in multiple nonsurgical patient populations. Therefore, this group of authors sought to examine the association between lower levels of preoperative CRP and outcomes in nonemergent coronary artery bypass graft (CABG) patients—a lower risk group for postoperative events. A subset of lower-acuity patients who were part of a large-scale prospective observational cohort study (CABG Genomics trial) was included in this analysis. To identify this lower-acuity subset, they excluded patients with an elevated preoperative troponin, evidence of a preoperative infection, concomitant valve, and/or emergency surgery. The authors have successfully demonstrated that after adjusting for other comorbidities, lower levels of CRP in nonemergent and lower-acuity patients are associated with a statistically significant increased risk of mortality at 7 years follow-up (Fig 2 in the original article). While it is important to note that the baseline characteristics of the patients differed significantly across multiple risk factors, such as there were more females, smokers, and patients with a greater body mass index in the higher CRP groups, these were accounted for in the regression analysis, and the conclusions remain important. These findings may improve our ability to risk stratify cardiac surgical patients and strengthen some of the current risk scores. However, the more important question is whether this is a modifiable risk factor. Future research is needed to identify whether this is a modifiable risk factor for this patient population, in addition to others.

E. A. Martinez, MD, MHS

Surgical "buy-in": The contractual relationship between surgeons and patients that influences decisions regarding life-supporting therapy
Schwarze ML, Bradley CT, Brasel KJ (Univ of Wisconsin, Madison; Med College of Wisconsin, Milwaukee)
Crit Care Med 38:843-848, 2010

Objective.—There is a general consensus by intensivists and nonsurgical providers that surgeons hesitate to withdraw life-sustaining therapy on their operative patients despite a patient's or surrogate's request to do so. The Objective of this study was to examine the culture and practice of surgeons to assess attitudes and concerns regarding advance directives for their patients who have high-risk surgical procedures.

Design.—A qualitative investigation using one-on-one, in-person interviews with open-ended questions about the use of advance directives during perioperative planning. Consensus coding was performed using a grounded theory approach. Data accrual continued until theoretical saturation was achieved. Modeling identified themes and trends, ensuring maximal fit and faithful data representation.

Setting.—Surgical practices in Madison and Milwaukee, WI.

Subjects.—Physicians involved in the performance of high-risk surgical procedures.

Interventions.—None.

Measurements and Main Results.—We describe the concept of surgical "buy-in," a complex process by which surgeons negotiate with patients a commitment to postoperative care before undertaking high-risk surgical procedures. Surgeons describe seeking a commitment from the patient to abide by prescribed postoperative care, "This is a package deal, this is what this operation entails," or a specific number of postoperative days, "I will contract with them and say, 'look, if we are going to do this, I am going to need 30 days to get you through this operation.'" "Buy-in" is grounded in a surgeon's strong sense of responsibility for surgical outcomes and can lead to surgeon unwillingness to operate or surgeon reticence to withdraw life-sustaining therapy postoperatively. If negotiations regarding life-sustaining interventions result in treatment limitation, a surgeon may shift responsibility for unanticipated outcomes to the patient.

Conclusions.—A complicated relationship exists between the surgeon and patient that begins in the preoperative setting. It reflects a bidirectional contract that is assumed by the surgeon with distinct implications and consequences for surgeon behavior and patient care.

▶ "The right to do something does not mean that doing it is right"—William Safire

Considering advanced directives outlined by the patient can be ethically challenging for surgeons in intensive care units (ICUs). There may be difficulty balancing the surgeon's opinion of what is deemed to be good versus best outcomes. More care may not be viewed by patients as best care.

Schwarze and colleagues completed a qualitative study of 10 physicians involved in high-risk surgical procedures to generate hypotheses regarding surgeons' views on advanced directives and end-of-life care. In this study, 2 scenarios were used to guide and assess the nature of the relationship between surgeons and patients.

A number of observations may be made from this study. First, the collaborative relationship between the patient, surgeon, family, and the nonsurgical clinical team is of significant importance, viewed as an informal contract. Second, the surgeons should consider the ethical position they may be placing the entire team in when committing a patient to therapies that may be above and beyond what they may have wished for in their advanced directive. Third, the surgeons describe an overwhelming feeling of responsibility for a poor patient outcome. Bearing a burden of this magnitude may interfere with the aggressiveness in postoperative interventions on future patients with potential disregard for patients' wishes for life-sustaining interventions.

As a staff nurse, I recall other nurses informing me that when a patient goes to surgery, the advanced directive is temporarily on hold. What did this represent? Does it mean that all measures will be endured while in the operating room or that once the patients consent to surgery, they are committed to all rescue efforts and postoperative interventions necessary to recover from the surgery.

In a study by Cassell and colleagues, the administrative model in the ICU, personal, professional, and national values affect how end-of-life decisions are carried out.[1] Collaborative efforts in decision making ought to include the patient, family, and members of the surgical and nonsurgical clinical ICU team. The ICU environment model may play more of a role in facilitating end-of-life decision making. A first step to doing what is right may be to evaluate the model in your ICU, creating an atmosphere of agreement that more care is not always the best care.

C. A. Schorr, RN, MSN

Reference

1. Cassell J, Buchman TG, Streat S, Stewart RM. Surgeons, intensivists, and the covenant of care: administrative models and values affecting care at the end of life–Updated. *Crit Care Med.* 2003;31:1551-1557.

Variability in data: The Society of Thoracic Surgeons National Adult Cardiac Surgery Database
Brown ML, Lenoch JR, Schaff HV (Univ of Alberta, Edmonton, Canada; Mayo Clinic, Rochester, MN)
J Thorac Cardiovasc Surg 140:267-273, 2010

Objective.—Since 1989, data have been reported to the Society of Thoracic Surgeons National Adult Cardiac Surgery Database for quality improvement. This information is also data mined for national quality indicators, policy initiatives, and research. Such use has important limitations, because data elements cannot be verified for accuracy. We determined variability of disease etiology and operative data database elements when abstracted by untrained physician abstractors.

Methods.—We selected 30 patients who underwent cardiovascular surgery from January to December 2005 (10 each of coronary artery bypass grafting, mitral valve repairs, and aortic valve and associated aortic procedures). Four abstractors (2 cardiothoracic residents and 2 fellows) abstracted 28 variables. Results were compared with abstraction performed by a professional abstractor.

Results.—Median percentage agreement among all cases was 89% (range, 42%–100%). Agreements were 94% (28%–100%) for mitral valve, 84% (18% 100%) for aortic valve, and 93% (35%–100%) for coronary artery bypass grafting. Among the aortic valve group, etiology of aortic valve disease had poor agreement (68%) because of cases in which multiple definitions could apply. Degree of valvular regurgitation also had poor agreement (median, 67%; range, 28%–95%). Number of internal thoracic artery grafts and absence of significant valvular disease were reported consistently. Agreements between types of aortic valve procedure and between methods of mitral valve repair (65% and 83%, respectively) were less than expected.

Conclusions.—We found variable agreement among untrained data abstractors. This has important implications regarding interpretation of database studies with de-identified data. Without good quality control and consistent standardized definitions, aggregate data in clinical databases may be suspect.

▶ The goal of performance measurement is to drive improvements in health care quality. This premise is that data can be used by hospitals and health care practitioners to identify variations in care, identify gaps in care, and to target improvement initiatives. The Society of Thoracic Surgeons (STS) and cardiac surgery has a long tradition of performance measurement with the STS National Adult Cardiac Surgery Database that was developed in 1989. This database was designed as a clinical database with prospectively collected data and is widely accepted as a credible reporting system that has driven significant improvements in cardiovascular care delivery. Although clinical data such as these are very expensive to capture, they are felt to be more accurate than administrative data. In this article, the authors identify potential gaps in the quality of the STS data. They found variable agreement in data abstraction by untrained data abstractors. The article highlights the need for the use of valid data to drive quality improvement and emphasizes that there must be good quality control. Electronic health records (EHRs) have the potential to improve and support broad reaching performance measurement and the comparative effectiveness research agenda.[1] As we implement EHR nationally, we must strive to have consistent definitions and good quality control—key elements identified by the authors of this article.[2] In addition, we need to consider interoperability, which will allow data exchange between multiple clinical networks if we are going to broadly improve care.

E. A. Martinez, MD, MHS

References

1. Buntin MB, Jain SH, Blumenthal D. Health information technology: laying the infrastructure for national health reform. *Health Aff (Millwood).* 2010;29: 1214-1219.
2. Brown ML, Lenoch JR, Schaff HV. Variability in data: the Society of Thoracic Surgeons National Adult Cardiac Surgery Database. *J Thorac Cardiovasc Surg.* 2010;140:267-273.

Miscellaneous

AVAS Best Clinical Resident Award (Tied): Management and outcomes of the open abdomen in nontrauma patients

Balentine C, Subramanian A, Palacio CH, et al (Michael E. DeBakey VA Med Ctr, Houston, TX)
Am J Surg 198:588-592, 2009

Background.—Little is known regarding the morbidity and mortality of the open abdomen technique in older nontrauma patients.

Methods.—A retrospective chart review identified cases of emergency laparotomy in which open abdomens were used.

Results.—Eighty-eight patients with open Acute Physiology and Chronic Health Evaluation (APACHE) abdomens were identified. An overall mortality rate of 34%, consistent with mortality predicted by APACHE IV score, was seen. Common complications included ventilator-associated pneumonia (30%) and acute renal failure (22%). A perioperative APACHE IV score of greater than 65 and an albumin level less than 2.5 g/dL were found to predict an increased likelihood of long-term assisted care placement after discharge from the acute care setting.

Conclusions.—The use of the open abdomen technique in older nontrauma patients carries acceptable morbidity and mortality given the acuity of disease. Focus on ventilator-associated pneumonia prevention and aggressive fluid resuscitation to avoid acute renal failure may improve outcomes. Need for long-term assisted care placement can be predicted early after admission based on the APACHE IV score or albumin level (Fig 1, Table 4).

▶ The authors present a realistic review of contemporary practice in elderly, debilitated, nontrauma patients requiring open abdomen technique for a variety of acute conditions.[1,2] Multiple operative procedures are frequently required. The incidence of complications is high, including death, pneumonia, and other organ dysfunction. I was disappointed to see that acute presentation of hernia was present in approximately 15% of the patients, and fistulas were

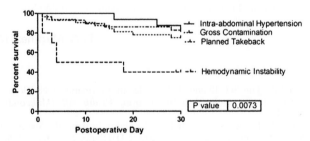

FIGURE 1.—Thirty-day survival by indication for open abdomen. (Reprinted from Balentine C, Subramanian A, Palacio CH, et al. AVAS Best Clinical Resident Award (Tied): management and outcomes of the open abdomen in nontrauma patients. *Am J Surg.* 2009;198:588-592, with permission from Elsevier.)

TABLE 4.—Predicting LTAC Placement

		Univariate			Multivariate	
Variable	OR	95% CI	*P*	OR	95% CI	*P*
Albumin level						
<2.5 g/dL	15.8	2.7–93	.002	12.5	1.8–88	.01
ASA 3 or 4	2.9	1.0–8.5	.05	1.9	.31–11.5	.49
Smoking	.47	.16–1.4	.17	.37	.07–2.1	.26
Hypertension	2.9	.98–8.5	.05	3.31	.52–21	.2
ICU stay >21 d	3.2	.97–10.3	.06	3.6	.44–29.4	.23
Age >60 y	1.6	.58–4.6	.35	.77	.15–4.1	.76
APACHE IV						
score >65	5.5	1.3–23.9	.02	8.6	1.4–52.7	.02

CI = confidence interval; ASA = American Society of Anesthesiology.

identified in 13 individuals.[3] While I do not believe that leaving the abdomen open caused all of these complications, the patient who requires an open abdomen technique clearly must be recognized as a patient at risk for multiple postoperative management problems.

Not surprisingly, markers consistent with severity of underlying disease predicted the likelihood of long-term institutional care (Table 4). Survival of patients based on indication for the open abdomen technique is consistent with other literature. Readers should note that the patient with hemodynamic instability has less than 50% survival. Unfortunately, we are not given additional information regarding the cause for hemodynamic instability.

This article represents a point of comparison for high-risk civilian populations where the open abdomen technique is used. Other than noting the surprisingly high risk of perioperative complications, I note that the tissue transfers and the technique of component separation are used much more frequently in the trauma and acute surgery population than that is reported here. Whether this change in technical focus would have any effect on complication patterns seen is unclear.[4]

D. J. Dries, MSE, MD

References

1. Shapiro MB, Jenkins DH, Schwab CW, Rotondo MF. Damage control: collective review. *J Trauma.* 2000;49:969-978.
2. Jansen JO, Loudon MA. Damage control surgery in a non-trauma setting. *Br J Surg.* 2007;94:789-790.
3. Fischer PE, Fabian TC, Magnotti LJ, et al. A ten-year review of enterocutaneous fistulas after laparotomy for trauma. *J Trauma.* 2009;67:924-928.
4. Ko JH, Wang EC, Salvay DM, Paul BC, Dumanian GA. Abdominal wall reconstruction: lessons learned from 200 "component separation" procedures. *Arch Surg.* 2009;144:1047-1055.

How far can we go with positive end-expiratory pressure (PEEP) in liver transplant patients?

Saner FH, Olde Damink SWM, Pavlaković G, et al (Univ Hosp Essen, Germany; Maastricht Univ, The Netherlands; Univ Clinic Göttingen, Germany)
J Clin Anesth 22:104-109, 2010

Study Objective.—To assess the effect of positive end-expiratory pressure (PEEP) up to 15 cm H_2O on blood flow throughput of the liver and its effects on systemic hemodynamics in patients following liver transplantation.

Design.—Prospective, interventional study.

Setting.—Intensive care unit (ICU) of a university hospital.

Patients.—74 consecutive liver transplant recipients with a regular allocated cadaveric graft.

Intervention.—The lungs of all study patients were postoperatively mechanically ventilated with biphasic positive airway pressure. Three different PEEP levels (5, 10, and 15 cm H_2O) were randomly set within 4 hours of admission to the ICU. Systemic hemodynamic parameters were recorded using a pulmonary artery catheter and flow velocities were measured of the hepatic artery, portal vein, and right hepatic vein using a Doppler.

Measurements and Main Results.—PEEP of 15 cm H_2O induced a significant increase in central venous pressure and pulmonary capillary wedge pressure versus PEEP 5 cm H_2O. Flow velocities of the right hepatic vein, portal vein, and hepatic artery were not influenced by PEEP. There also was no impact of increased PEEP on mean arterial pressure or cardiac index.

Conclusion.—PEEP up to 15 cm H_2O does not impair liver outflow or systemic hemodynamics in liver transplant patients (Table 3).

▶ Liver transplantation is being performed with increasing frequency, and these patients typically require at least some period of mechanical ventilatory support.

TABLE 3.—Hemodynamic Parameters, Resistive Index (RI) of Hepatic Artery, and Systolic-Diastolic Ratio (SD Ratio) of the Hepatic Vein at PEEP Levels of 5, 10, and 15 cm H_2O

	PEEP = 5 cm H_2O	PEEP = 10 cm H_2O	PEEP = 15 cm H_2O
Heart rate (bpm)	89 ± 20	88 ± 21	88 ± 21
MAP (mmHg)	87 ± 13	85 ± 12	84 ± 16
MPAP (mmHg)	24 ± 6	25 ± 6	$26 \pm 5^*$
CVP (mmHg)	9 ± 3	10 ± 4	$12 \pm 3^*$
PCWP (mmHg)	12 ± 4	13 ± 4	$15 \pm 4^*$
IVCP (mmHg)	13 ± 5	14 ± 5	15 ± 5
CI (L/min^1/m^2)	4.6 ± 1.6	4.6 ± 1.6	4.5 ± 1.8
RI	0.5 ± 0.1	0.5 ± 0.1	0.6 ± 0.2
S/D ratio	1.9 ± 1	1.9 ± 0.9	1.9 ± 0.6

All data are means ± SD.
PEEP = positive end-expiratory pressure, HR = heart rate, MAP = mean arterial pressure, MPAP = mean pulmonary arterial pressure, PCWP = pulmonary capillary wedge pressure, IVCP-inferior vena cava pressure, CI = cardiac index, CVP = central venous pressure.
*$P < 0.025$.

For those patients who have significant oxygenation abnormalities, positive end-expiratory pressure (PEEP) is typically used to remedy the problem. There has been some concern that higher levels of PEEP may adversely impact hemodynamic function and in particular, hepatic blood flow. This could have important consequences to a newly transplanted organ. Fortunately, these data suggest that PEEP levels up to 15 cm H_2O had minimal impact on hepatic blood flow and hemodynamic function. Obviously, there are many factors that influence hemodynamic function and organ perfusion, but these data suggest that with proper attention to proper volume status and with careful monitoring, higher levels of PEEP can be incorporated into our posttransplant support strategy with little adverse hemodynamic effect.

R. A. Balk, MD

Red Blood Cell Transfusion Threshold in Postsurgical Pediatric Intensive Care Patients: A Randomized Clinical Trial
Rouette J, Trottier H, Ducruet T, et al (Université de Montréal, QC; CHU Sainte-Justine, Montreal, QC)
Ann Surg 251:421-427, 2010

Background.—The optimal transfusion threshold after surgery in children is unknown. We analyzed the general surgery subgroup of the TRIPICU (Transfusion Requirements in Pediatric Intensive Care Units) study to determine the impact of a restrictive versus a liberal transfusion strategy on new or progressive multiple organ dysfunction syndrome (MODS).

Methods.—The TRIPICU study, a prospective randomized controlled trial conducted in 17 centers, enrolled a total of 648 critically ill children with a hemoglobin equal to or below 9.5 g/dL within 7 days of pediatric intensive care unit (PICU) admission to receive prestorage leukocyte-reduced red-cell transfusion if their hemoglobin dropped below either 7.0 g/dL (restrictive) or 9.5 g/dL (liberal). A subgroup of 124 postoperative patients (60 randomized to restrictive and 64 to the liberal group) were analyzed. This study was registered at http://www.controlled-trials.com and carries the following ID ISRCTN37246456.

Results.—Participants in the restrictive and liberal groups were similar at randomization in age (restrictive vs. liberal: 53.5 ± 51.8 vs. 73.7 ± 61.8 months), severity of illness (pediatric risk of mortality [PRISM] score: 3.5 ± 4.0 vs. 4.4 ± 4.0), MODS (35% vs. 29%), need for mechanical ventilation (77% vs. 74%), and hemoglobin level (7.7 ± 1.1 vs. 7.9 ± 1.0 g/dL). The mean hemoglobin level remained 2.3 g/dL lower in the restrictive group after randomization. No significant differences were found for new or progressive MODS (8% vs. 9%; $P = 0.83$) or for 28-day mortality (2% vs. 2%; $P = 0.96$) in the restrictive versus liberal group. However, there was a statistically significant difference between groups for PICU length of stay (7.7 ± 6.6 days for the restrictive group vs. 11.6 ± 10.2 days for the liberal group; $P = 0.03$).

Conclusions.—In this subgroup analysis of pediatric general surgery patients, we found no conclusive evidence that a restrictive red-cell transfusion strategy, as compared with a liberal one, increased the rate of new or progressive MODS or mortality.

▶ Abundant data exist in the adult population, suggesting that product transfusion is associated with increased infection risk and organ dysfunction.[1] This study suggests that in the pediatric setting, comparable risk does not exist. An interesting and positive finding that is not explained by the authors is the increased duration of ICU care in the liberal transfusion group.

A number of observations can be made. First, the age of blood in this study is relatively young. With units averaging 15 days in age, the risk of age-related product complications is reduced.[2] Second, we are not given the data regarding the use of plasma products. The risk of transfusion-related acute lung injury (TRALI) and other product-related complications increase in proportion to the amount of plasma in the blood products used.[3] Third, the authors use leukocyte-reduced blood. The value of leukocyte reduction is questioned, and TRALI, the most important complication of transfusion, is probably little affected by leukoreduction.[4]

This study is important, as it demonstrates an acceptable low hemoglobin level for pediatric patients.[5-7] In addition, as the authors appropriately conclude, the hemoglobin level should not determine a transfusion trigger. I suspect that the physiology of unnecessary transfusion in children is similar to that in adults. Oxygen extraction is reduced if unnecessary transfusion is provided.[8]

D. J. Dries, MSE, MD

References

1. Bernard AC, Davenport DL, Chang PK, Vaughan TB, Zwischenberger JB. Intraoperative transfusion of 1 U to 2 U packed red blood cells is associated with increased 30-day mortality, surgical-site infection, pneumonia, and sepsis in general surgery patients. *J Am Coll Surg.* 2009;208:931-939.
2. Weinberg JA, McGwin G Jr, Marques MB, et al. Transfusions in the less severely injured: does age of transfused blood affect outcomes? *J Trauma.* 2008;65:794-798.
3. Marik PE, Corwin HL. Acute lung injury following blood transfusion: expanding the definition. *Crit Care Med.* 2008;36:3080-3084.
4. Nathens AB, Nester TA, Rubenfeld GD, Nirula R, Gernsheimer TB. The effects of leukoreduced blood transfusion on infection risk following injury: a randomized controlled trial. *Shock.* 2006;26:342-347.
5. Corwin HL, Gettinger A, Pearl RG, et al. The CRIT Study: Anemia and blood transfusion in the critically ill-current clinical practice in the United States. *Crit Care Med.* 2004;32:39-52.
6. Hebert PC, Wells G, Blajchman MA, et al. A multicenter, randomized, controlled clinical trial of transfusion requirements in critical care. Transfusion Requirements in Critical Care Investigators, Canadian Critical Care Trials Group. *N Engl J Med.* 1999;340:409-417.
7. Bateman ST, Lacroix J, Boven K, et al. Anemia, blood loss, and blood transfusion in North American children in the intensive care unit. *Am J Respir Crit Care Med.* 2008;178:26-33.
8. Gramm J, Smith S, Gamelli RL, Dries DJ. Effect of transfusion on oxygen transport in critically ill patients. *Shock.* 1996;5:190-193.

Venous Thromboembolism Risk and Prophylaxis in the Acute Care Hospital Setting (ENDORSE Survey): Findings in Surgical Patients

Kakkar AK, for the ENDORSE Investigators (Barts and The London School of Medicine and Dentistry, UK; et al)
Ann Surg 251:330-338, 2010

Objective.—To evaluate venous thromboembolism (VTE) risk in patients who underwent a major operation, including the use of, and factors influencing, American College of Chest Physicians-recommended types of VTE prophylaxis.

Summary Background Data.—The Epidemiologic International Day for the Evaluation of Patients at Risk for Venous Thromboembolism in the Acute Hospital Care Setting (ENDORSE) survey, conducted in 358 hospitals in 32 countries, reported that globally, more than 40% of at-risk patients do not receive VTE prophylaxis. Limited data are available regarding VTE prophylaxis practices according to surgery type and patient characteristics.

Methods.—Patients aged ≥18 years undergoing major surgery were included in this prespecified subanalysis. VTE risk and use of prophylaxis were determined from hospital medical records according to the 2004 American College of Chest Physicians guidelines. Multivariable analyses were performed to identify factors associated with VTE prophylaxis use.

Results.—Of the 18,461 patients in ENDORSE who had undergone major surgery, 17,084 (92.5%) were at-risk for VTE and 10,638 (62.3%) received prophylaxis. Use of prophylaxis varied according to major surgery type from 86.0% for orthopedic surgery to 53.8% in urologic/gynecologic and 53.6% in other procedures. Major orthopedic surgery was most strongly associated with prophylaxis use (hip replacement: odds ratio 6.2, 95% confidence interval [CI] 5.0–7.6; knee replacement: odds ratio 5.9, 95% CI 4.6–7.8).

Conclusions.—The majority of surgical patients are at high-risk for VTE. Despite long-standing recognition of the high-risk for VTE in surgical patients, thromboprophylaxis remains underutilized.

▶ Venous thromboembolism (VTE) is an important clinical problem in surgical patients.[1] It is perhaps best studied in the orthopedic population where prophylaxis is provided aggressively and risk associated with prophylaxis appears to be low. The prevalence of VTE in the injured and perioperative patient appears to grow with the tendency of clinicians to be more aggressive in screening.[2]

This massive data set has a number of important epidemiologic lessons. First, a number of variables that increase risk for VTE are clearly identified (Fig 5).[3] Among these are obesity, placement of central venous catheters (an extremely common practice in high-risk patients), immobilization, underlying cardiovascular disease, gastrointestinal and hepatobiliary disorders, and increasing age. Second, even in patients with malignancy, bleeding risk was assessed at low or moderate in 85% to 90% of patients. This is far more patients than receive full prophylaxis. This statistic does not include patients with intracranial problems but is focused

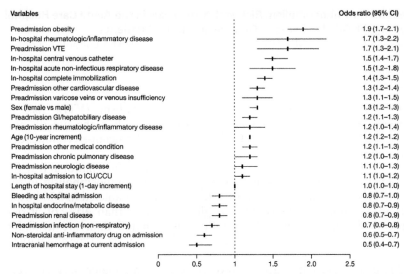

FIGURE 5.—Independent factors, excluding surgery type, associated with the use of ACCP-recommended VTE prophylaxis in surgical patients at-risk for VTE. ACCP indicates American College of Chest Physicians; CCU, critical care unit; CI, confidence interval; GI, gastrointestinal; ICU, intensive care unit; VTE, venous thromboembolism. (Reprinted from Kakkar AK, for the ENDORSE Investigators. Venous thromboembolism risk and prophylaxis in the acute care hospital setting (ENDORSE survey): findings in surgical patients. *Ann Surg.* 2010;251:330-338.)

on abdominal, urologic, or gynecologic procedures. Even if the patient is diagnosed with cancer, less than half of patients surveyed received chemical prophylaxis. These data become more startling when the limited role for mechanical prophylaxis in many settings is identified.

The rate of VTE will increase with aggressiveness in screening.[2] Examination of the wide range of prophylaxis utilization in this survey demonstrates inconsistency in practice, which can and should be addressed.[4]

D. J. Dries, MSE, MD

References

1. Collins R, Scrimgeour A, Yusuf S, Peto R. Reduction in fatal pulmonary embolism and venous thrombosis by perioperative administration of subcutaneous heparin. Overview of results of randomized trials in general, orthopedic, and urologic surgery. *N Engl J Med.* 1988;318:1162-1173.
2. Pierce CA, Haut ER, Kardooni S, et al. Surveillance bias and deep vein thrombosis in the national trauma data bank: the more we look, the more we find. *J Trauma.* 2008;64:932-937.
3. Cohen AT, Tapson VF, Bergmann JF, et al. Venous thromboembolism risk and prophylaxis in the acute hospital care setting (ENDORSE study): a multinational cross-sectional study. *Lancet.* 2008;371:387-394.
4. Geerts WH, Bergqvist D, Pineo GF, et al. Prevention of venous thromboembolism: American College of Chest Physicians Evidence-Based Clinical Practice Guidelines (8th Edition). *Chest.* 2008;133:381S-453S.

7   Sepsis/Septic Shock

A Comparison of Central and Mixed Venous Oxygen Saturation in Circulatory Failure

Ho KM, Harding R, Chamberlain J, et al (Royal Perth Hosp, Western Australia, Australia; et al)
J Cardiothorac Vasc Anesth 24:434-439, 2010

Objective.—The purpose of this study was to evaluate whether central venous oxygen saturation can be used as an alternative to mixed venous oxygen saturation in patients with cardiogenic and septic shock.

Design.—Prospective clinical study.

Setting.—A tertiary intensive care unit in a university hospital.

Participants.—Twenty patients with cardiogenic or septic shock requiring a pulmonary artery catheter and inotropic support.

Interventions.—None.

Measurements and Main Results.—The central venous oxygen saturation overestimated the mixed venous oxygen saturation by a mean bias (or an absolute difference) of 6.9%, and the 95% limits of agreement were large (−5.0% to 18.8%). The difference between central and mixed venous oxygen saturation appeared to be more significant when mixed venous oxygen saturation was <70%. The changes in central and mixed venous oxygen saturation did not follow the line of perfect agreement closely in different clinical conditions. The central or mixed venous oxygen saturation had a significant ability to predict the status of cardiac output state, but this ability was reduced when the effect of hyperoxia was not considered.

Conclusion.—Central and mixed venous oxygen saturation measurements are not interchangeable numerically.

▶ Mixed venous oxygen saturation (SvO_2) and central venous oxygen saturation ($ScvO_2$) have both been proposed as potential hemodynamic targets for critically ill patients with circulatory compromise. Targeting an $ScvO_2$ > 70% or an SvO_2 > 65% is thought to represent adequate oxygen delivery. Current guidelines recommend using an $ScvO_2$ > 70% or an SvO_2 > 65% as an end point for resuscitation in patients with sepsis-induced hypoperfusion and/or septic shock. However, SvO_2 and $ScvO_2$ are not the same and may not be interchangeable. Reports on how well these numbers correlate are mixed. Some studies have found poor correlation.[1] Other authors report a strong correlation.[2] The purpose of this study was to evaluate whether SvO_2 and $ScvO_2$ can be used interchangeably in the clinical setting. The authors studied a group of patients with cardiogenic or septic shock who had a pulmonary artery catheter and required inotropic support. In this study $ScvO_2$ overestimated the SvO_2. This difference was more pronounced when the SvO_2 was < 70%. Finally, the authors report that the changes in $ScvO_2$ and SvO_2 did not follow a line of perfect agreement in several clinical conditions. Based on their results, the authors concluded that $ScvO_2$ and SvO_2 are not interchangeable. Although the results of this study are important, it is difficult to reach a definitive answer to the question. (Are $ScvO_2$ and SvO_2 interchangeable?) It is important to understand the limitations of these as it is other hemodynamic monitoring tools we use in the intensive care unit. Finally, perhaps the most important message is to treat hemodynamic instability early and use predefined end points. As our knowledge about these specific end points changes, we will be better suited to change current guidelines.

S. L. Zanotti-Cavazzoni, MD

References

1. Dueck MH, Klimek M, Appenrodt S, Weigand C, Boerner U. Trends but not individual values of central venous oxygen saturation agree with mixed venous oxygen saturation during varying hemodynamic conditions. *Anesthesiology.* 2005;103:249-257.
2. Reinhart K, Kuhn HJ, Hartog C, Bredle DL. Continuous central venous and pulmonary artery oxygen saturation monitoring in the critically ill. *Intensive Care Med.* 2004;30:1572-1578.

Characteristics of plasma NOx levels in severe sepsis: high interindividual variability and correlation with illness severity, but lack of correlation with cortisol levels

Ho JT, Chapman MJ, O'Connor S, et al (The Univ of Adelaide, North Terrace, Australia; Royal Adelaide Hosp, North Terrace, Australia; et al)
Clin Endocrinol 73:413-420, 2010

Objectives.—Nitric oxide (NO) concentrations are elevated in sepsis and their vasodilatory action may contribute to the development of hyperdynamic circulatory failure. Hydrocortisone infusion has been reported to reduce nitric oxide metabolite (NOx) concentrations and facilitate vasopressor withdrawal in septic shock. Our aim was to determine whether NOx concentrations relate to (i) protocol-driven vasopressor initiation and withdrawal and (ii) plasma cortisol concentrations, from endogenous and exogenous sources. Demonstration of a relation between NOx, cortisol and vasopressor requirement may provide an impetus towards the study of hydrocortisone-mediated NOx suppression as a tool in sepsis management.

Design.—A prospective study of 62 patients with severe sepsis admitted to the intensive care unit.

Measurements.—Plasma NOx, total and free cortisol, and corticosteroid-binding globulin (CBG) concentrations were measured and related to protocol-driven vasopressor use for 7 days following admission.

Results.—Patients who developed septic shock ($n - 35$) had higher plasma NOx, total and free cortisol, and lower CBG concentrations than the nonseptic shock group ($n = 27$). Cortisol, CBG and NOx concentrations correlated with illness severity. Free cortisol, and to a lesser extent total cortisol, but not NOx concentrations, predicted septic shock. NOx concentrations were higher in nonsurvivors, and the concentrations were characteristically stable within individuals but marked interindividual differences were only partly accounted for by illness severity or renal dysfunction. NOx concentrations did not correlate with cortisol, did not relate to vasopressor requirement and did not fall after standard dose hydrocortisone, given for clinical indications.

Conclusions.—Nitric oxide production increased with sepsis severity but did not correlate with plasma cortisol or vasopressor requirement. NOx levels were not suppressed reproducibly by hydrocortisone. High interindividual variability of NOx levels suggests that absolute NOx levels may not be a suitable target for individualized hydrocortisone therapy.

▶ Nitric oxide (NO) and hydrocortisone have been studied and discussed within the context of sepsis for several decades. Previous research has established that overproduction of NO causes microvascular abnormalities in patients with sepsis, suggesting that blocking NO production may be a potential therapeutic target in septic patients. Hydrocortisone has been shown in vitro to inhibit inducible NO synthase, while hydrocortisone has been shown in vivo to increase rate of vasopressor withdrawal in patients with sepsis. The authors hypothesized that NO metabolite (NOx) concentration correlated with both vasopressor and glucocorticoid requirements in patients with sepsis. If such correlation was found, NOx could possibly be used to guide glucocorticoid use and dosage in individual patients with sepsis. The authors designed a prospective observational study and collected daily plasma cortisol, free cortisol, corticosteroid-binding globulin, and plasma NOx levels in 62 patients with sepsis. As in previous studies, the authors found that both plasma NOx and cortisol levels correlated with severity of sepsis; however, the authors were unable to show correlation between plasma NOx levels and vasopressor requirement or plasma NOx and cortisol levels. The authors observed that the patients had high interindividual variability in plasma NOx levels and concluded that this makes plasma NOx concentration an unsuitable marker to guide glucocorticoid treatment.

S. L. Zanotti-Cavazzoni, MD

Effect of Preinjury Statin Use on Mortality and Septic Shock in Elderly Burn Patients

Fogerty MD, Efron D, Morandi A, et al (Vanderbilt Univ School of Medicine, Nashville, TN; Johns Hopkins Univ School of Medicine, Baltimore, MD; et al)
J Trauma 69:99-103, 2010

Background.—Premorbid statin use has been associated with decreased mortality in septic and trauma patients. This has been ascribed to the pleiotropic, anti-inflammatory effects of HMG-CoA reductase inhibitors. This association has not been investigated in burn victims.

Methods.—A retrospective review of 223 consecutive patients, aged 55 years and older admitted to Vanderbilt University Regional Burn Center from January 2006 to December 2008, was performed. Multivariate regression analysis determined odds ratios of death and sepsis by statin use, adjusting for cardiovascular comorbidities.

Results.—Of 223 patients, 70 (31.4%) were taking statins before admission. Mean age and mean total body surface area burn were not significantly different by statin use. The odds ratio of inhospital death was 0.17 (95% confidence interval 0.05–0.57; $p = 0.004$) if on statins. The odds ratio of mortality when stratified by cardiovascular comorbidities did not change. Sepsis developed in 30 patients (13.5%), with an odds ratio in statin users of 0.50 (95% confidence interval 0.20–1.30; $p = 0.155$).

Conclusion.—Preinjury statin use was associated with an 83% reduction in the odds of death after thermal injury. The odds of sepsis decreased by 50%, although not statistically significant. Further study is warranted to investigate the potential benefits of statin therapy in the management of burn victims.

▶ While multiple previous studies have reported protective effects of 3-hydroxy-3-methyl-glutaryl-coenzyme A reductase inhibitors (statins) on nonburn critically ill patients, these effects had not been verified in patients with burns. The authors observed reduced rates of mortality and sepsis in patients with burns taking statins before admission to the burn unit. Statins have been shown to reduce cardiovascular events in the outpatient setting through their cholesterol-lowering effects; however, the mechanism of their protective effects on critically ill patients has not been fully elucidated. Statins have been shown to interfere at multiple levels in cell signaling, resulting in downregulation of the inflammatory response. Laboratory studies have shown statins to impair lymphocyte adhesion to the endothelium and downregulate the expression of major histocompatibility complex class II. Animal studies have shown statins to improve microvascular circulation by increasing concentrations of endothelial nitric oxide synthase (eNOS) while decreasing concentrations of inducible NOS. In human studies, statins have been shown to reduce levels of interleukin-6 and tumor necrosis factor-α in patients with sepsis receiving statins compared with patients receiving placebos. Furthermore, the timing of statin use needs to be further elucidated to determine if these medications need to be continued during hospitalization to gain protective effects and if patients starting statins during the hospitalization obtain the same protective effects as patients on statins at preadmission. Given the low cost and side-effect profile of this drug class, the use of statins on critically ill patients needs to be fully studied.

S. L. Zanotti-Cavazzoni, MD

Etiology of Illness in Patients with Severe Sepsis Admitted to the Hospital from the Emergency Department
Heffner AC, Horton JM, Marchick MR, et al (Carolinas Med Ctr, Charlotte, NC)
Clin Infect Dis 50:814-820, 2010

Background.—Patients identified with sepsis in the emergency department often are treated on the basis of the presumption of infection; however, various noninfectious conditions that require specific treatments have clinical presentations very similar to that of sepsis. Our aim was to describe the etiology of illness in patients identified and treated for severe sepsis in the emergency department.

Methods.—We conducted a prospective observational study of patients treated with goal-directed resuscitation for severe sepsis in the emergency department. Inclusion criteria were suspected infection, 2 or more criteria for systemic inflammation, and evidence of hypoperfusion. Exclusion criteria were age of <18 years and the need for immediate surgery. Clinical data on eligible patients were prospectively collected for 2 years. Blinded observers used a priori definitions to determine the final cause of hospitalization.

Results.—In total, 211 patients were enrolled; 95 (45%) had positive culture results, and 116 (55%) had negative culture results. The overall mortality rate was 19%. Patients with positive culture results were more likely to have indwelling vascular lines ($P = .03$), be residents of nursing homes ($P = .04$), and have a shorter time to administration of antibiotics in the emergency department (83 vs 97 min; $P = .03$). Of patients with negative culture results, 44% had clinical infections, 8% had atypical infections, 32% had noninfectious mimics, and 16% had an illness of indeterminate etiology.

Conclusion.—In this study, we found that >50% of patients identified and treated for severe sepsis in the emergency department had negative culture results. Of patients identified with a sepsis syndrome at presentation, 18% had a noninfectious diagnosis that mimicked sepsis, and the clinical characteristics of these patients were similar to those of patients with culture-positive sepsis.

▶ Mortality in severe sepsis and septic shock (SS/SS) remains high; however, the early detection and treatment of SS/SS using an early quantitative resuscitation strategy imparts a significant reduction in mortality.[1] This strategy is particularly effective if a definitive source of the inflammatory syndrome can be expeditiously identified and targeted therapy applied. However, current international guidelines for management of the septic patient include aggressive resuscitative efforts within the first 6 hours of recognition of septic parameters.[2] Even under ideal circumstances, meeting the time constraints for providing early therapy often prohibits establishing a definitive infectious source.

This article proposes to delineate the various etiologies of the illness, infectious and otherwise, as well as hospital outcomes in patients diagnosed and treated for sepsis in the emergency department of a large urban medical center.

The authors did a secondary analysis of data on 211 patients treated with an institutional standard-of-care protocol for early quantitative resuscitation of severe sepsis. Diagnoses were assigned by 2 independent physician observers who categorized patients into 1 of 2 groups: culture-positive or culture-negative. Culture-negative patients were then categorized into 1 of 4 groups: clinical infections, atypical infections, noninfectious mimics, and indeterminate. They found that 55% of patients were culture-negative; however, most of them (52%) had clinical infections as per their predefined criteria.

Of note, the resuscitative interventions were statistically similar among culture-negative and culture-positive patients, and the patients with no infection identified had lower hospital mortality. This suggests no harm in resuscitating patients with noninfectious disease processes.

Although a percentage of patients initially assessed to have diagnostic criteria consistent with SS/SS will ultimately be found to have noninfectious illnesses, the benefits of early goal-directed therapy appear to outweigh the risks. Continued evaluation for alternative or contributing factors in any sepsis syndrome is always warranted.

S. L. Zanotti-Cavazzoni, MD

References

1. Westphal GA, Koenig A, Filho MC, et al. Reduced mortality after the implementation of a protocol for the early detection of severe sepsis. [published online ahead of print October 29, 2010]. J Crit Care. doi:10.1016/j.jcrc.2010.08.001.
2. Dellinger RP, Levy MM, Carlet JM, et al. Surviving Sepsis Campaign: international guidelines for management of severe sepsis and septic shock: 2008. *Crit Care Med.* 2008;36:296-327.

Evaluation of a modified early goal-directed therapy protocol
Crowe CA, Mistry CD, Rzechula K, et al (Advocate Christ Med Ctr, Oak Lawn, IL)
Am J Emerg Med 28:689-693, 2010

Objectives.—The study aimed to determine mortality in septic patients 2 years after introduction of a modified early goal-directed therapy (EGDT) protocol and to measure compliance with the protocol.

Design.—This was an observational study of prospectively identified patients treated with EGDT in our emergency department (ED) from May 2007 through May 2008 and compared with retrospectively obtained data on patients treated before protocol implementation, from May 2004 to May 2005.

Setting.—This study was conducted at a large tertiary-care suburban community hospital with more than 85 000 ED visits annually and 700 inpatient beds.

Patients.—Patients with severe sepsis or septic shock were included in the study.

Interventions.—A modified EGDT protocol was implemented.

Measurements and Main Results.—A total of 216 patients were treated with our EGDT protocol, with 32.9% mortality (95% confidence interval [CI], 26.6%-39.2%); 183 patients (84.7%) had septic shock, with a mortality of 34.4% (95% CI, 28%-41%). Our control group of 205 patients had a 27.3% mortality (95% CI, 21.2%-33.5%), of which 123 had septic shock with a mortality of 43.1% (95% CI, 34%-52%). Early goal-directed therapy protocol compliance was as follows: 99% received adequate intravenous fluids, 99% had a central line, 98% had antibiotics in the first 6 hours, 28% had central oxygen saturation measured, 3.7% received dobutamine, and 19% were transfused blood.

Conclusions.—Although we found a trend toward decreased mortality in patients with septic shock treated with EGDT, with an absolute difference of 8.7%, this difference was not statistically significant. Compliance with individual elements of the protocol was variable.

▶ Outcomes in septic shock have been associated with multiple factors, many of which have a time-sensitive component. Early hemodynamic support using early goal-directed therapy (EGDT) protocol has been effective in improving outcomes in patients with severe sepsis and septic shock. Early antibiotic treatment has also been proposed as an important determinant of survival in patients with severe sepsis. The surviving sepsis campaign (SSC) has incorporated these concepts into its evidence based guidelines for the treatment of patients with severe sepsis. The SSC bundles have goals to target mean arterial pressure (MAP) > 65 and central venous oxygen saturation ($ScvO_2$) of 70%. Since the first study of Rivers et al, and also after implementing the SSC guidelines, several investigators demonstrated a decrease in mortality rate using EGDT when compared with outcomes of historical controls. The association with decreased mortality typically correlates with greater crystalloid volume infusion and earlier administration of vasopressors.

Crowe et al conducted an observational study at a large tertiary-care suburban community hospital emergency department using a modified EGDT protocol. The authors looked at mortality rates for patients with severe sepsis and septic shock pre- and postimplementation of the protocol. The study concluded that there was no difference in mortality rates between the protocol group and the control group, despite a trend toward decreased mortality. At the same time, the study noted that compliance with the protocol was variable, and the use of several of its components was low.

Although the overall result of the study failed to demonstrate a mortality benefit, a few observations are worth discussing:

1. A crucial point in the management of patients with severe sepsis is early identification. The percentage of patients with septic shock in this study (84.7% in the protocol group and 60% in the control group) is much higher when compared with other populations of patients with sepsis. This may reflect the fact that these patients had arrived late in their process of illness and raises a question about the time of identification of illness at the nursing homes from which most of these patients were transferred.

2. The demographic data lack important components such as comorbidities and the number of end-organ dysfunctions, which could play an important role in determining outcome.[1]

3. The lactate level was higher in the protocol group when compared with that in the control group (35% had lactate > 4, vs 12%). This correlates with a sicker group of patients in the first and would have clinical implications regarding survival. Trzeciak et al have shown that when lactate levels were measured in patients with infection and possible sepsis, the probability of acute-phase mortality (< 3 days) and in-hospital mortality (> 3 days) increased significantly and in a linear fashion with increasing range of initial lactate levels.[2]

4. The goal of treatment to target specific MAP, central venous pressure (CVP), and $ScvO_2$ is not mentioned clearly. Only 7.1% of protocol patients received an arterial line, despite the fact that 84% of them had septic shock. Around 18% had no CVP monitoring and in some, 2 L of fluids were given after which vasopressor therapy was initiated. $ScvO_2$ was only used in 28% of the cases. These elements reflect major deviation from the EGDT protocol and hence can affect the results of the study. The EGDT study and the SSC guidelines identified the first 6 hours as the golden hours of resuscitation for sepsis-induced hypoperfusion during which specific targeted MAP, CVP, and $ScvO_2$ should be met. Varpula et al demonstrated that during the first 48 hours of management of septic shock, the strongest correlates with mortality were an MAP < 65 and $ScvO_2 < 70\%$.[3]

From the above discussion, the findings of this study regarding survival outcomes do not present strong conclusions, and its results cannot be generalized. On the other hand, it highlights the challenges and barriers that exist for implementation of a protocol for early identification and intervention in severe sepsis. Some of the difficulties were discussed by the authors, such as the need for ongoing education and increased staffing. This remains an important topic of discussion. A core component to address such an issue is putting in place a team that can drive a cultural change through establishing an organized approach, continuous training, ongoing efforts to tackle problems, and implementation of a performance improvement program that continues to review results and provide feedback to health care providers.

S. L. Zanotti-Cavazzoni, MD

References

1. Levy MM, Macias WL, Vincent JL, et al. Early changes in organ function predict eventual survival in severe sepsis. *Crit Care Med.* 2005;33:2194-2201.

2. Trzeciak S, Dellinger RP, Chansky ME, et al. Serum lactate as a predictor of mortality in patients with infection. *Intensive Care Med.* 2007;33:970-977.
3. Varpula M, Tallgren M, Saukkonen K, Voipio-Pulkki LM, Pettilä V. Hemodynamic variables related to outcome in septic shock. *Intensive Care Med.* 2005; 31:1066-1071.

Inferior vena cava diameter correlates with invasive hemodynamic measures in mechanically ventilated intensive care unit patients with sepsis

Schefold JC, Storm C, Bercker S, et al (Charité Univ Medicine Berlin, Germany; Univ Hosp Leipzig, Germany)
J Emerg Med 38:632-637, 2010

Early optimization of fluid status is of central importance in the treatment of critically ill patients. This study aims to investigate whether inferior vena cava (IVC) diameters correlate with invasively assessed hemodynamic parameters and whether this approach may thus contribute to an early, non-invasive evaluation of fluid status. Thirty mechanically ventilated patients with severe sepsis or septic shock (age 60 ± 15 years; APACHE-II score 31 ± 8; 18 male) were included. IVC diameters were measured throughout the respiratory cycle using transabdominal ultrasonography. Consecutively, volume-based hemodynamic parameters were determined using the single-pass thermal transpulmonary dilution technique. This was a prospective study in a tertiary care academic center with a 24-bed medical intensive care unit (ICU) and a 14-bed anesthesiological ICU. We found a statistically significant correlation of both inspiratory and expiratory IVC diameter with central venous pressure ($p = 0.004$ and $p = 0.001$, respectively), extravascular lung water index ($p = 0.001$, $p < 0.001$, respectively), intrathoracic blood volume index ($p = 0.026$, $p = 0.05$, respectively), the intrathoracic thermal volume (both $p < 0.001$), and the PaO_2/FiO_2 oxygenation index ($p = 0.007$ and $p = 0.008$, respectively). In this study, IVC diameters were found to correlate with central venous pressure, extravascular lung water index, intrathoracic blood volume index, the intrathoracic thermal volume, and the PaO_2/FiO_2 oxygenation index. Therefore, sonographic determination of IVC diameter seems useful in the early assessment of fluid status in mechanically ventilated septic patients. At this point in time, however, IVC sonography should be used only in addition to other measures for the assessment of volume status in mechanically ventilated septic patients.

▶ In the days of early goal-directed therapy, optimization of fluid balance is key. Therefore, any noninvasive way of accurately estimating hemodynamic status certainly grabs the critical care community's attention. Although this study did not aim to replace invasive hemodynamic monitoring, it shines a light on an alternative way of assessing fluid status in ventilated intensive care unit patients with sepsis, especially during the initial resuscitation phase.

What is even more promising is that inferior vena cava diameter measurement does not seem to require extensive training or experience, potentially increasing its applicability. In addition, this study documented a low interobserver variability (14 ± 7%; 2.5 ± 1.2 mm), which could simplify the interpretation of measurements obtained. It is likely that the role of bedside ultrasound will continue to grow in the care of the critically ill. Studies such as this one illustrate the tremendous potential to use this technology at the bedside as an extension of our physical examination and monitoring techniques to provide point-of-care information with direct therapeutic implications.

S. L. Zanotti-Cavazzoni, MD

Long-term Cognitive Impairment and Functional Disability Among Survivors of Severe Sepsis

Iwashyna TJ, Ely EW, Smith DM, et al (Univ of Michigan Med School, Ann Arbor; Vanderbilt Univ, Nashville, TN; Stony Brook Univ Med Ctr, NY)
JAMA 304:1787-1794, 2010

Context.—Cognitive impairment and functional disability are major determinants of caregiving needs and societal health care costs. Although the incidence of severe sepsis is high and increasing, the magnitude of patients' long-term cognitive and functional limitations after sepsis is unknown.

Objective.—To determine the change in cognitive impairment and physical functioning among patients who survive severe sepsis, controlling for their presepsis functioning.

Design, Setting, and Patients.—A prospective cohort involving 1194 patients with 1520 hospitalizations for severe sepsis drawn from the Health and Retirement Study, a nationally representative survey of US residents (1998-2006). A total of 9223 respondents had a baseline cognitive and functional assessment and had linked Medicare claims; 516 survived severe sepsis and 4517 survived a nonsepsis hospitalization to at least 1 follow-up survey and are included in the analysis.

Main Outcome Measures.—Personal interviews were conducted with respondents or proxies using validated surveys to assess the presence of cognitive impairment and to determine the number of activities of daily living (ADLs) and instrumental ADLs (IADLs) for which patients needed assistance.

Results.—Survivors' mean age at hospitalization was 76.9 years. The prevalence of moderate to severe cognitive impairment increased 10.6 percentage points among patients who survived severe sepsis, an odds ratio (OR) of 3.34 (95% confidence interval [CI], 1.53-7.25) in multivariable regression. Likewise, a high rate of new functional limitations was seen following sepsis: in those with no limits before sepsis, a mean 1.57 new limitations (95% CI, 0.99-2.15); and for those with mild to moderate limitations before sepsis, a mean of 1.50 new limitations (95% CI, 0.87-2.12). In contrast, nonsepsis general hospitalizations were associated

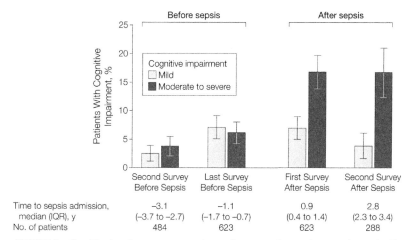

FIGURE 2.—Cognitive impairment among survivors of severe sepsis at each survey time point. Error bars indicate 95% confidence intervals (CIs); IQR, interquartile range. Interpretive Example: Compared with stable rates before severe sepsis, the prevalence of moderate to severe cognitive impairment increased from 6.1% (95% CI, 4.2%-8.0%) before severe sepsis to 16.7% (95% CI, 13.8%-19.7%) at the first survey after severe sepsis (*P*<.001 by χ² test; Table 2). (Reprinted from Iwashyna TJ, Ely EW, Smith DM, et al. Long-term cognitive impairment and functional disability among survivors of severe sepsis. *JAMA.* 2010;304:1787-1794, with permission from the American Medical Association.)

with no change in moderate to severe cognitive impairment (OR, 1.15; 95% CI, 0.80-1.67; *P* for difference vs sepsis=.01) and with the development of fewer new limitations (mean among those with no limits before hospitalization, 0.48; 95% CI, 0.39-0.57; *P* for difference vs sepsis <.001 and mean among those with mild to moderate limits, 0.43; 95% CI, 0.23-0.63; *P* for difference=.001). The declines in cognitive and physical function persisted for at least 8 years.

Conclusions.—Severe sepsis in this older population was independently associated with substantial and persistent new cognitive impairment and functional disability among survivors. The magnitude of these new deficits was large, likely resulting in a pivotal downturn in patients' ability to live independently (Fig 2).

▶ Severe sepsis is the most common cause of mortality and morbidity in the intensive care unit. Hundreds of thousands are admitted to hospitals each year with severe sepsis in the United States. Some reports have suggested long-term impact on quality of life in survivors of severe sepsis. However, the long-term impact of severe sepsis on cognitive and physical functioning is unknown. Physical and cognitive impairment after acute illness have significant implications for patients, their families, and ultimately the health care system.

The objective of this study was to evaluate whether an episode of severe sepsis increases the incidence of sequent worsening cognitive impairment and function disabilities among survivors. The authors took advantage of an ongoing national cohort study of older Americans that included detailed information from personal surveys and medical claims. They specifically evaluated the long-term impact of severe sepsis on cognitive and functional status. The authors report a clinically and statistically significant increase in moderate to severe cognitive impairment among survivors after having an episode of severe sepsis (Fig 2). They also identified a significant increase in functional disabilities of survivors of sepsis. These changes in physical and cognitive function noted with severe sepsis were greater than those noted in survivors of hospitalizations for other clinical diagnoses. Perhaps the greatest value of this landmark study is the identification of severe long-term sequelae for older patients who survive severe sepsis. With an aging population and increasing estimates of the burden of sepsis, this finding clearly has important health care implications. From an individual patient standpoint, the level of cognitive impairment found in the patients from this cohort after sepsis was associated with significant increases in informal care provided by families and worsening overall health outcomes. The study emphasizes the importance of understanding the long-term implications of a growing problem in critical care such as severe sepsis. It also forces intensivists to think of better ways to minimize these effects and work on preventive strategies and better treatment modalities for sepsis. In summary, this large study followed a representative cohort of older adults and has shown that the odds of acquiring moderate to severe cognitive impairment were 3.3 times higher after an episode of sepsis, with an additional mean increase of 1.5 new functional limitation per person among those with no or mild to moderate pre-existing functional limitations. Further research is needed in this area.

S. L. Zanotti-Cavazzoni, MD

Sepsis and Endothelial Permeability

Lee WL, Slutsky AS (St Michael's Hosp, Toronto, Ontario, Canada; Univ of Toronto, Ontario, Canada)
N Engl J Med 363:689-691, 2010

Background.—Sepsis refers to the widespread inflammatory response brought on by microbial infections. Its clinical manifestations have been recognized for millennia but treatment is lacking. Currently sepsis cases are increasing in frequency, causing considerable financial impact and leading to death in up to 70% of patients. Nonspecific supportive care is the primary therapeutic approach, showing the inadequacy of medicine's understanding of sepsis.

Current Views.—Leukocytes are the focus of research efforts traditionally. It is believed that sepsis causes immunosuppression manifest by lymphocyte apoptosis and susceptibility to nosocomial infections. Progressive subcutaneous and body cavity edema develop commonly in patients with sepsis, indicating increased vascular permeability. An accumulation of parenchymal and interstitial fluid inhibits organ function by increasing the distance needed for oxygen diffusion and compromising microvascular perfusion because of elevated interstitial pressure. Recovery from septic shock is often heralded by spontaneous diuresis as the body rids itself of the excess fluid. The blood vessels are all lined by endothelial cells, so the vascular leakage and tissue edema seen in septic shock may well indicate endothelial dysfunction. Widespread microvascular endothelial damage would be capable of producing vascular leaking and edema as well as shock, microvascular thrombosis, and organ failure, which often occur in patients with severe sepsis shortly before death. The significance of endothelial impairment remains unclear, but if it contributes to disease and death related to sepsis, new treatment approaches may be suggested.

Research.—London et al studied the role of a signaling pathway involving the Slit and Robo proteins in regulating vascular permeability. These proteins play a role in neuronal development, but also contribute to angiogenesis. The London et al study showed that recombinant Slit can attenuate the endothelial permeability caused by endotoxin activity and cytokines in vitro. The Robo4 receptor was required for this protective effect, and enhanced localization to the cell membrane of a key adhesion molecule, VE-cadherin, served as a necessary mediator. VE-cadherin is the principal component of adherens junctions, which are tightly regulated protein complexes that link adjacent endothelial cells and prevent the egress of leukocytes and vascular leak. Displacing VE-cadherin from the cell membrane into the cell's interior causes gaps between endothelial cells and increased permeability. The protein p120-catenin binds to and stabilizes VE-cadherin at the membrane. Dissociation of p120-catenin and VE-cadherin is prevented by the Slit protein, thus reducing the incidence of vascular leakage. These findings held in three different mouse models of infection. Giving an intravenous injection of Slit before inducing disease dramatically reduced the mortality in infected animals without lowering the high levels of lung and serum cytokines in infected animals, indicating that enhanced vascular integrity and reduced mortality could be achieved even in animals with extensive inflammation.

Conclusions.—The results of the London et al study require confirmation in humans, but it appears that the endothelium is critical to vascular integrity in patients with sepsis. Understanding the endothelial barrier's function, endothelial repair, and endothelial regeneration may lead to new therapies for sepsis.

▶ Animal models could be disproving the old adage that edema in sepsis is purely an aesthetic concern. London and colleagues have been working to elucidate the role of endothelial permeability in sepsis. When studying vascular endothelial (VE)-cadherin, the major component of adherens junctions, they found that a protein (Slit) binds to the Robo4 receptor on the plasma membrane, which then binds VE-cadherin to p120-catenin, thus stabilizing the cell junction. London et al's work in mouse models showed that recombinant Slit is also effective in preventing endothelial cell dissociation. More importantly, when injected before induction of disease, it also decreases mortality in infected animals (3 different mouse models: gram-negative bacterial pneumonia, intra-abdominal sepsis, and H5N1 influenza) without decreasing circulating cytokines. This stresses that the endothelial barrier might be a pivotal therapeutic target in the treatment of human sepsis.

S. L. Zanotti-Cavazzoni, MD

The Association of Race and Survival from Sepsis after Injury
Plurad DS, Lustenberger T, Kilday P, et al (Los Angeles County + Univ of Southern California Med Ctr)
Am Surg 76:43-47, 2010

Genetic variation is associated with outcome disparity in critical illness. We sought to determine if race is independently associated with the development of posttraumatic sepsis and subsequent related mortality. Our Intensive Care Unit database was queried for admissions from January 1, 2000 to June 30, 2007. Patients were prospectively followed for sepsis (Any four of the following symptoms: temperature $\geq 38°$ C, heart rate (HR) ≥ 90 b/m, RR ≥ 20 b/m (or $PaCO_2 \leq 32$ mm Hg), white blood cell count (WBC) ≥ 12, or vasopressor requirement all with an infectious source). White, Black, Hispanic, and Asian groups were defined. "Other" race was excluded. Most of the 3998 study patients were male (3157, 79.0%). Blunt trauma (2661, 66.6%) predominated. Six hundred seventy-seven (16.9%) met sepsis criteria. Mortality was 14.0 per cent (560). Sepsis was increased in Asians *versus* all others combined (23.7% *vs* 16.1%). Race was independently associated with sepsis (adjusted odds ratio (OR) 1.12 (1.01–1.24), P value = 0.03). Sepsis associated mortality was 36.9 per cent (250/677). Black race demonstrated an increased survival *versus* all others after sepsis (25.4% *vs* 37.7%) but this was not statistically significant (adjusted OR 0.96 (0.73–1.18), P value = 0.71). Race is independently associated with posttraumatic sepsis and possibly subsequent sepsis associated mortality. Further related study is needed with the ultimate goal of genetically based treatments for the prevention and treatment of sepsis after injury.

▶ Genetic variation has long been attributed as one of the causes of outcome disparity among critically ill patients. In this study, the author's objective was to evaluate whether race was associated with the development of posttraumatic sepsis and outcome. The authors reported a significant association between race and the incidence of posttraumatic sepsis. There was also an association with increased survival in patients whose race was classified as black. Although these findings are of interest, it is important to remember that the interactions between genes and the environment are complex. It is certainly interesting to discover that particular genotypes regulate inflammatory responses, but there is no congruity between identified genotypes and readily identifiable phenotypic traits used to determine race. Further studies are needed to fully understand the relationship between race, genetic makeup, disease, and ultimately critical illness outcomes. Understanding these relationships is the cornerstone to achieving the ultimate goal of genetically based treatments for the prevention and treatment of sepsis.

S. L. Zanotti-Cavazzoni, MD

Validation of a Screening Tool for the Early Identification of Sepsis
Moore LJ, Jones SL, Kreiner LA, et al (The Methodist Hosp, Houston, TX; Univ of Texas Health Science Ctr, Houston)
J Trauma 66:1539-1547, 2009

Background.—Sepsis is the leading cause of mortality in noncoronary intensive care units. Recent evidence based guidelines outline strategies for the management of sepsis and studies have shown that early implementation of these guidelines improves survival. We developed an extensive logic-based sepsis management protocol; however, we found that early recognition of sepsis was a major obstacle to protocol implementation. To improve this, we developed a three-step sepsis screening tool with escalating levels of decision making. We hypothesized that aggressive screening for sepsis would improve early recognition of sepsis and decrease sepsis-related mortality by insuring early appropriate interventions.

Methods.—Patients admitted to the surgical intensive care unit were screened twice daily by our nursing staff. The initial screen assesses the systemic inflammatory response syndrome parameters (heart rate, temperature, white blood cell count, and respiratory rate) and assigns a numeric score (0–4) for each. Patients with a score of ≥ 4 screened positive proceed to the second step of the tool in which a midlevel provider attempts to identify the source of infection. If the patients screen positive for both systemic inflammatory response syndrome and an infection, the intensivist was notified to determine whether to implement our sepsis protocol.

Results.—Over 5 months, 4,991 screens were completed on 920 patients. The prevalence of sepsis was 12.2%. The screening tool yielded a sensitivity of 96.5%, specificity of 96.7%, a positive predictive value of 80.2%, and a negative predictive value of 99.5%. In addition, sepsis-related mortality decreased from 35.1% to 23.3%.

Conclusions.—The three step sepsis screening tool is a valid tool for the early identification of sepsis. Implementation of this tool and our logic-based sepsis protocol has decreased sepsis-related mortality in our SICU by one third.

▶ Sepsis is one of the most important causes of death in patients admitted to the intensive care unit. Although criteria for the diagnosis of sepsis have been proposed, it is still a difficult task to recognize sepsis at the bedside, especially in the early phases of the disease. Furthermore, there is growing evidence that early intervention with time-sensitive therapies, such as antibiotics and hemodynamic support, is critical in determining patients' outcomes. In this study, the authors did an excellent job in bringing to the forefront a system that recognizes and categorizes all patients who might become septic. Through the use of a custom-built computerized program, early parameters of systemic inflammatory response syndrome (SIRS) and sepsis could be identified, thus allowing the implementation of institution-specific sepsis protocols. The process itself is simple and nonarduous. The first step entails analysis of the SIRS criteria and deriving a scoring system; if a threshold of 4 or more is achieved, escalation to the next step occurs. The second step focuses on finding a source of infection; if such was found, then step 3, the institution-specific sepsis protocol, is initiated.

The results of this study highlight the fact that a simple process, using commonly obtained vital signs, can improve our ability to recognize an often complex disease. Earlier identification would hopefully lead to earlier treatment and improved outcomes.

S. L. Zanotti-Cavazzoni, MD

Ventricular Dilation Is Associated With Improved Cardiovascular Performance and Survival in Sepsis

Zanotti Cavazzoni SL, Guglielmi M, Parrillo JE, et al (Cooper Univ Hosp, Camden, NJ)
Chest 138:848-855, 2010

Objectives.—Myocardial dysfunction in sepsis may be associated with changes in left ventricular (LV) size. The goal of this study was to evaluate the impact of myocardial dysfunction and changes in LV diameter on hemodynamics and survival in a murine model of sepsis.

Methods.—C57Bl/6 mice (n = 30) were used. Septic mice (n = 24) had cecal ligation and puncture (CLP) followed by fluid and antibiotic resuscitation and control mice (n = 6) received sham ligation. Echocardiography with a 30-mHz probe was performed at baseline and at frequent predefined time points after CLP. Stroke volume (SV), cardiac output (CO), LV internal diameter in diastole (LVIDd), and fractional shortening (FS) were measured. LV dilation was prospectively defined as an increase in LVIDd $\geq 5\%$ from baseline values. Septic animals were classified as dilators or nondilators.

Results.—Among septic animals, 37% were dilators and 63% were nondilators. After CLP, SV and CO decreased early in both groups. With resuscitation, SV and CO improved to a greater extent in dilators than nondilators (for SV, 46.0 ± 8.2 vs 36.1 ± 12.7 µL at 24 h, $P = .05$; for CO, 20.4 ± 4.8 vs 14.8 ± 6.7 mL/min, $P = .04$). Survival at 72 h was significantly improved in dilators compared with nondilators (88% vs 40%, $P = .01$).

Conclusions.—In a clinically relevant murine model of sepsis, animals with LV dilation had better cardiovascular performance and increased survival. Our results suggest that LV dilation is associated with improved

SV and CO, a pattern resulting in greatly improved survival. These studies highlight the importance of diastolic function in septic shock.

▶ Over the past decade, a growing body of evidence both experimental and clinical has shed light on the role of diastolic function as an essential component in determining cardiac function after years of focusing only on the systolic component. Left ventricular (LV) diastolic dysfunction is now well recognized in 40% to 50% of patients with congestive heart failure (CHF) who have normal or increased LV ejection fraction. Diastolic dysfunction had also been described in sepsis, both in animals and humans; however, similar to its counterpart in CHF, it has been ignored. This was in part secondary to the lack of recognition of the importance of diastolic dysfunction, heterogeneity of the septic population in which such an observation was not always easily recognized, and the need for invasive techniques to quantify the myocardial function. Fortunately, advances in echocardiography, including Doppler tissue imaging, have improved the assessment of LV dysfunction.

In this article, the authors use an established murine model of sepsis to evaluate the impact of myocardial dysfunction and changes in LV diameter and survival. Of importance, LV dilation, defined as an increase in LV internal diameter in diastole (LVIDd) >5% of baseline, was noted in 37% of the septic animals (named dilators), whereas 63% did not show any LV dilation (named nondilators). Dilators had better hemodynamics after resuscitation when compared with nondilators. This improvement in hemodynamics was thought to be driven by effect of LV dilation on restoration of stroke volume. Interestingly, survival at 72 hours was significantly improved in dilators compared with nondilators (88% vs 40%, $P = .01$). To capture these subtle changes of LV dilation, the authors had to perform periodic echocardiography studies through specific intervals of time.

Given the complexity and heterogeneity of the septic population that is associated with multiple variables, this study is very helpful as it provides a reproducible animal model of sepsis with which myocardial dysfunction can be further characterized in a more controlled setting. The method used for serial echocardiography studies to monitor diastolic function and LV dilation is a key element that needs to be considered in any future animal studies or human clinical trials that address diastolic dysfunction in patients with sepsis. More importantly, its findings highlight the prominent role of diastolic function in patients with severe sepsis and septic shock, which would probably have prognostic and therapeutic implications.

S. L. Zanotti-Cavazzoni, MD

8 Metabolism/ Gastrointestinal/ Nutrition/ Hematology-Oncology

A Randomized, Clinical Trial of Frozen Versus Standard Nasogastric Tube Placement
Chun D-H, Kim NY, Shin Y-S, et al (CHA Univ, Sungnam, Korea; Yonsei Univ College of Medicine, Seoul, Korea)
World J Surg 33:1789-1792, 2009

Background.—Insertion of a nasogastric tube (NGT) in an anesthetized, paralyzed, and intubated patient is difficult, and many methods have been proposed to aid in the procedure. We present a simple insertion technique.

Methods.—A silicone NGT was made rigid by filling it with distilled water and freezing it. Patients were randomized into either the control or the frozen group, and an NGT was inserted after intubation.

Results.—A total of 100 patients (50 in each group) were included in this study. The success rate increased significantly by making the tube more rigid (control:frozen = 58%:88%; $p = 0.001$). There was no difference between groups in the incidence of nasal bleeding.

Conclusions.—A simple method of freezing an NGT with distilled water increased the success rate of insertion for intubated patients.

▶ Placing a nasogastric tube (NGT) is frequently more difficult than desired for both the proceduralist and the patient. When the patient cannot contribute by swallowing, the task remains difficult and this is true whether intraoperatively or in an ICU. Not placing a NGT in many patients is simply bad care, and so a tension exists between the need to place a NGT and the difficulty in so doing with the potential for coincidental harm. These authors studied the impact of prefreezing a NGT on success rate of placement intraoperatively after intubation, a scenario analogous to an intubated and sedated patient in an ICU. As can be seen in Table 1, they had a higher successful placement rate achieved at a faster interval. These are important findings, but significant

TABLE 1.—Patient Characteristics

	Control (n = 50)	Frozen (n = 50)
Patient characteristics		
Age (yr)	59.2 (9.8)	59.1 (13.1)
Male/female ratio	29/21	32/18
Height (cm)	161.4 (16.2)	161.9 (16.9)
Weight (kg)	64.4 (9.4)	65.1 (16.4)
Effect of frozen NGT		
Successful insertion	29/50	44/50[*]
Active nasal bleeding	0	0
Mucosal bleeding	6	3
Total time for insertion (sec)	120 (133)	83 (43)

Values are mean (SD) or number
[*]$p = 0.001$ vs. control group

limitations persist. The study is underpowered to identify harm. The authors did evaluate for bleeding and found no difference, but by being underpowered for all significant complications the reader is left not knowing enough about the safety of such an approach. In addition, perforation rates of the retropharynx are quite small but positive, and thus could be higher with a stiffer tube. In addition and importantly in litigious environments like the United States, freezing the tube may vacate any product protection as it is not approved by the manufacturer and could lead to unknown consequences including material failure. Such failure could conceivably lead to the NGT fracturing after placement, requiring potentially an endoscopic retrieval procedure or even distal mucosal harm. This liability seems unwarranted without further study. It might also be prudent for investigators to work with the manufacturer to seek approval for such an approach if further investigation indeed demonstrates safety.

T. Dorman, MD

Inflammation, vitamin deficiencies and organ failure in critically ill patients
Corcoran TB, O'Neill MP, Webb SAR, et al (Royal Perth Hosp, Western Australia)
Anaesth Intensive Care 37:740-747, 2009

It is unknown whether biochemical vitamin deficiencies in critical illness are associated with severity of illness, organ dysfunction, inflammation or mortality. This nested cohort study recruited 98 patients admitted as emergencies to the intensive care unit, who had a stay of greater than 48 hours. Patient data were prospectively collected. Within the first 48 hours of admission, concentrations of C-reactive protein, vitamins A, E, B_1, B_{12} and folate were measured on arterial blood. These measures were then repeated at least once during the later (>48 hours) period of their stay. Seventy patients (71%) had completed vitamin studies eligible for inclusion in the analysis. Ten patients died (14.3%) during their hospital stay

TABLE 2.—Change in Vitamin Status and Hospital Mortality

	Total[†]	Died[‡]	Survived[‡]	P value[§]
Vitamin A, n = 67				
Entire cohort	67	10	57	0.504
R-R	12 (17.9)	2 (16.7)	10 (83.3)	
R-D	16 (23.9)	4 (25)	12 (75)	
D-D	35 (52.2)	4 (11.4)	31 (88.6)	
D-R	4 (6)	0	4 (100)	
Vitamin E, n = 62	Total	Died	Survived	P value[§]
Entire cohort	62	9	53	0.225
R-R	32 (51.6)	4 (12.5)	28 (87.5)	
R-D	4 (6.5)	2 (50)	2 (50)	
D-D	18 (29)	2 (11.1)	16 (88.9)	
D-R	8 (12.9)	1 (12.5)	7 (87.5)	
Thiamine (B$_1$)*, n = 38	Total	Died	Survived	P value[§]
Entire cohort	38	7	31	0.164
R-R	31 (81.6)	5 (16.1)	26 (83.9)	
R-D	4 (10.5)	1 (25)	3 (75)	
D-D	2 (5.3)	0	2 (100)	
D-R	1 (2.6)	1 (100)	0	
Folate*, n = 23	Total	Died	Survived	P value[§]
Entire cohort				N/A
R-R	23	5 (21.7)	18 (78.3)	
R-D	0	0	0	
D-D	0	0	0	
D-R	0	0	0	
Vitamin B$_{12}$, n = 70	Total	Died	Survived	P value[††]
Entire cohort	70	10	60	0.146
R-R	65 (92.9)	8 (12.3)	57 (87.7)	
R-D	0	0	0	
D-D	0	0	0	
D-R	5 (7.1)	2 (40)	3 (60)	

R-R = replete on admission and remained so during intensive care unit (ICU) stay, R-D = replete on admission but subsequently became deficient during ICU stay, D-R = deplete on admission but subsequently became replete during ICU stay, D-D = deplete on admission and remained so during ICU stay.
[†]Percentage refers to total group number.
[‡]Percentage refers to row percentage within the individual vitamin status group.
[§]Pearson χ^2 value.
[††]Fisher's exact test.
*Analysis restricted to those patients who did not receive thiamine or folate supplementation during their stay.

and mortality was associated with age, admission source and severity of illness scores. Vitamin B$_{12}$ concentration was weakly associated with C-reactive protein concentrations on admission to the intensive care unit (r on days one and two = 0.4 [P = 0.002], 0.36 [P = 0.04], respectively) and with the Sequential Organ Failure Assessment score between days two and four (Spearman's r = 0.361 [P = 0.04], 0.42 [P = 0.02] and 0.48 [P = 0.02], respectively). Vitamin A concentration was weakly associated with the C-reactive protein concentrations on days one and five (Spearman's r = −0.5 [P = 0.001], −0.4 [P = 0.03], respectively). Change in deficiency status of any of the vitamins over time in the first week of intensive care admission did not appear to influence mortality. We conclude that while weak correlations were identified between vitamins A and B$_{12}$ and C-reactive protein and Sequential Organ Failure

Assessment scores, the importance of these associations and their relationship to hospital mortality remain to be determined.

▶ Nutritional support of patients who are critically ill or injured is complex. Route, dose, and timing are just a few of the concerns and controversial topics. Supplement administration is mostly based on pathophysiologic principles and not solid data. Changes in vitamin status and particular deficiencies of important vitamins during critical illness might be quite important in some patients. At present, very little is known. This article sets the stage for further investigations into this potentially important topic by assessing serially vitamin levels in patients who stay longer than 48 hours, and the authors look for associations with inflammatory markers and mortality. As can be seen in Table 2, there are some potentially important associations. For instance, when one considers vitamin A, the highest mortality is seen in the population that started with levels considered normal but then subsequently fell to levels considered deficient. In truth, this small study does not have many positive findings, but the idea is intriguing, and further study with a larger number of patients is needed. Future studies should include a higher number of serial measurements and more information about nutritional support and organ dysfunction, as both have a significant impact on a clinician's ability to interpret such data.

T. Dorman, MD

A Prospective Study on Evaluating the Diagnostic Yield of Video Capsule Endoscopy Followed by Directed Double-Balloon Enteroscopy in Patients with Obscure Gastrointestinal Bleeding
Li X, Dai J, Lu H, et al (Shanghai Jiaotong Univ School of Medicine, China)
Dig Dis Sci 55:1704-1710, 2010

Aims.—Video capsule endoscopy (VCE) and double-balloon enteroscopy (DBE) are two novel methods for examining the small bowel and could be complementary to each other. The aim of the present study is to prospectively evaluate the diagnostic yield of VCE followed by a directed DBE in patients with obscure gastrointestinal (GI) bleeding.

Methods.—Patients with obscure gastrointestinal bleeding for a complete VCE examination were involved in the study. DBE was recommended after a negative or indeterminate finding of VCE. The diagnostic and follow-up data were collected for analysis.

Results.—A total of 190 patients with a complete VCE examination were enrolled in the study. The overall positive detection rate for small-bowel disease in the VCE group was 86.8% (165/190), while 63.7% (121/190) patients were definitely diagnosed. Fifty-one patients with indeterminate (44 cases) and negative (seven cases) findings of first VCE underwent DBE procedures. A total of 18 patients with negative VCE findings refused the further examination. DBE demonstrated a positive finding in 66.7% (34/51) patients, 33 from indeterminate group and one from the negative group. Following an unrevealing DBE, at surgical follow-up, three further negative DBE procedures were documented. The overall diagnostic yield was 88.9%, including 121 diagnoses made by VCE alone and 48 by both VCE and DBE (confirmed at surgery or other treatments). The negative predictive value (NPV) and positive predictive value (PPV) of DBE in indeterminate VCE were 81.8 and 100%, respectively.

Conclusions.—Capsule endoscopy followed by directed double-balloon enteroscopy is a good strategy for investigating the causes of obscure GI bleeding and especially in confirming indeterminate and negative findings from VCE.

▶ Obscure gastrointestinal bleeding is defined as hemorrhage that persists despite a thorough negative evaluation with an upper endoscopy and a colonoscopy. Direct visualization methods include video capsule endoscopy (VCE), push enteroscopy, and double-balloon enteroscopy (DBE). Radiographic studies such as the small-bowel follow-through and enteroclysis have largely been replaced with more sensitive modalities. VCE completion rates are generally higher than enteroscopy methods, but both have yielded superior results when compared with the X-ray studies.

The design of the study was to evaluate the diagnostic accuracy and clinical efficacy of VCE followed by DBE in patients with obscure gastrointestinal bleeding. One hundred ninety patients were prospectively enrolled in this study. One hundred twenty-one out of 190 had a definitive diagnosis by VCE alone. Forty-four patients had indeterminate findings and 7 patients had a negative examination. DBE demonstrated a positive test in 34 out of 51 patients. Follow-up was provided for a year, longer in some cases. All patients with a positive VCE were stable after definitive therapy was used. The final diagnostic yield for VCE followed by DBE was 88.9%. DBE that followed an indeterminate VCE had high positive predictive and negative predictive values. There were no significant adverse effects in the DBE cases.

This study demonstrated an effective way to evaluate and treat obscure gastrointestinal bleeding. The DBE enhances the sensitivity of small intestinal evaluation. The VCE provides a location that can be targeted by the enteroscope. This technology may also obviate the need for surgical intervention.

VCE is a technology that is widely available. However, there are fewer centers that provide excellence in DBE. The demand for this procedure will increase as more of these cases remain in the domain of the gasteroenterologist.

C. W. Deitch, MD

Duration of red blood cell storage and survival of transfused patients

Edgren G, Kamper-Jørgensen M, Eloranta S, et al (Karolinska Institutet, Stockholm, Sweden; Copenhagen Univ Hosp, Denmark; Univ of California, San Francisco; et al)

Transfusion 50:1185-1195, 2010

Background.—Disquieting reports of increased complication and death rates after transfusions of red blood cells (RBCs) stored for more than 14 days prompted us to perform an observational retrospective cohort study of mortality in relation to storage time.

Study Design and Methods.—We conducted a cohort study utilizing data on all recipients of at least one RBC transfusion in Sweden and Denmark between 1995 and 2002, as recorded in the Scandinavian Donations and Transfusions (SCANDAT) database. Relative risks of death in relation to storage time were estimated using Cox regression, adjusted for several possible confounding factors.

Results.—After various exclusions, 404,959 transfusion episodes remained for analysis. The 7-day risk of death was similar in all exposure groups, but a tendency for a higher risk emerged among recipients of blood stored for 30 to 42 days (hazard ratio, 1.05; 95% confidence interval [CI], 0.97-1.12), compared to recipients of blood stored for 10 to 19 days. With 2-year follow-up, this excess remained at the same level (hazard ratio, 1.05; 95% CI, 1.02-1.08). No dose-response pattern was revealed and no differential effect was seen when the analyses were restricted to recipients of leukoreduced units only.

Conclusion.—Although a small excess mortality was noted in recipients of the oldest RBCs, the risk pattern was more consistent with weak confounding than with an effect of the momentary exposure to stored RBCs. It seems, thus, that any excess mortality conferred by older RBCs in the combined Swedish and Danish transfusion recipient population is likely less than 5%, which is considerably smaller than in the hitherto largest investigation.

▶ Limitations in the utility and efficacy of packed red cell transfusion, as a result of various biochemical and morphological changes that occur during the storage process, are becoming increasingly well recognized not only by blood bankers but also by clinicians. In addition, in recent years numerous studies have appeared indicating that older blood (ie, blood stored for longer periods of time) is associated with a variety of complications in critically ill patient populations, ranging from infection to organ failures to death. In this study, these investigators reviewed the records of over 400 000 transfusions in 2 Scandinavian countries and assessed the relationship between the storage time of the blood and mortality. A very small (5%) increased risk of mortality was found to be associated with the oldest blood (storage time 30-42 days), but this effect was felt to be significantly lesser than that reported by many previous studies. Overall, the investigators found no association between storage time and mortality in most subgroups evaluated. A major difference between this study and most of the previous literature, despite the size of the sample evaluated, is the general nature of the population studied. Most, if not all, of the previous studies reported have been of critically/acutely ill patients, whose responses to the potential effects of transfusion may be more pronounced than that of a less sick population. A second difference is that this study looked at mortality only. Several previous studies looked at other adverse outcomes. Even if it is ultimately confirmed that there is little or no mortality effect associated with prolonged storage time, the issue of other adverse effects remains an open question.

D. R. Gerber, DO

Duration of red cell storage before transfusion and in-hospital mortality
Eikelboom JW, Cook RJ, Liu Y, et al (McMaster Univ, Ontario, Canada; Univ of Waterloo, Ontario, Canada)
Am Heart J 159:737-743.e1, 2010

Background.—Red cell transfusions are lifesaving in severely anemic or acutely bleeding patients but may be associated with an increased risk of cardiovascular events in critically ill patients. The objective of the study was to examine the association between duration of pretransfusion storage of red cells and in-hospital mortality.

Methods.—We used multivariable Cox regression modeling with time-dependent stratification to assess the effect of age of transfused red blood cells on risk of in-hospital mortality in a registry of consecutive patients admitted to an acute care facility with a major diagnosis of cardiovascular disease.

Results.—Four thousand nine hundred thirty-three consecutive patients with a major diagnosis of cardiovascular disease admitted to acute care facilities in Hamilton, Canada, received 21,435 units of red cells. The median number of units received was 3 (interquartile range 2-5), and the median age of transfused blood was 17 (interquartile range 13-22) days. After adjustment for demographics, clinical characteristics, and time-dependent covariates and stratification by the number of units transfused, the relative risk for death was 1.02 for every 1-day increase in maximum age of blood. The adjusted relative risk for death increased with each increasing quartile of maximum age of blood, with patients in the highest quartile having a relative risk for death of 1.48 (95% CI 1.07-2.05) compared with those in the lowest (reference) quartile.

Conclusions.—In hospitalized patients with a major diagnosis of cardiovascular disease, there is a modest independent association between increasing duration of storage of red cells and risk of in-hospital mortality that appears to be continuous and graded.

▶ Numerous studies have appeared over the past several years indicating that transfusion may be associated with increased mortality in many patients with ischemic heart disease, even in the setting of active coronary ischemia, despite the proven adverse impact of anemia in these patients. These outcomes may be attributable to the so-called storage lesion, which occurs in banked blood, resulting in impaired microcirculatory blood flow and offloading of oxygen at the tissue level, among other defects. These investigators sought to evaluate whether the duration of red blood cell storage time before transfusion was related to mortality in patients with cardiovascular disease. Records of nearly 5000 patients, of whom approximately 85% had ischemic heart disease, were reviewed. The authors found a relative risk of mortality of 1.02 for every 1-day increase in the maximum age of blood that was transfused in this patient population. These findings are consistent with the overall body of literature, suggesting that older blood is associated with more complications and worse outcomes than is fresher blood. Standard criteria have not been used from 1 study to another to define these terms; however, it is commonly accepted that significant degradation of stored red cells begins after approximately 14 days. The median age of the blood transfused in this study was 17 days, similar to the national average in the United States. These findings may help explain the literature reporting an increased mortality in patients with ischemic heart disease who receive transfusions and lend further support to the idea that a relatively restrictive transfusion strategy may be a beneficial approach in this patient population, even though it is contrary to long-standing practice.

D. R. Gerber, DO

Effective reduction of transfusion-related acute lung injury risk with male-predominant plasma strategy in the American Red Cross (2006-2008)
Eder AF, Herron RM Jr, Strupp A, et al (American Red Cross, Rockville, MD; Southern California Region, Pomona, CA; Lewis and Clark Region, Salt Lake City, UT; et al)
Transfusion 50:1732-1742, 2010

Background.—Plasma components from female donors were responsible for most cases of transfusion-related acute lung injury (TRALI) reported to the American Red Cross (ARC) between 2003 and 2005. Consequently, we began preferentially distributing plasma from male donors for transfusion in 2006 and evaluated the effect on reported TRALI cases in the ensuing 2 years.

Study Design and Methods.—Suspected TRALI cases reported to the ARC Hemovigilance Program in calendar years (CY) 2006, 2007, and 2008 are described. Any case involving a fatality was also independently reviewed by three ARC physicians and classified as probable TRALI or not TRALI.

Results.—The percentage of plasma collected from male donors and distributed for transfusion increased each year from 55% in CY2006 to 79% in CY2007 and 95% in CY2008. Independent medical review of the 77 reported TRALI cases involving a fatality identified 38 cases as probable TRALI. Plasma was the only component transfused in six of these cases in 2006, five in 2007, and zero in 2008. Overall, the analysis of reported fatalities and nonfatal cases demonstrates that TRALI involving only plasma transfusion was significantly reduced in 2008 compared to 2006 (32 vs. 7 cases; odds ratio [OR] = 0.21; 95% confidence interval [CI] = 0.08-0.45), to a level that was no longer different from the rate of TRALI observed for RBC transfusion (4.0 vs. 2.3 per 10^6 distributed components; OR = 1.78; 95% CI = 0.67-4.36).

Conclusions.—Reported TRALI cases from plasma transfusion decreased in 2008 compared to the prior 2 years simultaneously with the conversion to male-predominant plasma for transfusion.

▶ Transfusion-associated acute lung injury (TRALI) has become, at least among critical care practioners and blood banking professionals, a well-recognized complication of the use of various blood component therapies. Although often ascribed to packed red blood cell (PRBC) transfusions, it has been historically and more commonly linked to the use of plasma. The data from early 2000 clearly demonstrated that plasma obtained from multiparous female donors, primarily on the basis of increased levels of human leukocyte antigen antibodies, was associated with a significantly higher incidence of this complication, leading to policies in many countries to limit the donor pool for plasma for transfusion to men. In this article, the authors report on the results of a donor-restriction strategy in the United States for the period from 2006-2008 on the incidence of TRALI. Over the period evaluated, since the restrictions have been implemented, nonfatal cases of plasma-related instances of TRALI have declined significantly and now occur at a rate similar to that of PRBC. Fatalities have also declined significantly. Similar efforts will now be extended to the arena of platelet apheresis, to recruit more male donors for this process in an effort to bring down the overall and fatality-associated TRALI rates identified with it.

D. R. Gerber, DO

Transfusion Requirements After Cardiac Surgery: The TRACS Randomized Controlled Trial

Hajjar LA, Vincent J-L, Galas FRBG, et al (Hospital das Clinicas da Faculdade de Medicina da Universidade de São Paulo, Brazil; Université Libre de Bruxelles, Brussels, Belgium)
JAMA 304:1559-1567, 2010

Context.—Perioperative red blood cell transfusion is commonly used to address anemia, an independent risk factor for morbidity and mortality after cardiac operations; however, evidence regarding optimal blood transfusion practice in patients undergoing cardiac surgery is lacking.

Objective.—To define whether a restrictive perioperative red blood cell transfusion strategy is as safe as a liberal strategy in patients undergoing elective cardiac surgery.

Design, Setting, and Patients.—The Transfusion Requirements After Cardiac Surgery (TRACS) study, a prospective, randomized, controlled clinical noninferiority trial conducted between February 2009 and

February 2010 in an intensive care unit at a university hospital cardiac surgery referral center in Brazil. Consecutive adult patients (n = 502) who underwent cardiac surgery with cardiopulmonary bypass were eligible; analysis was by intention-to-treat.

Intervention.—Patients were randomly assigned to a liberal strategy of blood transfusion (to maintain a hematocrit ≥30%) or to a restrictive strategy (hematocrit ≥24%).

Main Outcome Measure.—Composite end point of 30-day all-cause mortality and severe morbidity (cardiogenic shock, acute respiratory distress syndrome, or acute renal injury requiring dialysis or hemofiltration) occurring during the hospital stay. The noninferiority margin was predefined at −8% (ie, 8% minimal clinically important increase in occurrence of the composite end point).

Results.—Hemoglobin concentrations were maintained at a mean of 10.5 g/dL (95% confidence interval [CI], 10.4-10.6) in the liberal-strategy group and 9.1 g/dL (95% CI, 9.0-9.2) in the restrictive-strategy group ($P < .001$). A total of 198 of 253 patients (78%) in the liberal-strategy group and 118 of 249 (47%) in the restrictive-strategy group received a blood transfusion ($P < .001$). Occurrence of the primary end point was similar between groups (10% liberal vs 11% restrictive; between-group difference, 1% [95% CI, −6% to 4%]; $P = .85$). Independent of transfusion strategy, the number of transfused red blood cell units was an independent risk factor for clinical complications or death at 30 days (hazard ratio for each additional unit transfused, 1.2 [95% CI, 1.1-1.4]; $P = .002$).

Conclusion.—Among patients undergoing cardiac surgery, the use of a restrictive perioperative transfusion strategy compared with a more liberal strategy resulted in noninferior rates of the combined outcome of 30-day all-cause mortality and severe morbidity.

Trial Registration.—clinicaltrials.gov Identifier: NCT01021631.

▶ Transfusion of packed red blood cells (PRBCs) is an extremely common practice in patients undergoing cardiothoracic (CT) surgical procedures. The Society of Thoracic Surgeons/Society of Cardiovascular Anesthesiologists' (STS-SCA) joint recommendations, issued in 2007, suggested that transfusion in this population is generally appropriate when the hemoglobin is less than 6 gm/dL and not unreasonable if it is less than 7 gm/dL. The overwhelming preponderance of literature to date that has examined the relationship between transfusion and outcomes in patients undergoing CT surgical procedures has indicated an adverse impact, but the great majority of these studies have been either retrospective or observational in nature. This is the first, prospective, randomized study performed to directly assess the impact of PRBC transfusion on outcomes in patients undergoing CT surgical procedures. After patients were randomized to a liberal transfusion arm (transfused to keep hematocrit over 30%) or a restrictive transfusion arm (transfused to keep hematocrit over 24%), the investigators determined that there were no differences in the primary outcome measurement between the 2 groups. In the multiple regression analysis, the number of units of blood transfused was independently associated with a number of adverse outcomes, including, but not limited to, pulmonary, cardiac, and infectious complications and death. This is a potentially landmark study, similar to the original Transfusion Requirements in Critical Care Study, which first established that a restrictive transfusion strategy is not only safe but perhaps also beneficial in a broad range of critically ill patients. In a similar fashion, this study seems to establish that patients undergoing CT surgical procedures are likely to do at least as well and may in many cases benefit from a restrictive approach to PRBC transfusion. It should serve as a strong impetus to readdress transfusion strategies in this patient population, particularly in institutions or by clinicians who still tend to adhere to more liberal transfusion strategies, despite the STS-SCA recommendations.

D. R. Gerber, DO

Gastric versus transpyloric feeding in severe traumatic brain injury: a prospective, randomized trial
Acosta-Escribano J, Fernández-Vivas M, Grau Carmona T, et al (Hospital General Universitario de Alicante, Spain; Hospital Universitario Virgen de la Arrixaca, Murcia, Spain; Hospital Universitario Doce de Octubre, Madrid, Spain)
Intensive Care Med 36:1532-1539, 2010

Purpose.—To evaluate the efficacy of transpyloric feeding (TPF) compared with gastric feeding (GF) with regard to the incidence of ventilator-associated pneumonia in severe traumatic brain injury patients (TBI).

Design and Setting.—Prospective, open-label, randomized study in an intensive care unit of a university hospital.

Patients.—One hundred and four CHI adult patients admitted for TBI between April 2007 and December 2008. Patients were included within the first 24 h after ICU admission and were followed until discharge or 30 days after admission.

Intervention.—Patients were randomized to TPF or GF groups. They received the same diet, with $25 \, \text{kcal} \, \text{kg}^{-1} \, \text{day}^{-1}$ of calculated energy requirements and a nitrogen intake of $0.2 \, \text{g} \, \text{N} \, \text{kg}^{-1} \, \text{day}^{-1}$. Primary outcome was the incidence of early and ventilatory-associated pneumonia. Secondary outcomes were enteral nutrition-related gastrointestinal complications (GIC), days on mechanical ventilation, length of ICU stay and hospital stay, and sequential organ failure assessment score (SOFA).

Results.—The TPF group had a lower incidence of pneumonia, OR 0.3 (95% CI 0.1–0.7, $P = 0.01$). There were no significant differences in other nosocomial infections. The TPF group received higher amounts of diet compared to the GF group (92 vs. 84%, $P < 0.01$) and had lesser incidence of increased gastric residuals, OR 0.2 (95% CI 0.04–0.6, $P = 0.003$).

Conclusions.—Enteral nutrition delivered through the transpyloric route reduces the incidence of overall and late pneumonia and improves nutritional efficacy in severe TBI patients.

▶ Patients with traumatic brain injury have high metabolic demands. Early in the course of the disease process, energy consumption and protein catabolism increase. This consumptive process leads to an impaired immune response, which increases the susceptibility to nosocomial infections. The author notes that patients with traumatic brain injury who are fed early have improved outcomes. However, this approach is potentially problematic. Patients with neurologic trauma experience gastrointestinal complications such as decreased motility, which potentially may lead to reflux and aspiration. Providing enteral nutrition distal to the pylorus may decrease this risk, although it is not standard procedure in the trauma unit. The aim of this prospective study was to compare the efficacy of nutritional delivery in patients fed beyond the pylorus with that of standard gastric feeds and determine the rate of pulmonary complications in both groups of patients.

The study randomized 54 patients to receive gastric feeds and 50 patients to receive transpyloric feeds. The sites of the tubes were verified, the head of the bed elevated, and the target nutrition was delivered within 48 hours. Variables that were collected included the incidence of early compared with late development of pneumonia, gastrointestinal adverse effects, neurologic sequelae, hospital stay, and mortality at 30 days.

The rate of pneumonia was significantly higher in the patients with gastric feeds (57%) compared with those fed distally (32%). The difference was noted primarily in late-onset pulmonary infections. The overall volume of tube feeds was higher in the transpyloric feeding group, and as would be expected, the gastric residuals were lower. There were no statistical differences in the length of stay in the intensive care unit, overall hospital stay, the length of mechanical ventilation, or mortality.

This study was not designed to look at overall costs during the patient stay. Despite having similar hospital courses, were the costs lower in the patients fed distally? Potentially, there were fewer diagnostic studies and less utilization of antibiotics and prokinetics. However, the study did demonstrate that transpyloric feeding in this patient setting was a safe and an effective way to deliver a high percentage of the nutritional requirement. The overall decrease in pneumonia may have been related to the lower risk of aspiration. This feeding paradigm may offer significant benefits in the future, especially if this method is shown to be associated with morbidity benefits and cost-effectiveness.

C. W. Deitch, MD

Glucose variability is associated with intensive care unit mortality

Hermanides J, Vriesendorp TM, Bosman RJ, et al (Academic Med Ctr, Amsterdam, The Netherlands, Onze Lieve Vrouwe Gasthuis, Amsterdam, The Netherlands)
Crit Care Med 38:838-842, 2010

Objective.—Mounting evidence suggests a role for glucose variability in predicting intensive care unit (ICU) mortality. We investigated the association between glucose variability and intensive care unit and in-hospital deaths across several ranges of mean glucose.

Design.—Retrospective cohort study.

Setting.—An 18-bed medical/surgical ICU in a teaching hospital.

Patients.—All patients admitted to the ICU from January 2004 through December 2007.

Interventions.—None.

Measurements and Main Results.—Two measures of variability, mean absolute glucose change per hour and SD, were calculated as measures of glucose variability from 5728 patients and were related to ICU and in-hospital death using logistic regression analysis. Mortality rates and adjusted odds ratios for ICU death per mean absolute glucose change per hour quartile across quartiles of mean glucose were calculated. Patients were treated with a computerized insulin algorithm (target glucose 72–126 mg/dL). Mean age was 65 ± 13 yrs, 34% were female, and 6.3% of patients died in the ICU. The odds ratios for ICU death were higher for quartiles of mean absolute glucose change per hour compared with quartiles of mean glucose or SD. The highest odds ratio for ICU death was found in patients with the highest mean absolute glucose change per hour in the upper glucose quartile: odds ratio 12.4 (95% confidence interval, 3.2–47.9; *p* < .001). Mortality rates were lowest in the lowest mean absolute glucose change per hour quartiles.

Conclusions.—High glucose variability is firmly associated with ICU and in-hospital death. High glucose variability combined with high mean glucose values is associated with highest ICU mortality. In patients treated with strict glycemic control, low glucose variability seemed protective, even when mean glucose levels remained elevated.

▶ Glycemic control in the intensive care unit (ICU) has been the subject of a major debate over the last decade with multiple studies leading to conflicting results. The optimal glucose range remains unclear. Considering that existing studies have been unsuccessful in establishing the optimal glucose level, more recently investigators have studied glucose variability (GV) in critically ill patients. There is emerging evidence that GV could have a role in predicting outcomes in critically ill patients.

In this elegant study, the authors evaluated glucose variability in a group of critically ill patients. The authors concluded that high GV is firmly associated with ICU and in-hospital death. Although this study possibly sheds light on the importance of studying GV rather than individual glucose readings, it assumes that tight glucose control is beneficial. Some investigators would not agree with this assumption based on recent trial results. However, the evaluation of glucose variability seems to be an area of great potential in terms of further improvements in our understanding of the complex effects of hyperglycemia in critical illnesses. A prospective randomized controlled study targeting GV rather than a specific glucose range is needed. Until then, it is probably wise to target a blood glucose range of 110 to 180 and avoid hypoglycemia in our ICU practice.

S. L. Zanotti-Cavazzoni, MD

Infectious Complications in Patients with Severe Acute Pancreatitis
Xue P, Deng L-H, Zhang Z-D, et al (West China Hosp, Chengdu, Sichuan Province)
Dig Dis Sci 54:2748-2753, 2009

This study aims to investigate the clinical characteristics of infectious complications in severe acute pancreatitis (SAP). From September 2003 to March 2005, 140 patients with SAP were retrospectively identified. SAP was defined by the diagnostic criteria formulated for SAP at the 2002 Bangkok World Congress of Gastroenterology in Thailand. Clinical data of the infected and non-infected patients was compared and the characteristics of infection were also analyzed. There were 44 patients who developed infectious complications with a rate of 31.4% (44/140). The severity index, the incidence of complications and mortality, was significantly higher in the infected patients than in the non-infected patients ($P < 0.05$). Of 65 episodes of infection, infected (peri) pancreatic necrosis accounted for 47.7% (31/65), pneumonia for 27.7% (18/65), bacteremia for 10.8% (7/65), urinary tract infection for 6.1% (4/65), and gastrointestinal tract infection for 7.7% (5/65). The earliest infection was observed in pneumonia (10.7 ± 2.5 days), followed by bacteremia (13.7 ± 1.5 days), gastrointestinal tract infection (16.8 ± 3.9 days), infected (peri)pancreatic necrosis (17.6 ± 2.9 days), and urinary tract infection (20.5 ± 4.8 days). Gram-negative bacteria were preponderantly found, comprising 56.6% (64/113) of the isolated strains. Gram-positive bacteria and fungus accounted for 22.1% (25/113) and 21.2% (24/113) of the isolated strains, respectively. Infectious complications in patients with SAP occurred in those who had severe episodes, and consequently complicated the clinical courses. Infected (peri)pancreatic necrosis is the most susceptible and pneumonia is the earliest. Gram-negative bacteria were predominant in multi-microorganisms.

▶ This retrospective analysis focuses on the infectious complications that lead to increases in the morbidity and mortality of severe acute pancreatitis. Infection in this setting is a trigger of multiorgan dysfunction. Patients who die from severe pancreatitis usually succumb to sepsis. This study further characterizes the etiologic pathogens, anatomic sites, and the timing of such involvement during the course of their disease.

The authors included patients with severe acute pancreatitis defined by contrasted CT, elevations of the serum amylase and lipase, and history, using accepted scoring systems. Prophylactic antibiotics were given for 7 to 14 days. This intervention falls in line with the American Gastroenterological Association guidelines but differs from the American College of Gastroenterology guidelines. The topic of prophylactic antibiotics has been the subject of much study over the past decade, but there is still no consensus among gastroenterologists. Microbiologic studies were indicated in the presence of fever, elevated leukocyte count, and clinical deterioration.

Higher Ranson score and Acute Physiology and Chronic Health Evaluation and Balthazar CT scores were noted in the infection group. Not entirely unexpected was that this group also had a higher need for mechanical ventilation, higher incidence of gastrointestinal complications, and an overall increased mortality. The common sites of infection were in the necrotic tissues of the peripancreatic region, the lungs, the gastrointestinal tract, and the urinary tract.

The retrospective design of this study is appropriate for such an observational analysis. This article re-emphasizes the feared complication of infection in severe acute pancreatitis and its negative outcome in terms of morbidity and mortality. It is interesting that the lung is the site of the earliest infection. This raises the question whether aggressive interventions directed at preserving or improving lung function may prevent such complications. There is a large body of evidence that underscores the need to quickly identify, or even better, prevent infection in these patients. This study helps further characterize the timing and sites of infectious complications. The future must focus on prevention of these complications.

C. W. Deitch, MD

Nutrition therapy in the critical care setting: What is "best achievable" practice? An international multicenter observational study
Cahill NE, Dhaliwal R, Day AG, et al (Queen's Univ, Kingston, Ontario, Canada; Kingston General Hosp, Ontario, Canada, et al)
Crit Care Med 38:395-401, 2010

Objective.—To describe current nutrition practices in intensive care units and determine "best achievable" practice relative to evidence-based Critical Care Nutrition Clinical Practice Guidelines.

Design.—An international, prospective, observational, cohort study conducted January to June 2007.

Setting.—One hundred fifty-eight adult intensive care units from 20 countries.

Patients.—Two-thousand nine-hundred forty-six consecutively enrolled mechanically ventilated adult patients (mean, 18.6 per site) who stayed in the intensive care unit for at least 72 hrs.

Interventions.—Data on nutrition practices were collected from intensive care unit admission to intensive care unit discharge or a maximum of 12 days.

Measurements and Main Results.—Relative to recommendations of the Clinical Practice Guidelines, we report average, best, and worst site performance on key nutrition practices. Adherence to Clinical Practice Guideline recommendations was high for some recommendations: use of enteral nutrition in preference to parenteral nutrition, glycemic control, lack of utilization of arginine-enriched enteral formulas, delivery of hypocaloric parenteral nutrition, and the presence of a feeding protocol. However, significant practice gaps were identified for other recommendations. Average time to start of enteral nutrition was 46.5 hrs (site average range, 8.2–149.1 hrs). The average use of motility agents and small bowel feeding in patients who had high gastric residual volumes was 58.7% (site average range, 0%–100%) and 14.7% (site average range, 0%–100%), respectively. There was poor adherence to recommendations for the use of enteral formulas enriched with fish oils, glutamine supplementation, timing of supplemental parenteral nutrition, and avoidance of soybean oil-based parenteral lipids. Average nutritional adequacy was 59% (site average range, 20.5%–94.4%) for energy and 60.3% (site average range, 18.6%–152.5%) for protein.

Conclusions.—Despite high adherence to some recommendations, large gaps exist between many recommendations and actual practice in intensive care units, and consequently nutrition therapy is suboptimal. We have identified "best achievable" practice that can serve as targets for future quality improvement initiatives.

▶ Guidelines for nutritional repletion in the critical care unit are not well established nor standardized from 1 center to another. It is clear that adequate and early institution of feeding is associated with improved outcomes in a variety of medical and trauma settings. Accordingly, inadequate nutrition in this setting potentially place patients' recovery and health at risk. The authors of this study had previously developed clinical practice guidelines for nutrition in the critical care setting, but adherence to such had not been established. This prospective study was designed to determine the nutritional practices among several intensive care settings.

Mechanically ventilated patients were enrolled from 158 intensive care units from 20 countries and followed for a maximum of 12 days. The variables that were collected included all types of feeding, both enterally and parenterally, the use of motility agents, the use of recommended supplements, and the management of hyperglycemia. The authors discovered large variations with the compliance of their established practice guidelines. Despite their efforts in establishing these potential standards, there are clearly differing views regarding nutrition in the intensive care unit (ICU) setting. In many cases, nutrition is viewed as a supportive rather than a therapeutic intervention.

This is an excellent observational study. There are no defined outcomes; however, it serves to emphasize the need for acceptable nutritional standards that can be used in any ICU setting, regardless of the size or level of expertise. The authors must show that widespread adherence to clinical guidelines is associated with positive outcomes, and deviation from those established criteria is associated with deleterious effects. Nutritional education must be emphasized at all levels of training and must be viewed as a primary therapeutic intervention. There are defined guidelines for stroke, myocardial infarction, and gastrointestinal bleeding. It is time to develop and adhere to a structure for nutrition in the critical care setting.

C. W. Deitch, MD

9 Renal

Acute kidney injury in non-severe pneumonia is associated with an increased immune response and lower survival

Murugan R, on behalf of the Genetic and Inflammatory Markers of Sepsis (GenIMS) Investigators (Univ of Pittsburgh School of Medicine, PA; et al)
Kidney Int 77:527-535, 2010

While sepsis is a leading cause of acute kidney injury in critically ill patients, the relationship between immune response and acute kidney injury in less severely ill patients with infection is not known. Here we studied the epidemiology, 1-year mortality, and immune response associated with acute kidney injury in 1836 hospitalized patients with community-acquired severe and non-severe pneumonia. Acute kidney injury developed in 631 patients of whom 329 had severe and 302 had non-severe sepsis. Depending on the subgroup classification, 16–25% of the patients with non-severe pneumonia also developed acute kidney injury. In general, patients with acute kidney injury were older, had more comorbidity, and had higher biomarker concentrations (interleukin-6, tumor necrosis factor, D-dimer) even among patients without severe sepsis. The risk of death associated with acute kidney injury varied when assessed by Gray's survival model and after adjusting for differences in age, gender, ethnicity, and comorbidity. This risk was significantly higher immediately after hospitalization but gradually fell over time in the overall cohort and in those with non-severe pneumonia. A significantly higher risk of death (hazard ratio 1.29) was also present in those never admitted to an intensive care unit. Hence acute kidney injury is common even among patients with non-severe pneumonia and is associated with higher immune response and an increased risk of death (Fig 2, Table 2).

▶ Acute kidney injury is common in sepsis and is associated with increased mortality.[1,2] This study evaluated the impact of acute kidney injury on survival and hospital course in a population of patients with community-acquired pneumonia, whether or not they met the definition of severe sepsis or septic shock. As you might expect, just as in severe sepsis and septic shock, the presence of acute kidney injury, either at the onset of infection or as a complication during the period of infection, was associated with increased risk for hospital, 90-day, and 1-year mortality. In addition, the presence of acute kidney injury was associated with increased need for intensive care unit care and use of mechanical ventilatory support. These findings support the important impact of acute kidney injury on infection in general, similar to its major impact on severe sepsis

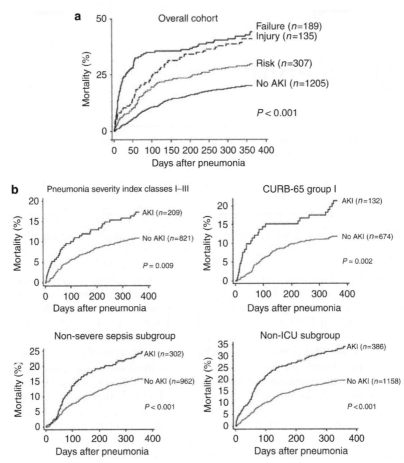

FIGURE 2.—One-year mortality in patients with and without AKI in the overall cohort and within non-severe CAP subgroups. (a) The Kaplan–Meier failure plots by maximum RIFLE stage for probability of death in the entire CAP cohort, which at 1 year was higher in patients with AKI than in patients without AKI (log rank $P < 0.001$). (b) Failure plots for probability of death at 1 year within the four non-severe CAP subgroups. Non-severe CAP patients with AKI in each of the four subgroups had higher probability of death associated with AKI at 1 year compared to those without AKI (log rank $P < 0.01$ for all subgroups). AKI, acute kidney injury; CAP, community-acquired pneumonia; RIFLE, Risk, Injury, and Failure criteria. (Reprinted with permission from Macmillan Publishers Ltd: Murugan R, on behalf of the Genetic and Inflammatory Markers of Sepsis (GenIMS) Investigators. Acute kidney injury in non-severe pneumonia is associated with an increased immune response and lower survival. *Kidney Int.* 2010;77:527-535.)

and septic shock. This observation also supports our emphasis on early goal-directed resuscitative efforts in an attempt to preserve and maintain organ system function, decreasing risk for developing acute kidney injury.[3]

R. A. Balk, MD

TABLE 2.—Hospital Course and Outcomes in Patients with and without AKI in the Overall Cohort

	No. (%)		
Characteristic[a]	AKI	No AKI	*P*-value
Developed severe sepsis	329 (52.1)	243 (20.1)	<0.001
Intensive care unit admission	245 (39)	47 (4)	<0.001
Mechanical ventilation	116 (18.4)	13 (1)	<0.001
Length of hospital stay, median (IQR)	8 (12–5)	5 (7–4)	<0.001
Hospital mortality	70 (11.1)	16 (1.3)	<0.001
90-day mortality	151 (24)	118 (9.8)	<0.001
1-year mortality	229 (36.3)	242 (20.1)	<0.001

Abbreviations: AKI, acute kidney injury; IQR, interquartile range.
[a]Hospital course and outcome in the entire cohort of 1836 patients with community-acquired pneumonia.

References

1. Schrier RW, Wang W. Acute renal failure and sepsis. *N Engl J Med.* 2004;351: 159-169.
2. Chen YC, Jenq CC, Tian YC, et al. Rifle classification for predicting in-hospital mortality in critically ill sepsis patients. *Shock.* 2009;31:139-145.
3. Rivers E, Nguyen B, Havstad S, et al. Early goal-directed therapy in the treatment of severe sepsis and septic shock. *N Engl J Med.* 2001;345:1368-1377.

Atrial fibrillation in hemodialysis patients: clinical features and associations with anticoagulant therapy

Wizemann V, Tong L, Satayathum S, et al (Georg Haas Dialysezentrum, Giessen, Germany; Arbor Res Collaborative for Health, Ann Arbor, MI; et al)
Kidney Int 77:1098-1106, 2010

Using data from the international Dialysis Outcomes and Practice Patterns Study (DOPPS), we determined incidence, prevalence, and outcomes among hemodialysis patients with atrial fibrillation. Cox proportional hazards models, to identify associations with newly diagnosed atrial fibrillation and clinical outcomes, were stratified by country and study phase and adjusted for descriptive characteristics and comorbidities. Of 17,513 randomly sampled patients, 2188 had preexisting atrial fibrillation, with wide variation in prevalence across countries. Advanced age, non-black race, higher facility mean dialysate calcium, prosthetic heart valves, and valvular heart disease were associated with higher risk of new atrial fibrillation. Atrial fibrillation at study enrollment was positively associated with all-cause mortality and stroke. The CHADS2 score identified approximately equal-size groups of hemodialysis patients with atrial fibrillation with low (less than 2) and higher risk (more than 4) for subsequent strokes on a per 100 patient-year basis. Among patients with atrial fibrillation, warfarin use was associated with a significantly higher stroke risk, particularly in those over 75 years of age. Our study shows that atrial fibrillation

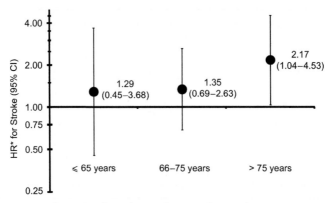

FIGURE 2.—Hazard ratio (HR) for stroke according to warfarin use, by age categories among patients with a diagnosis of atrial fibrillation at DOPPS enrollment. The numbers of patients (strokes) were 1001 (35), 1137 (61), and 1107 (49) for age groups $\leq$65, 66 to 75, and >75 years, respectively. The numbers (%) of patients on warfarin were 146 (15%), 192 (17%), and 171 (15%) for age groups $\leq$65, 66 to 75, and >75 years, respectively. Patients with prosthetic heart valves ($N = 177$) were excluded. Separate Cox models for each age category were used to estimate the hazard ratio and 95% confidence interval (whiskers) of first stroke after study entry, adjusted for age within the restricted category, sex, black race, years with ESRD, study phase, history of stroke, comorbid conditions as listed in Table 2, permanent pacemaker implanted, previous history of cardiac arrest, left ventricular hypertrophy, and valvular heart disease, stratified by region and study phase and accounting for effects of facility clustering. In addition to warfarin use, the following variables were statistically significant ($P < 0.05$) in a model including all age categories: neurologic disease ($P = 0.02$), diabetes ($P = 0.03$), and previous history of stroke ($P = 0.002$). (Reprinted from Wizemann V, Tong L, Satayathum S, et al. Atrial fibrillation in hemodialysis patients: clinical features and associations with anticoagulant therapy. *Kidney Int.* 2010;77:1098-1106, with permission from the International Society of Nephrology.)

is common and associated with elevated risk of adverse clinical outcomes, and this risk is even higher among elderly patients prescribed warfarin. The effectiveness and safety of warfarin in hemodialysis patients require additional investigation (Fig 2 and Table 4).

▶ Atrial fibrillation (AF) is one of the most frequently encountered cardiac arrhythmias, and its prevalence increases with age, male gender, and presence of other comorbid conditions.[1,2] In the intensive care unit (ICU), the incidence of AF ranges from 5% in medical patients up to 60% following valvular heart surgery.[2,3] In those patients, AF is associated with an increased ICU and hospital length of stay as well as a higher mortality.[4,5] While AF may be a marker of severity of illness,[6] there are clearly several adverse consequences attributable to this arrhythmia, per se.

One of the most feared complications of AF is embolic stroke. Anticoagulation is known to reduce the risk of stroke in AF, but it also raises the risk of bleeding. Thus, several scoring systems have been developed to identify patients whose risk:benefit ratio with anticoagulation is the most favorable. The most widely used risk stratification tool, the Congestive Heart Failure, Hypertension, Age, Diabetes Mellitus, prior Stroke (CHADS2), compounds 5 commonly recorded variables (congestive heart failure, hypertension, age, diabetes, and previous

TABLE 4.—Stroke Rates Among HD Patients with History of Atrial Fibrillation, By CHADS2 score[a]

CHADS2 Score[c]	(A) Patients with History of Non-Valvular AF— Prescribed Aspirin But Not Warfarin[b]			(B) All Patients with History of Non-Valvular AF[b]		
	Patients (n)	Stroke Events (n)	Stroke Rate Per 100 Patient-Years[d]	Patients (n)	Stroke Events (n)	Stroke Rate Per 100 Patient-Years[d]
0	16	0	0.0	141	1	0.5
1	114	1	0.6	568	18	2.1
2	174	6	2.3	875	23	1.9
3	167	8	3.8	882	45	3.9
4	92	6	5.6	403	27	6.0
5	70	6	6.1	311	25	6.5
6	10	2	19.0	70	9	12.7
Overall	643	29	3.3	3250	148	3.4

[a]Stroke rates during DOPPS follow-up among patients with history of atrial fibrillation (AF) at DOPPS enrollment, excluding 177 patients with mechanical heart valves.
[b]Column A includes dialysis patients generally comparable with those used to evaluate CHADS2 in the general population; 27 patients on heparin between dialysis sessions but not warfarin were also excluded; column B includes all AF patients without a mechanical heart valve.
[c]Based on stroke risk according to CHADS2 score in the general population: 0=low, 1 or 1–2=moderate, and ≥ 2 or 3=high risk. Among a non-dialysis Medicare population with non-valvular AF and not receiving warfarin, stroke rates for CHADS2 score=0, 1–2, and ≥ 3 were 0.8, 2.7, and 5.3 per 100 patient-years, respectively (refs. 11–13).
[d]Column A=891 patient-years; column B=4348 patient-years.

stroke) into a numerical score ranging from 0 to 6. Consensus guidelines recommend initiating anticoagulation for a score of 2 or more.[7]

Patients with end-stage renal disease (ESRD) have a very high prevalence of AF, but they were either excluded from, or underrepresented in, studies that were used to generate the aforementioned guidelines. Furthermore, because patients with ESRD also have a heightened tendency to bleed, standard scoring systems may not accurately assess their risk:benefit ratio with anticoagulation for AF.

Wizemann et al studied 17 513 hemodialysis patients from 12 countries (including the United States and Europe) as part of the Dialysis Outcomes and Practice Patterns Study. They showed that AF was much more common in patients with ESRD than in the general population. AF was associated with all-cause mortality and stroke. In this study, the CHADS2 score appeared to accurately stratify patients by stroke rate (Table 4). Nonetheless, in patients with AF over 75 years of age, warfarin use was associated with a higher risk of stroke.

The finding of a high stroke rate among older patients with AF on warfarin has a number of possible explanations. First, to the extent that warfarin predisposes to intracranial hemorrhage, the finding may be valid. Such a conclusion would tend to greatly inhibit the use of warfarin in this population, a position endorsed by some experts.[8] It should be noted, however, that the study was unable to distinguish between hemorrhagic stroke and embolic stroke. Second, there is likely to be confounding by assignment to warfarin, in that patients deemed by their physicians to be at the highest risk of stroke will be prescribed warfarin.

In summary, CHADS2 appears to accurately stratify patients on hemodialysis according to their stroke risk with AF. Patients with ESRD and a CHADS2 score less than 2 appear to be at a low risk of stroke and should not receive warfarin.

Management of patients with higher CHADS2 scores must be individualized. This article emphasizes the need for future prospective studies of the use of anticoagulants in this setting.

L. S. Weisberg, MD

References

1. Walsh SR, Oates JE, Anderson JA, Blair SD, Makin CA, Walsh CJ. Postoperative arrhythmias in colorectal surgical patients: incidence and clinical correlates. *Colorectal Dis.* 2006;8:212-216.
2. Jongnarangsin K, Oral H. Postoperative atrial fibrillation. *Med Clin North Am.* 2008;92:87-99.
3. Christian SA, Schorr C, Ferchau L, Jarbrink ME, Parrillo JE, Gerber DR. Clinical characteristics and outcomes of septic patients with new-onset atrial fibrillation. *J Crit Care.* 2008;23:532-536.
4. Valentine RJ, Rosen SF, Cigarroa JE, Jackson MR, Modrall JG, Clagett GP. The clinical course of new-onset atrial fibrillation after elective aortic operations. *J Am Coll Surg.* 2001;193:499-504.
5. Kohno H, Koyanagi T, Kasegawa H, Miyazaki M. Three-day magnesium administration prevents atrial fibrillation after coronary artery bypass grafting. *Ann Thorac Surg.* 2005;79:117-126.
6. Brathwaite D, Weissman C. The new onset of atrial arrhythmias following major noncardiothoracic surgery is associated with increased mortality. *Chest.* 1998;114:462-468.
7. Estes NA 3rd, Halperin JL, Calkins H, et al. ACC/AHA/Physician Consortium 2008 Clinical Performance measures for Adults with Nonvalvular Atrial Fibrillation or Atrial Flutter: a report of the American College of Cardiology/American heart Association Task Force on Performance measures and the Physician Consortium for Performance Improvement (Writing Committee to Develop Clinical Performance Measures for Atrial Fibrillation) Developed in Collaboration with the Heart Rhythm Society. *J Am Coll Cardiol.* 2008;51:865-884.
8. Bennett WM. Should dialysis patient ever receive warfarin and for what reasons? *Clin J Am Soc Nephrol.* 2006;1:1357-1359.

Catheter dysfunction and dialysis performance according to vascular access among 736 critically ill adults requiring renal replacement therapy: A randomized controlled study
Parienti J-J, for Members of the Cathedia Study Group (Côte de Nacre Univ Hosp Ctr, Caen, France; et al)
Crit Care Med 38:1118-1125, 2010

Objective.—To compare dialysis catheter function according to catheter site.

Design.—Multicenter, open, randomized controlled trial.

Setting.—Nine university-affiliated hospitals and three general hospitals in France.

Patients.—Seven hundred thirty-six patients in intensive care units who required a first venous catheterization to perform either intermittent hemodialysis (470 patients with 1275 sessions) or continuous renal replacement therapy (266 patients with 1003 days).

Intervention.—Patients randomly received either femoral (n = 370) or jugular (n = 366) catheterization. For the jugular site, right-side position (n = 252) was recommended.

Measurements and Main Results.—Time to catheter ablation for dysfunction, urea reduction ratio (intermittent hemodialysis), and down-time (continuous renal replacement therapy) were assessed for all participants and evaluated by randomly assigned catheterization site (femoral or jugular). Baseline demography and dialysis prescriptions were similar between the site arms. In modified intent-to-treat, catheter dysfunction occurred in 36 of 348 (10.3%) and 38 of 342 (11.1%) patients in the femoral and jugular groups, respectively. The risk of catheter dysfunction did not significantly differ between randomized groups (hazard ratio, 1.06; 95% confidence interval, 0.67–1.68; $p = .80$). Compared to the femoral site, the observed risk of dysfunction decreased in the right jugular position (15 of 226; 6.6%; adjusted hazard ratio, 0.58; 95% confidence interval, 0.31–1.07; $p = .09$) and significantly increased in the left jugular position (23 of 118; 19.5%; adjusted hazard ratio, 1.89; 95% confidence interval, 1.12–3.21; $p < .02$). The postintermittent hemodialysis mean urea reduction ratio per session was 50.8% (standard deviation, 16.1) for femoral vs. 52.8% (standard deviation, 15.8) for jugular ($p = .30$) sites, and the median continuous renal replacement therapy downtime per patient-day was 1.17 hrs (interquartile range, 0.75–1.50) for both sites ($p = .98$).

Conclusions.—In terms of catheter dysfunction and dialysis performance among critically ill adults requiring acute renal replacement therapy, jugular site did not significantly outperform femoral site placement.

▶ Despite recent advances in the practice of critical care nephrology, several controversial questions remain unanswered. Particularly vexing are those pertaining to renal replacement therapy, such as timing of initiation of hemodialysis, type of therapy (intermittent vs continuous), and intensity of treatment.

On the other hand, until recently, there was an agreement over the matters relating to vascular access, with the jugular site favored over the femoral site for its lower rate of catheter dysfunction and nosocomial infections.[1,2] That consensus, however, was based on sparse evidence from observational studies[3] and was recently shaken by the findings of a large randomized controlled trial showing that femoral catheters had no greater rate of infectious complications and were actually superior to jugular catheters in patients with low body mass indexes.[4]

This study is the first to our knowledge to compare dialysis catheter performance in a randomized controlled fashion. The investigators showed that catheter dysfunction was the lowest in the right internal jugular position, followed by femoral, and then left jugular, although the advantage of the right jugular position over the femoral did not achieve statistical significance (Fig 2 in the original article).

Another interesting finding of this study is that when the femoral catheter length was 20 cm (as per current clinical practice guidelines),[5] it was outperformed by the jugular site, whereas when the length was 25 cm (and thereby able to reach the inferior vena cava), there was an equivalent performance.

Based on this study and on the absence of solid evidence to the contrary, critical care practitioners should place dialysis catheters in either the right jugular or the femoral position (ensuring a 25 cm length), using the left jugular as a last resort. Regardless of the position of the catheter, good practice requires that its performance be monitored closely and that it be replaced promptly for dysfunction to ensure adequate renal replacement therapy.

L. S. Weisberg, MD

References

1. Schetz M. Vascular access for HD and CRRT. *Contrib Nephrol.* 2007;156: 275-286.
2. Canaud B, Desmeules S, Klouche K, Leray-Moragués H, Béraud JJ. Vascular access for dialysis in the intensive care unit. *Best Pract Res Clin Anaesthesiol.* 2004;18:159-174.
3. Oliver MJ, Callery SM, Thorpe KE, Schwab SJ, Churchill DN. Risk of bacteremia from temporary hemodialysis catheters by site of insertion and duration of use: a prospective study. *Kidney Int.* 2000;58:2543-2545.
4. Parienti JJ, Thirion M, Megarbane B, et al. Femoral vs jugular venous catheterization and risk of nosocomial events in adults requiring acute renal replacement therapy: a randomized controlled trial. *JAMA.* 2008;299:2413-2422.
5. III. NKF-K/DOQI Clinical Practice Guidelines for Vascular Access: update 2000. *Am J Kidney Dis.* 2001;37:S137-S181.

Heparin versus prostacyclin in continuous hemodiafiltration for acute renal failure: Effects on platelet function in the systemic circulation and across the filter

Arcangeli A, Rocca B, Salvatori G, et al (Catholic Univ School of Medicine, Largo Francesco Vito, Rome, Italy)
Thromb Res 126:24-31, 2010

Continuous venovenous hemodiafiltration (CVVHDF) is the treatment of choice for critically-ill patients suffering from acute renal failure (ARF). One major problem of extracorporeal circuits is their thrombogenicity, which requires pharmacological blockade of primary (platelet-dependent) or secondary (plasmatic) haemostasis, increasing the patient's bleeding risk.

Our study assessed platelet function during CVVHDF, comparing anti-coagulant versus antiplatelet pharmacological strategies, commonly used to avoid circuit clotting. Twenty-three critically-ill patients with ARF, requiring CVVHDF were randomized to a prostacyclin analogue (PGI) or to unfractionated heparin (UFH). Ex vivo platelet function, assessed by optical aggregometry (OPA) induced by collagen or ADP, was studied in peripheral blood at baseline, 4 and 24 hrs after starting CVVHDF, and at 4 hrs within the circuit, before and after the filter (n = 9). Coagulation was also monitored.

PGI significantly inhibited ADP-induced OPA of peripheral platelets: maximal aggregation (T_{max}) was reduced at 4 and 24 hrs by 20%, while collagen-induced T_{max} was significantly reduced at 4 hrs only. In the UFH group, collagen-induced OPA in peripheral platelets was significantly inhibited: slopes of OPA tracings were decreased by 25%, lag time was prolonged by 22%, T_{max} decreased by 10% already at 4 hrs. ADP-induced OPA showed a similar, but non-significant trend. UFH expectedly prolonged aPTT. In the UFH group, platelet responsiveness to collagen was significantly increased by 30% in post-filter versus pre-filter samples. This effect was blunted in the PGI group.

UFH does not protect platelets from filter-induced activation and is associated with a reduced function of systemic platelets. Platelet-inhibiting agents might better prevent the activatory effect of the filter.

▶ Dialysis-requiring acute renal failure (ARF) often complicates the clinical course of many critically ill patients. When facing hemodynamic instability or in certain specific situations (such as intoxications that require prolonged duration of treatment), physicians often choose continuous renal replacement therapy (CRRT).

Because extracorporeal circuits are thrombogenic, anticoagulants often are used to prevent clotting in the circuit. Heparin is the most frequently used anticoagulant for CRRT.[1] Its use in critically ill patients, however, carries an increased risk of bleeding and the potential for developing heparin-induced thrombocytopenia. Some centers have tried to circumvent these risks by anticoagulating only the extracorporeal circuit with sodium citrate, which is called regional citrate anticoagulation. This methodology has its own considerable risks, including hyper- and hypocalcemia, hypernatremia, metabolic alkalosis, and hypercitratemia.[2] There is a need to develop alternative strategies to prevent clotting in the CRRT circuit.

In this interesting study, Arcangelli et al examined platelet function in 23 critically ill patients on CRRT for ARF, randomized to receive 1 of 2 anticoagulants: unfractionated heparin or epoprostenol (a prostacyclin analog), infused continuously pre-filter.

They found that heparin failed to prevent filter-induced platelet activation, which paradoxically caused peripheral platelet hypofunction. Epoprostenol, on the other hand, prevented filter-induced platelet activation briefly without any effect on coagulation. Filter life and efficiency, and complications, were reported. The authors speculate that heparin's inhibition of systemic platelet responsiveness, along with its anticoagulant effect, may raise its risk of bleeding compared with prostacyclin.

Any judgment about the clinical use of prostacyclin as an anticoagulant for CRRT will depend on the results of a large trial examining clinically relevant end points, such as filter life and bleeding complications. Alternatives in such a trial should be heparin and no anticoagulant at all. This last strategy may prove to have the lowest risk:benefit ratio, especially for patients in whom high blood flow rates can be achieved.

L. S. Weisberg, MD

References

1. Oudemans-van Straaten HM, Wester JP, de Pont AC, Schentz MR. Anticoagulation strategies in continous renal replacement therapy: can the choice be evidenced based? *Intensive Care Med.* 2006;32:188-202.
2. Tolwani AJ, Willie KM. Anticoagulation for continuous renal replacement therapy. *Semin Dial.* 2009;22:141-145.

10 Trauma and Overdose

Abdominal Trauma After Terrorist Bombing Attacks Exhibits a Unique Pattern of Injury
Bala M, Rivkind AI, Zamir G, et al (Hadassah-Hebrew Univ Med Ctr, Jerusalem, Israel)
Ann Surg 248:303-309, 2008

Background.—The recent growth in the volume of civilian blast trauma caused by terrorist bombings warrants special attention to the specific pattern of injury associated with such attacks.

Objective.—To characterize the abdominal injuries inflicted by terrorist-related explosions and to compare the pattern of injury with civilian, penetrating and blunt, abdominal trauma.

Methods.—Retrospective analysis of prospectively collected data from 181 patients with abdominal trauma requiring laparotomy, who were admitted to the Hadassah Hospital, Jerusalem, Israel, from October 2000 to December 2005. Patients were divided into 3 groups according to mechanism of injury: terror-related blast injury (n = 21), gunshot wounds (GSW) (n = 73) and blunt trauma (n = 87).

Results.—Median injury severity score in the blast group was significantly higher compared with GSW and blunt groups (34, 18, and 29, respectively, $P < 0.0001$). Injury to multiple body regions (≥ 3) occurred in 85.7% of blast group, 28.8% of GSW group, and 59.7% of blunt group ($P < 0.001$). The pattern of intra-abdominal injury was different between the groups. Bowel injury was found in 71.4% of blast victims, 64.4% of GSW, and 25.3% of blunt group ($P < 0.001$). Parenchymal injury was found in one third of patients in blast and GSW groups versus 60.9% of patients in blunt group ($P = 0.001$). Penetrating shrapnel was the cause of bowel injury in all but 1 patient in the blast group (94.4%).

Conclusions.—Terrorist attacks generate more severe injuries to more body regions than other types of trauma. Abdominal injury inflicted by terrorist bombings causes a unique pattern of wounds, mainly injury to hollow organs. Shrapnel is the leading cause of abdominal injury following terrorist bombings (Figs 1 and 2).

▶ Compared are victims of blast, standard blunt, and gunshot injuries collected at a major trauma center in Jerusalem from 2000-2005. Patients sustaining terrorist bombing attacks had higher injury severity scores reflecting increased number of body regions involved. The death rate, however, is not different. We are given relatively few details regarding the incidents that provided patients

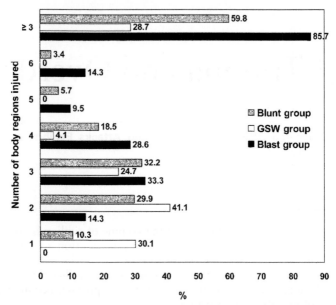

FIGURE 1.—The number of body regions involved in injury according to different mechanisms of trauma. *Significantly different, Kruskal-Wallis test, $P < 0.001$. (Courtesy of Bala M, Rivkind AI, Zamir G, et al. Abdominal trauma after terrorist bombing attacks exhibits a unique pattern of injury. *Ann Surg.* 2008;248:303-309.)

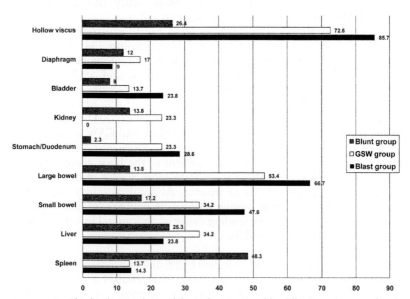

FIGURE 2.—The distribution of intra-abdominal injury caused by different mechanisms of trauma. *Significantly different, χ^2 test, $P < 0.001$. (Courtesy of Bala M, Rivkind AI, Zamir G, et al. Abdominal trauma after terrorist bombing attacks exhibits a unique pattern of injury. *Ann Surg.* 2008;248:303-309.)

for this study. For example, classic injuries associated with blast trauma, such as lung injury or neurologic injury, do not figure prominently as I might expect. Thus, I am not sure without details of the specific incidents that provided the patients whether the dataset is reflective of outcomes from terrorist incidents today.[1]

Nonetheless, the surgeon should be aware that patients sustaining terrorist injury will have a high frequency of bowel injury, although findings may be subtle as the missiles causing this injury (shrapnel) proceed at relatively low speed relative to gunshots. Gunshots are marked by significant local tissue trauma, while shrapnel from blast injury will have a more subtle presentation.

Resource consumption will also be higher in patients sustaining blast injury, probably due to the number of body regions involved. Significant solid organ injury is less likely in the setting of blast injury.

D. J. Dries, MSE, MD

Reference

1. Kashuk JL, Halperin P, Caspi G, Colwell C, Moore EE. Bomb explosions in acts of terrorism: evil creativity challenges our trauma systems. *J Am Coll Surg.* 2009;209: 134-140.

Blunt pancreatoduodenal injury: a multicenter study of the Research Consortium of New England Centers for Trauma (ReCONECT)
Velmahos GC, Tabbara M, Gross R, et al (Massachusetts General Hosp and Harvard Med School, Boston)
Arch Surg 144:413-419, 2009

Objectives.—To evaluate the safety of nonoperative management (NOM), to examine the diagnostic sensitivity of computed tomography (CT), and to identify missed diagnoses and related outcomes in patients with blunt pancreatoduodenal injury (BPDI).

Design.—Retrospective multicenter study.

Setting.—Eleven New England trauma centers (7 academic and 4 nonacademic).

Patients.—Two hundred thirty patients (>15 years old) with BPDI admitted to the hospital during 11 years. Each BPDI was graded from 1 (lowest) to 5 (highest) according to the American Association for the Surgery of Trauma grading system.

Main Outcome Measures.—Success of NOM, sensitivity of CT, BPDI-related complications, length of hospital stay, and mortality.

Results.—Ninety-seven patients (42.2%) with mostly grades 1 and 2 BPDI were selected for NOM: NOM failed in 10 (10.3%), 10 (10.3%) developed BPDI-related complications (3 in patients in whom NOM failed), and 7 (7.2%) died (none related to failure of NOM). The remaining 133 patients were operated on urgently: 34 (25.6%) developed BPDI-related complications and 20 (15.0%) died. The initial CT missed BPDI in

30 patients (13.0%); 4 of them (13.3%) died but not because of the BPDI. The mortality rate in patients without a missed diagnosis was 8.8% (P =.50). There was no correlation between time to diagnosis and length of hospital stay (Spearman r = 0.06; P =.43). The sensitivity of CT for BPDI was 75.7% (76% for pancreatic and 70% for duodenal injuries).

Conclusions.—The NOM of low-grade BPDI is safe despite occasional failures. Missed diagnosis of BPDI continues to occur despite advances in CT but does not seem to cause adverse outcomes in most patients.

▶ This is good multicenter data from several New England trauma centers. Various levels of trauma care are represented, which strengthens the quality of results obtained. A number of important observations are made. First, one is unlikely to see significant blunt pancreatoduodenal injury in the absence of other problems. These patients had high injury severity scores. Do not expect significant pancreatoduodenal trauma in someone with minimal or no signs of injury. Unfortunately, computed tomography (CT) scan is not the optimal imaging modality. Later-generation scanners are somewhat better than early machines, but none is perfect. Another remarkable aspect of this data is that early and later-generation scanners are compared.

As the authors establish that CT scanning is not ideal, we must acknowledge that false-negative studies may be present at these centers. The good news is that it usually does not matter. Patients will develop clinical changes, which lead to additional imaging or operation. In this series, those changes appear within hours.

Perhaps the greatest shortcoming in this study is the failure to distinguish between pancreatic and duodenal injury.[1,2] Patterns of management are different in each. The good news, once again, is that rapid intervention generally is not warranted unless there is obvious bleeding.

D. J. Dries, MSE, MD

References

1. Kao LS, Bulger EM, Parks DL, Byrd GF, Jurkovich GJ. Predictors of morbidity after traumatic pancreatic injury. *J Trauma.* 2003;55:898-905.
2. Cuddington G, Rusnak CH, Cameron RD, Carter J. Management of duodenal injuries. *Can J Surg.* 1990;33:41-44.

Complications of recombinant activated human coagulation factor VII
Howes JL, Smith RS, Helmer SD, et al (The Univ of Kansas School of Medicine-Wichita; The Virginia Tech Carilion School of Medicine, Roanoke; et al)
Am J Surg 198:895-899, 2009

Background.—Recombinant factor VIIa (rFVIIa) frequently is used for treatment of life-threatening hemorrhage in trauma.

Methods.—A retrospective review of injured patients receiving rFVIIa at an American College of Surgeons–verified Level 1 trauma center was performed. Controls were matched for age, sex, Injury Severity Score, and traumatic brain injury. Thrombotic complications in patients administered rFVIIa, including deep venous thrombosis (DVT), pulmonary embolus, acute myocardial infarction, ischemic stroke, mesenteric ischemia, arterial thromboembolism, and death, were determined.

Results.—Thirty-six patients were given rFVIIa, of whom 5 (13.8%) had thrombotic complications. Indications for rFVIIa were life-threatening intracranial bleeding in the presence of pre-injury anticoagulation or hemorrhage. The incidences of DVT (n = 4) and acute myocardial infarction (n = 1) were noted. In the control group, there were fewer thrombotic complications (DVT, 1; pulmonary embolus, 1). The mortality rate (52.8%) was higher in patients receiving rFVIIa compared with the control group (22.2%; $P = .014$). Pre-injury anticoagulation was common in the treatment group.

Conclusions.—Pre-injury anticoagulation is frequently the indication for rFVIIa administration. Thrombotic complications occur with rFVIIa administration. The mortality rate of injured patients who receive rFVIIa is high (Table 4).

▶ The authors compare patients matched by standard trauma criteria where recombinant activated human coagulation factor VII was used in the management of acute intracranial hemorrhage or uncontrolled bleeding in the setting of massive transfusion.[1] The control group has similar demographics, but does not receive recombinant activated human factor VII. A dramatic decrease in survival is noted where factor VII is given. The incidence of thromboembolic complications also appears to be higher though treatment groups are small.[2]

Patients receiving recombinant activated factor VII were on a variety of anticoagulant agents, including aspirin, Plavix, and warfarin. While not specifically discussed by the authors, I believe that the use of these agents is a marker for severity of vascular disease. Treatment patients (received factor VII) had a higher incidence of atrial fibrillation and coronary artery disease. While a similar distribution of injury types is seen between groups, progression of hemorrhage can be very different where anticoagulants have been administered. This is not discussed by the authors.

TABLE 4.—Complications and Mortality

| Parameter | Study Group | | |
	Treatment	Control	*P* value
Complications			
DVT	4 (11.1%)	1 (2.8%)	.357
Pulmonary embolus	0 (0%)	1 (2.8%)	1.0
Myocardial infarction	1 (2.8%)	0 (0%)	1.0
Ischemia	0 (0%)	0 (0%)	1.0
Cerebrovascular event	0 (0%)	0 (0%)	1.0
All thrombotic events	5 (13.8%)	2 (5.6%)	.279
Death	19 (52.8%)	8 (22.2%)	.014

Number (percentage) shown.

Deep venous thrombosis (DVT) occurred more frequently in patients who had received recombinant factor VII. When did these patients receive DVT prophylaxis? DVT prophylaxis may be given as early 48 hours to 72 hours after head injury. It is unclear when DVT prophylaxis was given here.

Since demographics suggest similarity in treatment groups, I am concerned that factors not adequately described after randomization contribute to the significant difference in mortality in control and treatment arms of this small study.

D. J. Dries, MSE, MD

References

1. Boffard KD, Riou B, Warren B, et al. Recombinant factor VIIa as adjunctive therapy for bleeding control in severely injured trauma patients: two parallel randomized, placebo-controlled, double-blind clinical trials. *J Trauma*. 2005;59: 8-18.
2. Thomas GO, Dutton RP, Hemlock B, et al. Thromboembolic complications associated with factor VIIa administration. *J Trauma*. 2007;62:564-569.

Computed Tomography Grading Systems Poorly Predict the Need for Intervention after Spleen and Liver Injuries
Cohn SM, Arango JI, Myers JG, et al (Univ of Texas Health Science Ctr at San Antonio)
Am Surg 75:133-139, 2009

Computed tomography (CT) grading systems are often used clinically to forecast the need for interventions after abdominal trauma with solid organ injuries. We compared spleen and liver CT grading methods to determine their utility in predicting the need for operative intervention or angiographic embolization. Abdominal CT scans of 300 patients with spleen injuries, liver injuries, or both were evaluated by five trauma faculty members blinded to clinical outcomes. Studies were graded by American Association for the Surgery of Trauma criteria, a novel splenic injury CT grading system, and a novel liver injury grading system. The sensitivity and specificity of each methodology in predicting the need for intervention were calculated. The kappa statistic was used to determine interrater variability. Twenty-one per cent (39/189) of patients with splenic injuries visible on CT scans required interventions, whereas 14 per cent (21/154) of patients with liver injuries visible on CT required interventions. The overall sensitivity of all grading systems in predicting the need for surgery or angioembolization of the spleen or liver was poor; the specificity seemed to be fairly good. When evaluators were compared, the strength of agreement for the various scoring systems was only moderate. Anatomic CT grading systems are ineffective screening tools for excluding the need for operation or embolization after splenic or hepatic trauma. Although insensitive, CT is a good predictor (highly specific) of the need for intervention if certain definitive abnormalities are identified. Considerable inconsistency exists in interpretation of abdominal CT scans after trauma, even among experienced clinicians.

▶ A large number of abdominal CT scans are read using the standard American Association for the Surgery of Trauma grading system and a hybrid grading system developed at the reporting institution.[1,2] In each case, limited sensitivity and somewhat better specificity are reported for identifying injuries requiring embolization or operative intervention. A number of general comments can be made. At best, imaging provides a rough guide to the need for an intervention. Imaging cannot effectively predict the need for interventions in the absence of other clinical data. The hemodynamically unstable patient with a lesser pattern of change on the CT scan may require angiography and/or operation. The novel CT grading systems identified by the reporting institution not only clearly include markers of severe injury but also include subjectivity. For example, each CT grading system moves to intervention with a large hemoperitoneum. What is a large hemoperitoneum?

CT imaging has taken us far beyond the general data provided by diagnostic peritoneal lavage. However, this modality must be placed in the context of coexisting injuries that affect the willingness to observe patients with abdominal trauma and physiologic assessment of the patient.[3] This study is based on interventions performed on involved patients. The decision to intervene may not be an appropriate gold standard and is not consistently applied across surgical groups or among institutions.

D. J. Dries, MSE, MD

References

1. Peitzman AB, Heil B, Rivera L, et al. Blunt splenic injury in adults: multi-institutional study of the Eastern Association for the surgery of trauma. *J Trauma*. 2000;49:177-189.
2. Kozar RA, Moore FA, Moore EE, et al. Western Trauma Association critical decisions in trauma: nonoperative management of adult blunt hepatic trauma. *J Trauma*. 2009;67:1144-1149.
3. Plurad DS, Green DJ, Inaba K, et al. Blunt assault is associated with failure of nonoperative management of the spleen independent of organ injury grade and despite lower overall injury severity. *J Trauma*. 2009;66:630-635.

Critical Evaluation of Pulmonary Contusion in the Early Post-Traumatic Period: Risk of Assisted Ventilation
Hamrick MC, Duhn RD, Ochsner MG (Memorial Health Univ Med Ctr, Savannah, GA)
Am Surg 75:1054-1058, 2009

This study attempts to accurately quantify pulmonary contusion and predict those patients most likely to require assisted ventilation early in their hospital course. Patients admitted to a Level I trauma center were evaluated for pulmonary contusion by helical CT scan. Scans were

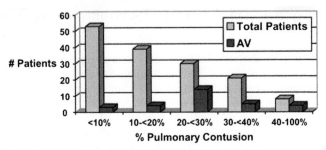

FIGURE 2.—AV refers to those patients who required assisted ventilation. This represents the percentage of each contusion group who required assisted ventilation. (Reprinted from Hamrick MC, Duhn RD, Ochsner MG. Critical evaluation of pulmonary contusion in the early post-traumatic period: risk of assisted ventilation. *Am Surg.* 2009;75:1054-1058.)

reviewed by a single radiologist who attempted to accurately quantify contusion as a percentage of total lung volume. These patients were then followed for 48 hours in an attempt to use CT measurements of contusion to predict those that would require assisted ventilation early in their hospital course. After using numerous exclusion criteria, 152 patients were included in the study. Of these, 31 patients (20%) required assisted ventilation within 48 hours of hospital admission. Twenty per cent pulmonary contusion proved to be a highly predictive variable leading to need for assisted ventilation. Of patients sustaining <20 per cent contusion, only 7 of 92 (8%) required assisted ventilation *versus* 24 of 60 (40%) sustaining >20 per cent contusion. Pulmonary contusion is a significant injury especially when contusion volume exceeds 20 per cent of total lung volume. With accurate measurement of contusion, we can identify those patients at high risk of requiring assisted ventilation early in their hospital course (Fig 2).

▶ This article complements a study performed a number of years ago by the Memphis Group at the Elvis Presley Trauma Center.[1] Again, early computed tomography (CT) scanning is a valuable modality to predict the need for mechanical ventilation and acute respiratory distress syndrome (ARDS) following pulmonary contusion. I was disappointed that these authors did not follow patients for more than 48 hours. CT imaging and clinical evolution of pulmonary contusion may occur for more than 48 hours and immediate scans may, therefore, underestimate the need for mechanical ventilation.[2]

On the positive side, these authors were very aggressive in obtaining scanning. Minimal plain radiographic or clinical criteria were necessary to motivate chest CT. Thus, I believe from this standpoint, the data are good. In addition, the authors were very careful to exclude patients who would require significant resuscitation. Therefore, transfusion-related acute lung injury (TRALI) and other comorbid conditions that could confound the diagnosis of pulmonary contusion are absent.[3]

The value of CT scanning in both diagnosis and prognostication for chest trauma is reinforced.

D. J. Dries, MSE, MD

References

1. Miller PR, Croce MA, Bee TK, et al. ARDS after pulmonary contusion: accurate measurement of contusion volume identifies high risk patients. *J Trauma*. 2001;51: 223-230.
2. Hoff SJ, Shotts SD, Eddy VA, Morris JA Jr. Outcome of isolated pulmonary contusion in blunt chest trauma. *Am Surg*. 1994;60:138-142.
3. Marik PE, Corwin HL. Acute lung injury following blood transfusion: expanding the definition. *Crit Care Med*. 2008;36:3080-3084.

Evaluation of Renal Function After Major Renal Injury: Correlation With the American Association for the Surgery of Trauma Injury Scale

Tasian GE, Aaronson DS, McAninch JW (Univ of California, San Francisco; San Francisco General Hosp, CA)
J Urol 183:196-200, 2010

Purpose.—In this study we evaluated the effect of major kidney injury on renal function.

Materials and Methods.—A retrospective cross-sectional analysis was conducted of all patients who sustained renal trauma between 1977 and 2008 at San Francisco General Hospital, and underwent post-injury dimercapto-succinic acid renal scan (67). Decrease in renal function was defined as the absolute percentage difference between the affected and unaffected kidney on dimercapto-succinic acid scan. Univariate (Spearman rank correlation) and multivariate (linear regression) analyses of the American Association for the Surgery of Trauma renal injury grade, patient age, mechanism of injury (blunt vs penetrating), side of injury, treatment used (nonoperative vs surgery), shock, gender, presence of gross hematuria, serum creatinine on hospital admission, postoperative complications and associated injuries were performed.

Results.—Of the 67 renal injuries 23 (34%) were managed nonoperatively. There were 43 (64%) injuries due to penetrating trauma and 24 (36%) due to blunt injury. Mean decrease in renal function for grade III, IV and V injuries was 15%, 30% and 65%, respectively. Univariate analysis demonstrated a significant association between decrease in renal function and injury grade (rho 0.43, p < 0.005). There was no difference in the decrease in kidney function between parenchymal and vascular causes for grade IV and V injuries. Although the right kidney demonstrated a greater decrease in function (rho 0.26, p = 0.033) on univariate analysis, multivariate analysis showed that only American Association for the Surgery of Trauma injury grade correlated with decreased function (correlation coefficient 14.3, 95% CI 4.7–24.8, p < 0.005).

Conclusions.—Decrease in kidney function is directly correlated with American Association for the Surgery of Trauma renal injury grade (Fig 1).

▶ This is a large data set obtained from the center with the largest recent academic contribution to the understanding of renal trauma. The link between

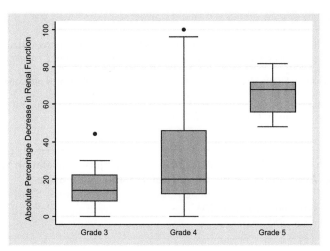

FIGURE 1.—Box plot of decrease in renal function as function of injury grade. Lower and upper limits of box represent 25th and 75th percentiles, respectively, and line through box represents median. (Reprinted from Tasian GE, Aaronson DS, McAninch JW. Evaluation of renal function after major renal injury: correlation with the American Association for the Surgery of Trauma injury scale. *J Urol*. 2010;183:196-200, with permission from the American Urological Association.)

anatomic and physiologic outcome is an interesting one. Usually, clinical decisions are based on physiologic rather than anatomic parameters. Given these authors and the quality of their work, I am inclined to believe these results.

The conclusions of this article hinge, however, on the relevance of dimercapto-succuinic acid (DMSA) scans obtained at a wide range of intervals after renal injury.[1,2] There is no dialysis or other long-term renal function data given. The key references arguing in favor of the DMSA scanning technique used are cited below. Clearly, additional validation data are required. The authors also note that comorbid conditions are not recorded here. In a typically young trauma patient, I do not see this as a limitation. For the most part, these patients should be without significant comorbidities.

D. J. Dries, MSE, MD

References

1. Moog R, Becmeur F, Dutson E, Chevalier-Kauffmann I, Sauvage P, Brunot B. Functional evaluation by quantitative dimercaptosuccinic acid scintigraphy after kidney trauma in children. *J Urol*. 2003;169:641-644.
2. Keller MS, Eric Coln C, Garza JJ, Sartorelli KH, Christine Green M, Weber TR. Functional outcome of nonoperatively managed renal injuries in children. *J Trauma*. 2004;57:108-110.

Functional and survival outcomes in traumatic blunt thoracic aortic injuries:
An analysis of the National Trauma Databank
Arthurs ZM, Starnes BW, Sohn VY, et al (Madigan Army Med Ctr, Tacoma, WA,
Univ of Washington)
J Vasc Surg 49:988-994, 2009

Objective.—Blunt thoracic aortic injury (BAI) remains a leading cause
of trauma deaths, and off-label use of endovascular devices has been
increasingly utilized in an effort to reduce the morbidity and mortality
in this population. Utilizing a nationwide database, we determined the
incidence of BAI, and analyzed both functional and survival outcomes at
discharge compared with matched controls.

Methods.—Patients with BAI were identified by International Classification of Disease-9 codes from the National Trauma Data Bank (Version
6.2), 2000-2005. Patients were analyzed based on aortic repair, associated
physiologic burden, and coexisting injuries. Control groups were matched
by age, mechanism, major thoracic Abbreviated Injury Scale score
(AIS $\geq$ 3), major head AIS, and major abdominal AIS. Outcomes were
assessed using the functional independence measure (FIM) score and overall mortality. FIM scores were scored from 1 (full assistance required) to 4
(fully independent) for three categories: feeding, locomotion, and
expression.

Results.—During the study period, 3,114 patients with BAI were identified among 1.1 million trauma admissions for an overall incidence of
0.3%. One hundred thirteen (4%) were dead on arrival, and 599 (19%)
died during triage. Of the patients surviving transport and triage
(n = 2402), 29% had a concomitant major abdominal injury and 31%
had a major head injury. Sixty-eight percent (1,642) underwent no repair,
28% (665) open aortic repair, and 4% (95) endovascular repair with associated mortality rates of 65%, 19%, and 18%, respectively ($P < .05$).
Aortic repair independently improved survival when controlling for associated injuries and physiologic burden (odds ratio (OR) = 0.36; 95%
confidence interval (CI), 0.24-0.54, $P < .05$). Compared with matched
controls, BAI resulted in a higher mortality (55% vs. 15%, $P < .05$), and
independently contributed to mortality (OR = 4.04; 95% CI, 3.53-4.63,
$P < .05$). In addition, BAI patients were less likely to be fully independent
for feeding (72% vs. 82%, $P < .05$), locomotion (33% vs. 55%, $P < .05$),
and expression (80% vs 88%, $P < .05$).

Conclusion.—This manuscript is the first to define the incidence of BAI
utilizing the NTDB. Remarkably, two-thirds of patients are unable to
undergo attempts at aortic repair, which portends a poor prognosis.
When controlling for associated injuries, blunt aortic injury independently
impacts survival and results in poor function in those surviving to
discharge.

▶ This is a remarkable study looking at the massive National Trauma Databank.
There are a number of technical concerns in this report, however. First, and most

important, most aortic repairs are currently done using endovascular technique.[1-3] Many of the functional results presented here may reflect a very small number of patients undergoing endograft placement. Second, within procedural groups, there is a difference in comorbidities.[4] Patients managed nonoperatively are more likely to have major head injury. Major head injury has been demonstrated to reflect poorer outcome. Third, among operative groups, the distribution of associated injuries was not consistent. Perhaps most important, the vast majority of blunt aortic injuries were not operated. Although some of these patients can be managed without an operation, most will require some procedure. It is unclear why so many patients were managed without endovascular or open vascular repairs.[5]

Patients with blunt aortic injury had significant morbidity and functional deficits. Why was this? Paraplegia rates between open and endovascular repair were both 2% or less. I must assume that morbidity associated with an operation and coexisting injuries are the best explanations for the diminished functional outcome in the setting of blunt aortic trauma. The authors note that patients with blunt aortic injury had poorer outcomes with respect to activities of daily living, including feeding, locomotion, and expression. It is unclear to me how these results can be explained simply on the basis of whether aortic injury is present or absent.

Thus, I am concerned that the pattern of care described in this article does not reflect contemporary practice. I do not have an anatomic or physiologic explanation for the observations made by these authors and conclude that morbidity associated with open repairs and associated injuries are the best explanations for outcomes reported.

D. J. Dries, MSE, MD

References

1. Nagy K, Fabian T, Rodman G, Fulda G, Rodriguez A, Mirvis S. Guidelines for the diagnosis and management of blunt aortic injury: an EAST Practice Management Guidelines Work Group. *J Trauma*. 2000;48:1128-1143.
2. Lebl DR, Dicker RA, Spain DA, Brundage SI. Dramatic shift in the primary management of traumatic thoracic aortic rupture. *Arch Surg*. 2006;141:177-180.
3. Demetriades D, Velmahos GC, Scalea TM, et al. Operative repair or endovascular stent graft in blunt traumatic thoracic aortic injuries: results of an American Association for the Surgery of Trauma Multicenter Study. *J Trauma*. 2008;64:561-571.
4. Demetriades D, Velmahos GC, Scalea TM, et al. Blunt traumatic thoracic aortic injuries: early or delayed repair—results of an American Association for the Surgery of Trauma prospective study. *J Trauma*. 2009;66:967-973.
5. Neschis DG, Scalea TM, Flinn WR, Griffith BP. Blunt aortic injury. *N Engl J Med*. 2008;359:1708-1716.

A national US study of posttraumatic stress disorder, depression, and work and functional outcomes after hospitalization for traumatic injury

Zatzick D, Jurkovich GJ, Rivara FP, et al (Univ of Washington School of Medicine, Seattle)

Ann Surg 248:429-437, 2008

Objective.—To examine factors other than injury severity that are likely to influence functional outcomes after hospitalization for injury.

Summary Background Data.—This study used data from the National Study on the Costs and Outcomes of Trauma investigation to examine the association between posttraumatic stress disorder (PTSD), depression, and return to work and the development of functional impairments after injury.

Method.—A total of 2707 surgical inpatients who were representative of 9374 injured patients were recruited from 69 hospitals across the US. PTSD and depression were assessed at 12 months postinjury, as were the following functional outcomes: activities of daily living, health status, and return to usual major activities and work. Regression analyses assessed the associations between PTSD and depression and functional outcomes while adjusting for clinical and demographic characteristics.

Results.—At 12 months after injury, 20.7% of patients had PTSD and 6.6% had depression. Both disorders were independently associated with significant impairments across all functional outcomes. A dose-response relationship was observed, such that previously working patients with 1 disorder had a 3-fold increased odds of not returning to work 12 months after injury odds ratio = 3.20 95% (95% confidence interval = 2.46, 4.16), and patients with both disorders had a 5-6 fold increased odds of not returning to work after injury odds ratio = 5.57 (95% confidence interval = 2.51, 12.37) when compared with previously working patients without PTSD or depression.

Conclusions.—PTSD and depression occur frequently and are independently associated with enduring impairments after injury hospitalization. Early acute care interventions targeting these disorders have the potential to improve functional recovery after injury.

▶ The authors paint a grim picture of the incidence of posttraumatic stress disorder (PTSD) and depression after injury in a large patient sample from multiple hospitals providing various levels of care across the United States.[1] Because of the characteristics of the study, a number of limitations should be noted. First, the diagnosis of depression is made simply on the basis of a telephone interview. Although a standard questionnaire is used, there is obvious room for inconsistency. Second, there is no accounting for premorbid state in this trauma population apart from survey data. Third, hospitals providing various levels of trauma care are reviewed.[2] It would be interesting to know whether hospitals with more mature or expansive trauma programs are similarly affected by depression and PTSD in involved patients.[3,4]

These authors highlight a major issue in trauma care that goes beyond mortality statistics. Because of the size of this database, it is difficult to appreciate hospital-specific opportunities for improvement. Clearly, better functional follow-up for patients sustaining injury must be considered even after the incisions have healed and fractures are stable.

The American College of Surgeons now requests alcohol screening at its trauma centers having level I designation. PTSD assessment is also recommended now. As we gather additional data on outcomes and innovation in management of these important but underappreciated problems, the bar for trauma care may be raised.

D. J. Dries, MSE, MD

References

1. Nirula R, Nirula G, Gentilello LM. Inequity of rehabilitation services after traumatic injury. *J Trauma*. 2009;66:255-259.
2. Cudnik MT, Newgard CD, Sayre MR, Steinberg SM. Level I versus Level II centers: an outcomes-based assessment. *J Trauma*. 2009;66:1321-1326.
3. Sorani MD, Lee M, Kim H, Meeker M, Manley GT. Race/ethnicity and outcome after traumatic brain injury at a single, diverse center. *J Trauma*. 2009;67:75-80.
4. Wutzler S, Maegele M, Marzi I, Spanholtz T, Wafaisade A, Lefering R, Trauma Registry of the German Society for Trauma Surgery. Association of preexisting medical conditions with in-hospital mortality in multiple-trauma patients. *J Am Coll Surg*. 2009;209:75-81.

A retrospective observational study examining the admission arterial to end-tidal carbon dioxide gradient in intubated major trauma patients
Hiller J, Silvers A, McIlroy DR, et al (Alfred Hosp, Melbourne, Victoria, Australia)
Anaesth Intensive Care 38:302-306, 2010

Major trauma patients who are intubated and ventilated are exposed to the potential risk of iatrogenic hypercapnic and hypocapnic physiological stress. In the pre-hospital setting, end-tidal capnography is used as a practical means of estimating arterial carbon dioxide concentrations and to guide the adequacy of ventilation. In our study, potentially deleterious hypercapnia (mean 47 mmHg, range 26 to 83 mmHg) due to hypoventilation was demonstrated in 49% of 100 intubated major trauma patients arriving at a major Australian trauma centre. A mean gradient of 15 mmHg arterial to end-tidal carbon dioxide concentration difference was found, highlighting the limitations of capnography in this setting. Moreover, 80% of the patients in the study had a head injury. Physiological deadspace due to hypovolaemia in these patients is commonly thought to contribute to the increased arterial to end-tidal carbon dioxide gradient in trauma patients. However in this study, scene and arrival patient hypoxia was more predictive of hypoventilation and an increased arterial to end-tidal carbon dioxide gradient than physiological markers of shock. Greater vigilance for hypercapnia in intubated trauma patients is required. Additionally, a larger study may confirm that lower end-tidal carbon dioxide levels could be safely targeted in the pre-hospital and emergency department ventilation strategies of the subgroup of major trauma patients with scene hypoxia.

▶ This single-center study at a large trauma hospital argues that there is a significant degree of hypoventilation in the setting of trauma and that end-tidal CO_2 measurements may not effectively describe the physiologic status of patients requiring respiratory support after injury.

The authors propose that physiologic dead space is associated with the wide discrepancy between arterial carbon dioxide partial pressure ($PaCO_2$) and end-tidal carbon dioxide partial pressure ($PetCO_2$), resulting in the increased $PaCO_2$-$PetCO_2$ gradient. A larger trial is proposed to confirm this suspicion. I suggest, rather, a smaller physiologic study with programmed resuscitation and carefully regulated blood loss. A large trial may fail to provide more than epidemiologic data. We will not obtain additional physiologic insight.

The authors also suggest that more aggressive ventilation may be appropriate in the setting of injury. I point out that multiple investigators warn of inappropriate hyperventilation with potential cerebral ischemia in the setting of injury.[1-3] Thus, the decision to use a more aggressive approach to ventilation should be made with caution.

Finally, the use of $PetCO_2$ monitoring is receiving increasing attention in the trauma community as part of an initial package for patient monitoring. These data confirm what intensivists already knew—$PetCO_2$ is less likely to be accurate in the unstable patient who has the greatest need for good monitoring data.

D. J. Dries, MSE, MD

References

1. Davis DP, Dunford JV, Poste JC, et al. The impact of hypoxia and hyperventilation on outcome after paramedic rapid sequence intubation of severely head injured patients. *J Trauma.* 2004;57:1-8.
2. Diringer MN, Videen TO, Yundt K, et al. Regional cerebrovascular and metabolic effects of hyperventilation after severe traumatic brain injury. *J Neurosurg.* 2002; 96:103-108.
3. Muizelaar JP, Marmarou A, Ward JD, et al. Adverse effects of prolonged hyperventilation in patients with severe head injury: a randomized clinical trial. *J Neurosurg.* 1991;75:731-739.

Autologous Blood Transfusion During Emergency Trauma Operations
Brown CVR, Foulkrod KH, Sadler HT, et al (Univ Med Ctr Brackenridge, Austin, TX; et al)
Arch Surg 145:690-694, 2010

Hypothesis.—Intraoperative cell salvage (CS) of shed blood during emergency surgical procedures provides an effective and cost-efficient resuscitation alternative to allogeneic blood transfusion, which is associated with increased morbidity and mortality in trauma patients.

Design.—Retrospective matched cohort study.

Setting.—Level I trauma center.

Patients.—All adult trauma patients who underwent an emergency operation and received CS as part of their intraoperative resuscitation. The CS group was matched to a no-CS group for age, sex, Injury Severity Score, mechanism of injury, and operation performed.

Main Outcome Measures.—Amount and cost of allogeneic transfusion of packed red blood cells and plasma.

Results.—The 47 patients in the CS group were similar to the 47 in the no-CS group for all matched variables. Patients in the CS group received an average of 819 mL of autologous CS blood. The CS group received fewer intraoperative (2 vs 4 U; $P = .002$) and total (4 vs 8 U; $P < .001$) units of allogeneic packed red blood cells. The CS group also received fewer total units of plasma (3 vs 5 U; $P = .03$). The cost of blood product transfusion (including the total cost of CS) was less in the CS group ($1616 vs $2584 per patient; $P = .004$).

Conclusion.—Intraoperative CS provides an effective and cost-efficient resuscitation strategy as an alternative to allogeneic blood transfusion in trauma patients undergoing emergency operative procedures.

▶ In data obtained from a trauma center in a city of moderate size, the authors suggest that cell salvage can be performed at acceptable risk and may be related to cost-benefit, particularly if patients were to require infusion of 2 units of autologous blood for operative therapy. Historical data suggest that complications arise with use of higher cell saver infusion volumes.[1] The cost difference between autologous and allogenic blood administration is small. No other epidemiologic data in the small patient population studied suggest a difference in outcome. We are given no data specifying the type and number of operations performed in patients of each group other than anatomic location.

The authors suggest that cell salvage included some contaminated red cells. The number of patients receiving contaminated red cells is unknown from these data. However, no difference in infectious complications is identified. Again, weak support of autologous blood transfusion is provided.

In summary, the financial argument provided here holds limited relevance in comparison with the overall cost of hospitalization of injured patients. It is not clear that the on-call expense for perfusionists is included in these calculations. We can be reassured that no new safety concerns relative to the use of autologous blood in emergency trauma operations have been identified. Given the risk of complications associated with allogenic transfusion, this technique warrants further study.[2]

D. J. Dries, MSE, MD

References

1. Horst HM, Dlugos S, Fath JJ, Sorensen VJ, Obeid FN, Bivins BA. Coagulopathy and intraoperative blood salvage (IBS). *J Trauma.* 1992;32:646-653.
2. Malone DL, Dunne J, Tracy JK, Putnam AT, Scalea TM, Napolitano LM. Blood transfusion, independent of shock severity, is associated with worse outcome in trauma. *J Trauma.* 2003;54:898-907.

Early Packed Red Blood Cell Transfusion and Acute Respiratory Distress Syndrome after Trauma

Chaiwat O, Lang JD, Vavilala MS, et al (Univ of Washington School of Medicine, Seattle; et al)
Anesthesiology 110:351-360, 2009

Background.—Transfusion of packed red blood cells (PRBCs) is a risk factor for acute respiratory distress syndrome (ARDS) in trauma patients. Yet, there is a paucity of information regarding the risk of ARDS with incremental PRBCs exposure.

Methods.—For this retrospective analysis, eligible patients from National Study on Costs and Outcomes of Trauma were included. Our main exposure was defined as units of PRBCs transfused during the first 24 h after admission. The main outcome was ARDS.

Results.—A total of 521 (4.6%) of 14070 patients developed ARDS, and 331 patients (63.5%) who developed ARDS received PRBCs transfusion. Injury severity, thoracic injury, polytrauma, and pneumonia receiving more than 5 units of fresh frozen plasma and 6–10 units of PRBCs were independent predictors of ARDS. Patients receiving more than 5 units of PRBCs had higher risk of developing ARDS (patients who received 6–10 units: adjusted odds ratio 2.5, 95% CI 1.12–5.3; patients who received more than 10 units: odds ratio 2.6, 95% CI 1.1–6.4). Each additional unit of PRBCs transfused conferred a 6% higher risk of ARDS (adjusted odds ratio 1.06; 95% CI 1.03–1.10).

Conclusions.—Early transfusion of PRBCs is an independent predictor of ARDS in adult trauma patients. Conservative transfusion strategies that decrease PRBC exposure by even 1 unit may be warranted to reduce the risk of ARDS in injured patients (Table 3).

▶ This is a careful analysis of a large database again demonstrating incremental increase in mortality associated with the administration of packed red blood cells after injury. Etiology of acute respiratory distress syndrome (ARDS) is unclear. Unfortunately, the timing of blood product administration is not provided. Thus, transfusion-related lung injury (TRALI) cannot be excluded or confirmed as the major cause of postinjury ARDS.[1] This is a severely injured patient group, and other cofactors have been demonstrated. It is encouraging to see that mortality in these patients is little more than 20% with ARDS. This is far less than what has been reported in the best of medical cohorts.[2]

In future studies, the combined effects of packed red blood cells, fresh frozen plasma, and platelets must be investigated. Unfortunately, despite having a robust data set, these investigators do not fully assess the possibility of synergistic effect based on blood product administration. If TRALI is the major cause of respiratory failure in these patients, careful data on fresh frozen plasma administration, platelet use, and timing of product provision are important. The authors also note that leukoreduction data are not available. I do not believe that this a technical concern, as leukoreduction probably will not have

TABLE 3.—Independent Predictors of ARDS

Risk Factor	Odds Ratio (95% CI)
Age, yr	1.02 (1.00–1.03)
NISS	1.02 (1.01–1.04)
Thoracic injury	1.57 (1.07–2.31)
Pneumonia	7.52 (4.48–12.60)
Polytrauma	2.77 (1.62–4.74)
PRBC transfusion units	
0	Ref
1–5	1.70 (0.72–4.03)
6–10	2.24 (1.06–4.73)
> 10	2.18 (0.93–5.11)
Fresh frozen plasma transfusion units	
0	Ref
1–5	1.66 (0.88–3.15)
> 5	2.55 (1.17–5.55)

ARDS = acute respiratory distress syndrome; NISS = New Injury Severity Scores; PRBC = packed red blood cell.

a significant effect on the incidence of TRALI. Table 3 reflects the incremental risk of ARDS associated with administration of fresh frozen plasma.

Finally, examining the product administration patterns reveals that these data do not reflect the blood product administration practice of many major trauma centers. At present, much greater amounts of fresh frozen plasma and platelets are given than is reflected in the data set here. Thus, if antibodies carried in plasma-based products are a major cause of TRALI and postinjury ARDS, this risk will be underestimated by this data set.

D. J. Dries, MSE, MD

References

1. Marik PE, Corwin HL. Acute lung injury following blood transfusion: expanding the definition. *Crit Care Med.* 2008;36:3080-3084.
2. Ventilation with lower tidal volumes as compared with traditional tidal volumes for acute lung injury and the acute respiratory distress syndrome. The Acute Respiratory Distress Syndrome Network. *N Engl J Med.* 2000;342:1301-1308.

Predefined Massive Transfusion Protocols are Associated With a Reduction in Organ Failure and Postinjury Complications

Cotton BA, Au BK, Nunez TC, et al (Vanderbilt Univ Med Ctr, Nashville, TN)
J Trauma 66:41-49, 2009

Introduction.—Massive transfusion (MT) protocols have been shown to improve survival in severely injured patients. However, others have noted that these higher fresh frozen plasma (FFP): red blood cell (RBC) ratios are associated with increased risk of organ failure. The purpose of this study was to determine whether MT protocols are associated with increased organ failure and complications.

Methods.—Our institution's exsanguination protocol (TEP) involves the immediate delivery of products in a 3:2 ratio of RBC:FFP and 5:1 for RBC:platelets. All patients receiving TEP between February 2006 and January 2008 were compared with a cohort (pre-TEP) of all patients from February 2004 to January 2006 that (1) went immediately to the operating room and (2) received MT (≥ 10 units of RBC in first 24 hours).

Results.—Two hundred sixty-four patients met inclusion (125 in the TEP group, 141 in the pre-TEP). Demographics and Injury Severity Score were similar. TEP received more intraoperative FFP and platelets but less in first 24 hours ($p < 0.01$). There was no difference in renal failure or systemic inflammatory response syndrome, but pneumonia, pulmonary failure, open abdomens, and abdominal compartment syndrome were lower in TEP. In addition, severe sepsis or septic shock and multiorgan failure were both lower in the TEP patients (9% vs. 20%, $p = 0.011$ and 16% vs. 37%, $p < 0.001$, respectively).

Conclusions.—Although MT has been associated with higher organ failure and complication rates, this risk appears to be reduced when blood products are delivered early in the resuscitation through a predefined protocol. Our institution's TEP was associated with a reduction in multiorgan failure and infectious complications, as well as an increase in ventilator-free days. In addition, implementation of this protocol was followed by a dramatic reduction in development of abdominal compartment syndrome and the incidence of open abdomens.

▶ Although massive transfusion protocols have been shown to improve outcomes in certain populations of patients with life-threatening hemorrhage, concerns remain about potential secondary complications associated with the use of large volumes of blood products because of their potential immunosuppressive and proinflammatory effects. Transfusion of packed red cells and other blood products has been associated with an increased risk of infection, organ failure, and other systemic complications. These authors investigated whether a massive transfusion protocol (which they designate an exsanguination protocol at their institution) would be associated with an increased incidence of such complications. This protocol differed from the commonly used 1:1:1 packed red blood cell (PRBC):fresh frozen plasma (FFP):platelet protocol used by the military and several other institutions; rather, their transfusion ratios used were 3:2 RBC:FFP and 5:1 RBC:platelets. One hundred twenty-five patients requiring at least 10 units of PRBC in the first 24 hours of admission after institution of the protocol were compared with 141 historical controls. The protocol group was more acutely ill, with higher injury scores than the control group but had lower 30-day mortality and lower overall use of blood products, despite the use of the aggressive transfusion protocol. The patients treated according to the protocol had significantly lower incidences of numerous organ failures including cardiac and hepatic failure, lower incidences of ventilator-associated pneumonia, and significantly less abdominal compartment syndrome/open abdomens. As the authors point out in the discussion, while these findings may seem paradoxical at first glance, they make sense upon deeper inspection. Although the patients treated on protocol received significant doses of blood and blood products, placing them at increased risk of the complications associated with transfusion, they still received less than the control group, so by comparison had proportionally better outcomes. They also received significantly less crystalloid than the control group, probably because of the large volume of colloid (FFP) they received as part of the resuscitation protocol, which was likely a significant factor in allowing for better early abdominal closure in that group. These findings lend further support to the general concept of the use of massive transfusion protocols. Not only do they appear to help with overall outcome and blood product utilization, but there is now evidence that they may also attenuate the incidence of organ dysfunction and other adverse outcomes, at least in patients with trauma. However, as the ratios of PRBC to FFP and platelets used in this protocol were so different from the more commonly used ratio of 1:1:1, it is clear that the optimal ratio of blood and other product replacement remains to be determined.

D. R. Gerber, DO

Changing paradigms in surgical resuscitation
Fouche Y, Sikorski R, Dutton RP (Univ of Maryland School of Medicine, Baltimore; Univ of Maryland Med System, Baltimore)
Crit Care Med 38:S411-S420, 2010

Patients undergoing emergency surgery typically require resuscitation, either because they are hemorrhaging or because they are experiencing significant internal fluid shifts. Intravascular hypovolemia is common at the time of anesthesia induction and can lead to hemodynamic collapse if not promptly treated. Central pressure monitoring is associated with technical complications and does not improve outcomes in this population. Newer modalities are in use, but they lack validation. Fluid resuscitation is different in bleeding and septic patients. In the former group, it is advisable to maintain a deliberately low blood pressure to facilitate clot formation and stabilization. If massive transfusion is anticipated, blood products should be administered from the outset to prevent the coagulopathy of trauma. Early use of plasma in a ratio approaching 1:1 with red blood cells (RBCs) has been associated with improved outcomes. In septic patients, early fluid loading is recommended. The concept of "goal-directed resuscitation" is based on continuing resuscitation until venous oxygen saturation is normalized. In either bleeding or septic patients, however, the most important goal remains surgical control of the source of pathology, and nothing should be allowed to delay transfer to the operating room. We review the current literature and recommendations for the resuscitation of patients coming for emergency surgery procedures.

▶ The authors provide an elegant review of many of the recent considerations in trauma and perioperative surgical resuscitation. This review comes from the R Adams Cowley Shock Trauma Center at the University of Maryland.

A variety of general observations can be summarized. First, central venous and pulmonary artery catheters probably have a limited role apart from drug infusion. Mixed venous or central venous oxygen saturation, while useful, has the limits of being a global parameter, which may not reflect the impact of resuscitation on individual tissues. Second, the authors appropriately emphasize the value of increasing ratios of fresh frozen plasma and platelets to packed red blood cells administered for hemorrhagic shock. They decline to mention the important work of Cotton and coworkers, which allows identification of appropriate patients for this type of resuscitation based on simple presentation characteristics. Administration of blood products in a 1:1:1 correspondence is probably appropriate for fewer than 10% and possibly under 5% of patients in civilian trauma practice.[1] A third strength of this article is identification of the importance of fluid selection relative to pathology. The recent work in blood product administration and hypotensive resuscitation where uncontrolled bleeding is possible are 2 examples of adapting the approach to resuscitation to the problem faced by the patient.[2] There is also discussion regarding vasoactive drugs. Again, vasoactive drug choices should reflect the patient pathology. Many basic scientists would agree that vasopressin could be replaced in physiologic amounts for hypovolemic or septic shock. The data on catecholamines and other vasoactive agents are not discussed in this article.[3]

Finally, what are clinical end points for resuscitation? End-organ function and tissue oxygen sensors are relatively insensitive and dependent on the type of shock encountered by the patient. Markers such as lactate are most effective when trends are available.

The reader on surgical resuscitation must also consider thromboelastography as a means to determine the propriety and type of blood product resuscitation, particularly in the setting of massive hemorrhage.[1]

D. J. Dries, MSE, MD

References

1. Cotton BA, Guy JS, Morris JA Jr, Abumrad NN. The cellular, metabolic, and systemic consequences of aggressive fluid resuscitation strategies. *Shock.* 2006; 26:115-121.
2. Dries DJ. Hypotensive resuscitation. *Shock.* 1996;6:311-316.
3. Dellinger RP, Levy MM, Carlet JM, et al. Survival Sepsis Campaign: international guidelines for management of severe sepsis and septic shock: 2008. *Crit Care Med.* 2008;36:296-327.

Complication Rates among Trauma Centers

Ang DN, Rivara FP, Nathens A, et al (Univ of Washington, Seattle; St Michael's Hosp, Toronto, Ontario, Canada; et al)
J Am Coll Surg 209:595-602, 2009

Background.—The goal of this study was to examine the association between patient complications and admission to Level I trauma centers (TC) compared with nontrauma centers (NTC).

Study Design.—This was a retrospective cohort study of data derived from the National Study on the Costs and Outcomes of Trauma (NSCOT). Patients were recruited from 18 Level I TCs and 51 NTCs in 15 regions encompassing 14 states. Trained study nurses, using standardized forms, abstracted the medical records of the patients. The overall number of complications per patient was identified, as was the presence or absence of 13 specific complications.

Results.—Patients treated in TCs were more likely to have any complication compared with patients in NTCs, with an adjusted relative risk (RR) of 1.34 (95% CI, 1.03, 1.74). For individual complications, only the urinary tract infection RR of 1.94 (95% CI, 1.07, 3.17) was significantly higher in TCs. TC patients were more likely to have 3 or more complications (RR, 1.83; 95% CI, 1.16, 2.90). Treatment variables that are surrogates for markers of injury severity, such as use of pulmonary artery catheters, multiple operations, massive transfusions (> 2,500 mL packed red blood cells), and invasive brain catheters, occurred significantly more often in TCs.

Conclusions.—Trauma centers have a slightly higher incidence rate of complications, even after adjusting for patient case mix. Aggressive treatment may account for a significant portion of TC-associated complications. Pulmonary artery catheter use and intubation had the most influence on overall TC complication rates. Additional study is needed to provide accurate benchmark measures of complication rates and to determine their causes.

▶ This study uses the large database from the National Study on Cost and Outcomes of Trauma (NSCOT) that was designed to determine the effectiveness of trauma centers in urban and suburban settings.[1] Patient recruitment occurred from July 2001 to November 2002. I note that we have already seen significant practice changes in the decade since the original data accrual occurred. Enrollment required the presence of at least 1 injury, with an Abbreviated Injury Scale (AIS) score of 3 or greater. This is a very broad enrollment criterion to gather patients for review.

However, there are a number of interesting observations consistent with recent work published by the ARDSNet Investigators. This review identified a significant risk of complications, including arrhythmias, pulmonary embolism, and cardiac arrest, in association with placement of pulmonary artery catheters.[2-4] Trauma centers were more likely to use low-molecular-weight heparin as part of deep venous thrombosis prophylaxis along with sequential compression devices. Trauma centers also screened for adverse events more commonly than nontrauma centers.[5] Surrogates of severity of injury, including pulmonary artery catheters, intracranial pressure monitors, massive transfusion, and operations per patient, were more common in trauma centers compared with nontrauma centers.

The authors argue that complications arise from differences in medical practice rather than the disease and suggest practice differences between the trauma and nontrauma centers. I suggest that despite the statistical methods, there were significant differences in disease as well. As noted in the Discussion section, the timing of complications related to the course of hospitalization and other coincident events cannot be determined from this database. If one concern is the increasing use of procedures at trauma centers, it is interesting to note that multiple operations, particularly reoperations for the abdomen, were not associated with increased risk of mortality in trauma centers but only in nontrauma centers.

In summary, I believe that it is important to examine the pattern of complications, particularly as they relate to procedures in trauma centers. Trauma centers need to consider risks involved in an aggressive procedural approach to injury. This comparison does not convince me that the study of care in trauma centers as opposed to nontrauma centers will improve our understanding.

D. J. Dries, MSE, MD

References

1. MacKenzie EJ, Rivara FP, Jurkovich GJ, et al. A national evaluation of the effect of trauma center care on mortality. *N Engl J Med*. 2006;354:366-378.
2. Friese RS, Shafi S, Gentilello LM. Pulmonary artery catheter use is associated with reduced mortality in severely injured patients: a National Trauma Data Bank analysis of 53,312 patients. *Crit Care Med*. 2006;34:1597-1601.
3. Connors AF Jr, Speroff T, Dawson NV, et al. The effectiveness of right heart catheterization in the initial care of critically ill patients. SUPPORT Investigators. *JAMA*. 1996;276:889-897.
4. National Heart, Lung, and Blood Institute Acute Respiratory Distress Syndrome (ARDS) Clinical Trials Network, Wheeler AP, Bernard GR, Thompson BT, et al. Pulmonary-artery versus central venous catheter to guide treatment of acute lung injury. *N Engl J Med*. 2006;354:2213-2224.
5. Pierce CA, Haut ER, Kardooni S, et al. Surveillance bias and deep vein thrombosis in the national trauma data bank: the more we look, the more we find. *J Trauma*. 2008;64:932-937.

Early predictors of morbidity and mortality in trauma patients treated in the intensive care unit

Brattström O, Granath F, Rossi P, et al (Karolinska Institutet, Stockholm, Sweden; Karolinska Univ Hosp, Stockholm, Sweden)
Acta Anaesthesiol Scand 54:1007-1017, 2010

Background.—We investigated the incidence and severity of post-injury morbidity and mortality in intensive care unit (ICU)-treated trauma patients. We also identified risk factors in the early phase after injury that predicted the later development of complications.

Methods.—A prospective observational cohort study design was used. One hundred and sixty-four adult patients admitted to the ICU for more than 24 h were included during a 21-month period. The incidence and severity of morbidity such as multiple organ failure (MOF), acute lung injury (ALI), severe sepsis and 30-day post-injury mortality were calculated and risk factors were analyzed with uni- and multivariable logistic regression analysis.

Results.—The median age was 40 years, the injury severity score was 24, the new injury severity score was 29, the acute physiology and chronic health evaluation II score was 15, sequential organ failure assessment maximum was 7 and ICU length of stay was 3.1 days. The incidences of post-injury MOF were 40.2%, ALI 25.6%, severe sepsis 31.1% and 30-day mortality 10.4%. The independent risk factors differed to some extent between the outcome parameters. Age, severity of injury, significant head injury and massive transfusion were independent risk factors for several outcome parameters. Positive blood alcohol was only a predictor of MOF, whereas prolonged rescue time only predicted death. Unexpectedly, injury severity was not an independent risk factor for mortality.

Conclusions.—Although the incidence of morbidity was considerable, mortality was relatively low. Early post-injury risk factors that predicted later development of complications differed between morbidity and mortality.

▶ Mortality after traumatic injury has traditionally been described as having a trimodal distribution. The first peak in mortality occurs from fatal injuries to the brain, spine, heart, or aorta or the development of acute respiratory distress. Progressive central nervous system injury or hemorrhage accounts for another peak in mortality in the first few hours after injury. While mortalities in the first peak are thought to be largely due to nonsurvivable injuries, improvements in prehospital care and the initial resuscitation have led to a reduction in mortality from traumatic injury.[1] Still, an additional 10% to 20% of trauma-related deaths occur during the third peak, 24 hours or more after injury.[2] Patients surviving the initial resuscitation in the trauma bay face a new set of challenges during care in the intensive care unit (ICU).

Not surprisingly, patients with trauma in the ICU share similar morbidities as medical patients in the ICU. As demonstrated by the authors, these patients develop multiple organ failure (MOF), acute lung injury (ALI), and sepsis resulting in significant morbidity. MOF, ALI, and sepsis were all shown to increase length of ICU stay while MOF and sepsis were shown to increase mortality. While the authors were unable to define independent risk factors aside from injury severity common to the development of all of these morbidities, age, fluid load, and blood transfusion were shown to be risk factors for multiple morbidities. This emphasizes that overaggressive initial resuscitation with large volumes of fluid or blood transfusion can have devastating consequences later in the ICU. As highlighted by the authors, further research needs to be done to improve the care of patients with trauma in the ICU to decrease the morbidity and mortality in this patient population.

S. L. Zanotti-Cavazzoni, MD

References

1. Probst C, Pape HC, Hiledebrand F, et al. 30 years of polytrauma care: an analysis of the change in strategies and results of 4849 cases treated at a single institution. *Injury.* 2009;40:77-83.
2. Acosta JA, Yang JC, Winchell RJ, et al. Lethal injuries and time to death in a level I trauma center. *J Am Coll Surg.* 1998;186:528-533.

Early *Versus* Late Stabilization of the Spine in the Polytrauma Patient
Dimar JR, Carreon LY, Riina J, et al (Norton Leatherman Spine Ctr, Louisville, KY; Ortholndy, Indianapolis, IN; et al)
Spine 35:S187-S192, 2010

Study Design.—Systematic review.

Objective.—To determine whether early spinal stabilization in the multiple trauma patient is safe and does not increase morbidity or mortality.

Summary of Background Data.—There is no consensus regarding the timing of surgical stabilization of the injured spine, especially in patients with multiple trauma. Designing and performing randomized clinical trials to evaluate early versus late surgery is difficult.

Methods.—Between January 1990 and July 2009, a computer-aided search using the keywords Spine or Spinal, Trauma, Spinal Cord Injury, and Surgery was done that included MEDLINE, EMBASE, HealthSTAR, Cumulative Index to Nursing and Allied Health Literature, Cochrane Database of Systematic Reviews, ACP Journal Club, Database of Abstracts of Reviews of Effects, Cochrane Central Register of Controlled Trials, PsycINFO, and PsychLit. Articles dealing only with neurologic improvement that did not mention other non-neurologic factors that were affected by early surgery were excluded. The authors selected and assessed the studies to be included in the analysis. An unblinded assessment of the quality of the study was done using the Grading of Recommendation, Assessment, Development and Evaluation approach to rank each article for its relevance to the topic.

Results.—Eleven articles directly comparing 2 cohorts that had early or late surgery were identified. All of the studies evaluated consistently demonstrated shorter hospital and intensive care unit length of stays, fewer days on mechanical ventilation, and lower pulmonary complications in patients who are treated with early spine decompression and stabilization. These advantages are more marked in patients with polytrauma. Data regarding morbidity and mortality rates are more variable.

Conclusion.—There is strong evidence within the literature that early surgical stabilization consistently leads to shorter hospital stays, shorter intensive care unit stays, less days on mechanical ventilation, and lower pulmonary complications. This effect is more evident in patients who have more severe injuries as measured by Injury Severity Score. This benefit is seen in both, spinal cord injured and noncord-injured patients. There is also some evidence that early stabilization does not increase the complication rates compared to late surgery.

▶ This study effectively summarizes the large amount of poorly controlled literature addressing an important question. Not surprisingly, data available support findings in other orthopedic literature, which favor early fracture stabilization in stable patients.[1] Because our knowledge of spinal cord protection is still in its infancy, the lack of obvious neurologic benefit with early spine stabilization should not be surprising.

An assumption in this work is that stable patients are taken to the operating room. However, there is little discussion regarding how a stable patient is defined. A recent German trial examining extremity fracture stabilization helps to identify patients where aggressive as opposed to limited operative therapy is appropriate.[2] Finally, the likelihood of benefit is greatest in patients with higher Injury Severity Scores. In some studies, patients with a lower injury burden tolerate delay in operation. Early spine stabilization can be justified from the perspective of resource use, even if consistent clinical benefit cannot be demonstrated.

D. J. Dries, MSE, MD

References

1. Scalea TM. Optimal timing of fracture fixation: have we learned anything in the past 20 years? *J Trauma.* 2008;65:253-260.
2. Harwood PJ, Giannoudis PV, van Griensven M, Krettek C, Pape HC. Alterations in the systemic inflammatory response after early total care and damage control procedures for femoral shaft fracture in severely injured patients. *J Trauma.* 2005;58:446-454.

Epidemiology of Traumatic Deaths: Comprehensive Population-Based Assessment

Evans JA, van Wessem KJP, McDougall D, et al (Univ of Newcastle, New South Wales, Australia)
World J Surg 34:158-163, 2010

Background.—The epidemiology of traumatic deaths was periodically described during the development of the American trauma system between 1977 and 1995. Recognizing the impact of aging populations and the potential changes in injury mechanisms, the purpose of this work was to provide a comprehensive, prospective, population-based study of Australian trauma-related deaths and compare the results with those of landmark studies.

Methods.—All prehospitalization and in-hospital trauma deaths occurring in an inclusive trauma system at a single Level 1 trauma center [400 patients with an injury severity score (ISS) >15/year] underwent autopsy and were prospectively evaluated during 2005. High-energy (HE) and low-energy (LE) deaths were categorized based on the mechanism of the injury, time frame (prehospitalization, <48 hours, 2–7 days, >7 days), and cause [which was determined by an expert panel and included central nervous system-related (CNS), exsanguination, CNS + exsanguination, airway, multiple organ failure (MOF)]. Data are presented as a percent or the mean ± SEM.

Results.—There were 175 deaths during the 12-month period. For the 103 HE fatalities (age 43 ± 2 years, ISS 49 ± 2, male 63%), the predominant mechanisms were motor vehicle related (72%), falls (4%), gunshots (8%), stabs (6%), and burns (5%). In all, 66% of the patients died during the prehospital phase, 27% died after <48 hours in hospital, 5% died after 3 to 7 days in hospital, and 2% died after >7 days. CNS (33%) and exsanguination (33%) were the most common causes of deaths, followed by CNS + exsanguination (17%) and airway compromise 8%; MOF occurred in only 3%. Six percent of the deaths were undetermined. All LE deaths ($n = 72$, age 83 ± 1 years, ISS 14 ± 1, male 45%) were due to low falls. All LE patients died in hospital (20% <48 hours, 32% after 3–7 days, 48% after 7 days). The causes of deaths were head injury (26%) and complications of skeletal injuries (74%).

Conclusions.—The HE injury mechanisms, time frames, and causes in our study are different from those in the earlier, seminal reports. The classic trimodal death distribution is much more skewed to early death. Exsanguination became as frequent as lethal head injuries, but the incidence of fatal MOF is lower than reported earlier. LE trauma is responsible for 41% of the postinjury mortality, with distinct epidemiology. The LE group deserves more attention and further investigation.

▶ Work from the 1970s and 1980s suggests a trimodal distribution of death following injury.[1] A large group died prior to hospital admission. There was a second group dying within hours and a third group dying within days to weeks due to multiple organ failure. Data presented here confirm the recent work of Sauaia et al in the 1990s, suggesting that the incidence of multiple organ failure in the setting of trauma is dramatically reduced from previous reports.[2] A number of important patterns persist. Bleeding and head injury are important contributors to early death. The relative contribution of head injury has decreased secondary to improved prehospital and hospital management. Bleeding, however, continues to be an important risk factor.[3]

The authors make an important comparison of low-energy and high-energy impact. Low-energy impact involves elderly patients and does not have prehospital mortality. Low-energy impact patients, however, have a significant pattern of death due to organ dysfunction and withdrawal of care after arrival at hospital. In this study, all patients sustaining low-energy trauma had a fall of less than 1 m. Twenty percent of low-energy trauma patients died within 48 hours of admission to hospital, while 31% of these individuals died between 2 and 7 days after hospitalization. Forty-nine percent of deaths occurred after 7 days of hospitalization. In a word, the low-energy and high-energy groups had a reversed pattern of mortality. Remarkably, the low-energy trauma, typically in the elderly, is responsible for a significant portion of overall postinjury mortality. We have historically focused on the young male trauma patient. These data argue that we must better understand injury in the elderly.

D. J. Dries, MSE, MD

References

1. Baker CC, Oppenheimer L, Stephens B, Lewis FR, Trunkey DD. Epidemiology of trauma deaths. *Am J Surg.* 1980;140:144-150.
2. Sauaia A, Moore FA, Moore EE, et al. Epidemiology of trauma deaths: a reassessment. *J Trauma.* 1995;38:185-193.

3. Kauvar DS, Lefering R, Wade CE. Impact of hemorrhage on trauma outcome: an overview of epidemiology, clinical presentations, and therapeutic considerations. *J Trauma*. 2006;60:S3-S11.

Evidence of Hormonal Basis for Improved Survival Among Females With Trauma-Associated Shock: An Analysis of the National Trauma Data Bank

Haider AH, Crompton JG, Chang DC, et al (Johns Hopkins Univ School of Medicine, Baltimore, MD; et al)
J Trauma 69:537-540, 2010

Background.—Basic science research suggests that sex hormones affect survival after traumatic shock. This study sought to determine the independent effect of gender on mortality among trauma patients in different hormone-related age groups.

Methods.—Review of severely injured trauma patients with shock included in the National Trauma Databank. Patients were stratified into three groups on the basis of likely hormonal status: prehormonal (age, 0–12 years), hormonal (age,13–64 years), and posthormonal (age, ≥65 years). Multiple logistic regression was used to analyze the independent effect of gender on mortality in each group, adjusting for anatomic and physiologic injury severity.

Results.—A total of 48,394 patients met our inclusion criteria (Injury Severity Score ≥16 and systolic blood pressure <90 mm Hg). Crude mortality was higher ($p < 0.05$) for males in all categories: prehormonal = 29% for males (n = 3,553) versus 24% for females (n = 1,831); hormonal = 34% for males (n = 26,778) versus 30% for females (n = 8,677) and posthormonal = 36% for males (n = 4,280) versus 31% for females (n = 3,275). After adjusting for covariates, women in the hormonally active group had a 14% decreased odds of death (0.86 [95% CI, 0.76–0.93) compared with men. Females did not exhibit this survival advantage in the prehormonal (odds of death = 0.92 [0.74–1.14) or posthormonal (odds of death = 0.90 [0.76–1.05) groups.

Conclusions.—Females aged between 13 and 64 years exhibit significantly lower mortality than males after trauma-associated shock. This outcome difference is lost at the extremes of age (preadolescent children and individuals aged ≥65 years) where the effects of sex hormones are absent or diminished. These findings suggest that hormonal differences play a role in the gender-based outcome disparities after traumatic shock.

▶ These authors query the massive National Trauma Data Bank. While this resource has the limitations of any administrative dataset, a number of messages seem clear.

First, the hormonal basis for improved survival is strongest among patients at greatest need for resuscitation. This is probably less than 5% to 10% of patients in civilian trauma practice. However, it is these patients who bear the greatest burden of mortality directly related to injury. Hemorrhage and shock are the common pathways to early mortality.[1]

An extensive animal literature suggests that primary sex hormones such as testosterone and estrogen play a significant role in host response after injury through regulation of cardiovascular, metabolic, and immune function.[2] Two effects may be important: the presence of female hormones and the absence of male hormones.

The impact of hormone manipulation on outcome is now being evaluated in the setting of traumatic brain injury in the Prophylaxis of Thromboembolism in Critical Care trial.[3] This multicenter National Institutes of Health work will set the stage for a next round of trials investigating hormonal manipulation in the setting of injury.

D. J. Dries, MSE, MD

References

1. Kauvar DS, Lefering R, Wade CE. Impact of hemorrhage on trauma outcome: an overview of epidemiology, clinical presentations, and therapeutic considerations. *J Trauma*. 2006;60:S3-S11.
2. Choudhry MA, Bland KI, Chaudry IH. Trauma and immune response—effect of gender differences. *Injury*. 2007;38:1382-1391.
3. Xiao G, Wei J, Yan W, Wang W, Lu Z. Improved outcomes from the administration of progesterone for patients with acute severe traumatic brain injury: a randomized controlled trial. *Crit Care*. 2008;12:R61.

Genetic Variation in Complement Component 2 of the Classical Complement Pathway is Associated With Increased Mortality and Infection: A Study of 627 Patients With Trauma

Morris JA Jr, Francois C, Olson PK, et al (Vanderbilt Univ Med Ctr, Nashville, TN; Potentia Pharmaceuticals, Louisville, KY; et al)

J Trauma 66:1265-1272, 2009

Background.—Trauma is a disease of inflammation. Complement Component 2 (C2) is a protease involved in activation of complement through the classical pathway and has been implicated in a variety of chronic inflammatory diseases. We hypothesized that genetic variation in C2 (E318D) identifies a high-risk subgroup of patients with trauma reflecting increased mortality and infection (ventilator-associated pneumonia [VAP]). Consequently, genetic variation in C2 may stratify patient risk and illuminate underlying mechanisms for therapeutic intervention.

Methods.—DNA samples from 702 patients with trauma were genotyped for C2 E318D and linked with covariates (age: mean 42.8 years, gender: 74% male, ethnicity: 80% white, mechanism: 84% blunt, injury severity score: mean 25.0, admission lactate: mean 3.13 mEq/L) and outcomes: mortality 9.9% and VAP: 18.5%). VAP was defined by quantitative bronchoalveolar lavage ($>10^4$). Multivariate regression analysis determined the relationship of genotype and covariates to risk of death

TABLE 2.—Univariate Analysis of C2 E318D Genotype With In-Hospital Mortality

	AA	GA	GG	Total
Survivors	0	48	568	616
Nonsurvivors	1	12 (20.0%)	73 (11.4%)	86(12.2%)
Total	1	60 (8.5%)	641 (91.3%)	702(100%)

Individuals with the GA genotype seemed to have a higher mortality rate than the GG genotype category. The p value for this using Pearson's χ^2 test was 0.05. The AA genotype was excluded from the analysis because only a single individual had this genotype.

TABLE 3.—Univariate Analysis of C2 E318D Genotype With VAP

	AA	GA	GG	Total
No VAP	1	40	507	548
VAP	0	20 (33.3%)	134 (20.9%)	154 (21.9%)
Total	0	60	641	702

Individuals with the GA genotype appeared to have a higher VAP rate than the GG genotype category. The p value for this using Pearson's χ^2 test was 0.06. The AA genotype was excluded from the analysis because only a single individual had this genotype.

and VAP. However, patients with injury severity score ≥ 45 were excluded from the multivariate analysis, as magnitude of injury overwhelms genetics and covariates in determining outcome.

Results.—Fifty-two patients (8.3%) had the high-risk heterozygous genotype, associated with a significant increase in mortality and VAP.

Conclusion.—In 702 patients with trauma, 8.3% had a high-risk genetic variation in C2 associated with increased mortality (odds ratio = 2.65) and infection (odds ratio = 2.00). This variation: (1) identifies a previously unknown high-risk group for infection and mortality; (2) can be determined at admission; (3) may provide opportunity for early therapeutic intervention; and (4) requires validation in a distinct cohort of patients (Tables 2 and 3).

▶ As our ability to identify various genetic polymorphisms increases, we are now entering an era of medicine where we can anticipate a different clinical response or enhanced susceptibility to a selected outcome based on the genetic profile of the individual. Some of these genetic predispositions will only be evident when in the setting of a specific type of stress response. This genetic association study attempted to determine if the C2 E318D genotype was associated with significant clinical impact on posttrauma patients. The finding of increased mortality and likelihood of developing ventilator-associated pneumonia in patients with this genetic polymorphism is interesting, but at this time we do not have specific interventions to use in patients known to have this genetic pattern that will prevent the development of pneumonia, other infections, or even ensure that their mortality rate is the same as the patient who does not have this genetic polymorphism. In the future, we may be able to provide personalized medical care that takes into account an individual patient's genetic polymorphisms and predispositions to various specific outcomes of interest. For now, it is business as usual, and this remains an interesting observation.

R. A. Balk, MD

Hematocrit, Systolic Blood Pressure and Heart Rate Are Not Accurate Predictors for Surgery to Control Hemorrhage in Injured Patients
Opreanu RC, Arrangoiz R, Stevens P, et al (Michigan State Univ, Lansing; Sparrow Health System, Lansing, MI)
Am Surg 76:296-301, 2010

Hematocrit (Hct), systolic blood pressure (SBP), and heart rate (HR) are considered to closely correlate with hypovolemia in injured patients. The clinical importance of these parameters in the early recognition of occult but clinically significant hemorrhage remains to be demonstrated. We undertook this study to assess the clinical importance of these parameters in the early recognition of occult hemorrhage in injured patients. A retrospective study of 7880 patients admitted to a Level I trauma center was carried out. Patients who underwent surgery were divided into the hemorrhage (n = 160) and no-hemorrhage group (n = 228). Hematocrit, SBP, and HR were correlated and receiver operating characteristic (ROC) curves were plotted. The ROC curves for Hct, SBP, and HR showed suboptimal areas under the graph. Even for different Hct thresholds and for hypotension and tachycardia, low predictive values were found. Although Hct, SBP, and HR levels were significantly altered among patients who require surgery for hemorrhage, the low predictive values of each parameter renders them as clinically unreliable individual tools for recognition of hemorrhagic patients who need surgery. Although useful in aggregate, as a pattern, or as indications for further diagnostic studies, these common parameters have limited usefulness individually.

▶ The classic stages of shock as reported by the American College of Surgeons and the Advanced Trauma Life Support algorithm for the management of injury include progressive changes in blood pressure and heart rate as part of the physiologic response to progressive bleeding.[1] These authors examine systolic blood pressure, hematocrit, and heart rate with operations performed to control hemorrhage as the gold standard. It is worthwhile to note that a growing percentage of hemorrhage is managed without operative procedures in the setting of injury. Nonetheless, these authors reinforce observations made by the University of California, Davis group that simple changes in vital signs do not necessarily reflect the degree of hemorrhage.[2]

While the authors do not address this point, this work indicates the need for careful use of technologies to provide timely identification of bleeding.

Bleeding, particularly in the early minutes to hours after trauma, is the critical link between survival and death.[3]

D. J. Dries, MSE, MD

References

1. American College of Surgeons Committee on Trauma. *Advanced Trauma Life Support for Doctors (ATLS)*. 8th ed. Chicago: American College of Surgeons; 2008.
2. Victorino GP, Battistella FD, Wisner DH. Does tachycardia correlate with hypotension after trauma? *J Am Coll Surg*. 2003;196:679-684.
3. Kauvar DS, Lefering R, Wade CE. Impact of hemorrhage on trauma outcome: an overview of epidemiology, clinical presentations, and therapeutic considerations. *J Trauma*. 2006;60:S3-S11.

Improved Characterization of Combat Injury
Champion HR, Holcomb JB, Lawnick MM, et al (Uniformed Services Univ of the Health Sciences, Bethesda, MD; Univ of Texas Health Science Ctr, Houston; SimQuest LLC, Silver Spring, MD; et al)
J Trauma 68:1139-1150, 2010

Background.—Combat injury patterns differ from civilian trauma in that the former are largely explosion-related, comprising multiple mechanistic and fragment injuries and high-kinetic-energy bullets. Further, unlike civilians, U.S. armed forces combatants are usually heavily protected with helmets and Kevlar body armor with ceramic plate inserts. Searchable databases providing actionable, statistically valid knowledge of body surface entry wounds and resulting organ injury severity are essential to understanding combat trauma.

Methods.—Two tools were developed to address these unique aspects of combat injury: (1) the Surface Wound Mapping (SWM) database and Surface Wound Analysis Tool (SWAT) software that were developed to generate 3D density maps of point-of-surface wound entry and resultant anatomic injury severity; and (2) the Abbreviated Injury Scale (AIS) 2005-Military that was developed by a panel of military trauma surgeons to account for multiple injury etiology from explosions and other high-kinetic-energy weapons. Combined data from the Joint Theater Trauma Registry, Navy/Marine Combat Trauma Registry, and the Armed Forces Medical Examiner System Mortality Trauma Registry were coded in AIS 2005-Military, entered into the SWM database, and analyzed for entrance site and wounding path.

Results.—When data on 1,151 patients, who had a total of 3,500 surface wounds and 12,889 injuries, were entered into SWM, surface wounds averaged 3.0 per casualty and injuries averaged 11.2 per casualty. Of the 3,500 surface wounds, 2,496 (71%) were entrance wounds with 6,631 (51%) associated internal injuries, with 2.2 entrance wounds and 5.8 associated injuries per casualty (some details cannot be given because of operational security). Crude deaths rates were calculated using Maximum AIS-Military.

Conclusion.—These new tools have been successfully implemented to describe combat injury, mortality, and distribution of wounds and associated injuries. AIS 2005-Military is a more precise assignment of severity to military injuries. SWM has brought data from all three combat registries together into one analyzable database. SWM and SWAT allow visualization of wounds and associated injuries by region on a 3D model of the body.

▶ Military practitioners have long suspected that standard civilian scoring systems were inadequate for grading multitrauma sustained by military personnel. Using analysis of internal injury patterns associated with characteristic surface changes, the authors built an outcome severity score for military trauma predicted by cutaneous findings.[1,2] Not surprisingly, the number of changes in severity of scoring between Abbreviated Injury Scale (AIS) 2005 and AIS 2005-Military was greatest in the head and neck. Approximately 230 of 360 severity increases in AIS 2005-Military relative to AIS 2005 came from changes in scoring of injuries to the head and neck. The vast majority of severity increment increases were single severity level when approximately 10% severity increases between AIS 2005 and AIS 2005-Military involved a 2-level increase. Remarkably, when actual data were obtained on more than 1100 military patients, surface wounds averaged 3.0 per casualty, but internal injuries averaged 11.2 per casualty. It should be noted that these scoring changes were heavily biased by the preponderance of explosion injuries. Maximum AIS-Military is strongly predictive of mortality.

D. J. Dries, MSE, MD

References

1. Kelly JR, Ritenour AE, McLaughlin DF, et al. Injury severity and causes of death from Operation Iraqi Freedom and Operation Enduring Freedom: 2003-2004 versus 2006. *J Trauma*. 2008;64:S21-S27.
2. Eastridge BJ, Jenkins D, Flaherty S, Schiller H, Holcomb JB. Trauma system development in a theater of war: experiences from Operation Iraqi Freedom and Operation Enduring Freedom. *J Trauma*. 2006;61:1366-1373.

Improvements in Early Mortality and Coagulopathy are Sustained Better in Patients With Blunt Trauma After Institution of a Massive Transfusion Protocol in a Civilian Level I Trauma Center

Dente CJ, Shaz BH, Nicholas JM, et al (Grady Memorial Hosp and Emory Univ School of Medicine, Atlanta, GA)

J Trauma 66:1616-1624, 2009

Introduction.—Transfusion practices across the country are changing with aggressive use of plasma (fresh-frozen plasma [FFP]) and platelets during massive transfusion with current military recommendations to use component therapy at a 1:1:1 ratio of packed red blood cells to FFP to platelets.

Methods.—A massive transfusion protocol (MTP) was designed to achieve a packed red blood cell:FFP:platelet ratio of 1:1:1 We prospectively gathered demographic, transfusion, and patient outcome data during the first year of the MTP and compared this with a similar cohort of injured patients (pre-MTP) receiving ≥ 10 red blood cell (RBC) in the first 24 hours of hospitalization before instituting the MTP.

Results.—One hundred sixteen MTP activations occurred. Twelve non-trauma patients and 31 who did not receive 10 RBC (15 deaths, 16 early bleeding controls) were excluded. Seventy-three MTP patients were compared with 84 patients with pre-MTP who had similar demographics and injury severity score (29 vs. 29, $p = 0.99$). MTP patients received an average of 23.7 RBC and 15.6 FFP transfusions compared with 22.8 RBC ($p = 0.67$) and 7.6 FFP ($p < 0.001$) transfusions in pre-MTP patients. Early crystalloid usage dropped from 9.4 L (pre-MTP) to 6.9 L (MTP) ($p = 0.006$). Overall patient mortality was markedly improved at 24 hours, from 36% in the pre-MTP group to 17% in the MTP group ($p = 0.008$) and at 30 days (34% mortality MTP group vs. 55% mortality in pre-MTP group, $p = 0.04$). Blunt trauma survival improvements were more marked and more sustained than victims of penetrating trauma. Early deaths from coagulopathic bleeding occurred in 4 of 13 patients in the MTP group vs. 21 of 31 patients in the pre-MTP group ($p = 0.023$).

Conclusions.—In the civilian setting, aggressive use of FFP and platelets drastically reduces 24-hour mortality and early coagulopathy in patients with trauma. Reduction in 30 day mortality was only seen after blunt trauma in this small subset.

▶ Exsanguinating hemorrhage is a leading cause of death in civilian and military trauma. Although clotting factors are lost in this process, resuscitation efforts have historically been targeted primarily at replacement of red blood cell losses, with correction of coagulopathies and thrombocytopenia only when they are clinically apparent or detected by laboratory evaluation. In recent years, the military has developed massive transfusion protocols, often using packed red cells, fresh frozen plasma, and platelets in a 1:1:1 ratio for injured patients with exsanguinating bleeding. Only a limited number of civilian institutions have adopted and evaluated the efficacy of such interventions to date. In this study, these investigators report on their experience with such a protocol in a level 1 trauma center, comparing 73 patients who were resuscitated using such a protocol with 84 patients who underwent resuscitation prior to the institution of the protocol. Although protocol patients received more blood components in the initial time period, prior to the establishment of the protocol, patients actually received more units of packed cells. Thirty-day mortality was significantly lower for victims of blunt trauma who were treated according to the protocol, while there was no difference in mortality for victims of penetrating trauma, regardless of transfusion method.

These data suggest that a more aggressive approach, as opposed to normal maintenance of hemostasis in massive hemorrhage, is likely to be of significant benefit. While these data are from a trauma population, they may be applicable to a medical population as well.

D. R. Gerber, DO

Management of Cervical Esophageal Injury After Spinal Surgery
Rueth N, Shaw D, Groth S, et al (Univ of Minnesota, Minneapolis)
Ann Thorac Surg 90:1128-1133, 2010

Background.—Esophageal injury is a rare but catastrophic complication of anterior cervical spine surgery. Cases of esophageal perforation may be discovered intraoperatively, or as late as 10 years after surgery. In the current study we aim to review the principles of care and provide an algorithm that can be employed for successful management of this complex problem.

Methods.—We performed a retrospective, Institutional Review Board-approved review of esophageal injuries resulting from anterior cervical spine surgery that were managed at our institution between January 1, 2007 and July 31, 2009. We collected demographic information, perioperative data, and final outcomes. Data were analyzed using descriptive statistics.

Results.—We identified 6 patients who met our criteria. All patients presented with esophageal leaks, neck abscesses, and osteomyelitis. Similarly, all had been treated prior to transfer, without resolution of their leak. After debridement, removal of hardware, long-term antibiotic therapy, maximization of nutrition, and supportive care, 80% of patients resumed oral intake (median time 66.5 days). Mortality was 16.7%.

Conclusions.—Neck exploration with removal of hardware, debridement, and open neck wound management are the basic principles of care. Management is often prolonged and requires multiple procedures; however, with persistence, closure is possible in the majority of patients. Our report serves as a guide for the treatment of this devastating problem (Fig 3).

▶ This brief case series incorporates a small number of important observations. Due to the relative rarity of this complication, I will summarize important messages.

Despite esophageal injury leading to leaks presenting at a variety of intervals after cervical spine stabilization procedures, most patients had successful fusion and stable spines. Patients presented with neck abscess and subsequent esophagocutaneous fistula. Initial management includes neck exploration, debridement, and removal of spine hardware as possible. In some cases, primary esophageal repair can be performed.

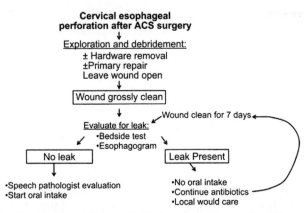

**Cervical esophageal
perforation after ACS surgery**
↓
Exploration and debridement:
± Hardware removal
±Primary repair
Leave wound open
↓
Wound grossly clean
↓
Wound clean for 7 days
Evaluate for leak:
•Bedside test
•Esophagogram

No leak

Leak Present

•Speech pathologist evaluation
•Start oral intake

•No oral intake
•Continue antibiotics
•Local would care

FIGURE 3.—Algorithm summarizing standardized management approach. (ACS = anterior cervical spine.) (Reprinted from Rueth N, Shaw D, Groth S, et al. Management of cervical esophageal injury after spinal surgery. *Ann Thorac Surg.* 2010;90:1128-1133, with permission from The Society of Thoracic Surgeons.)

Esophageal stents are another valuable adjunct in these patients. Neck wounds frequently are not closed. While hospitalization was lengthy in these patients, intensive care unit stay ranged from a few days to 2 weeks.

Perhaps the most important critical care intervention after source control for infection is identification and establishment of enteral nutrition access. This should be done as soon as possible after patient presentation, as adequate metabolic support is essential to healing and host defense in these patients.

D. J. Dries, MSE, MD

Neurological Effects of Blast Injury

Hicks RR, Fertig SJ, Desrocher RE, et al (National Insts of Health, Bethesda, MD)
J Trauma 68:1257-1263, 2010

Over the last few years, thousands of soldiers and an even greater number of civilians have suffered traumatic injuries due to blast exposure, largely attributed to improvised explosive devices in terrorist and insurgent activities. The use of body armor is allowing soldiers to survive blasts that would otherwise be fatal due to systemic damage. Emerging evidence suggests that exposure to a blast can produce neurologic consequences in the brain but much remains unknown. To elucidate the current scientific basis for understanding blast-induced traumatic brain injury (bTBI), the NIH convened a workshop in April 2008. A multidisciplinary group of neuroscientists, engineers, and clinicians were invited to share insights on bTBI, specifically pertaining to: physics of blast explosions, acute clinical observations and treatments, preclinical and computational models, and lessons from the international community on civilian exposures.

This report provides an overview of the state of scientific knowledge of bTBI, drawing from the published literature, as well as presentations, discussions, and recommendations from the workshop. One of the major recommendations from the workshop was the need to characterize the effects of blast exposure on clinical neuropathology. Clearer understanding of the human neuropathology would enable validation of preclinical and computational models, which are attempting to simulate blast wave interactions with the central nervous system. Furthermore, the civilian experience with bTBI suggests that polytrauma models incorporating both brain and lung injuries may be more relevant to the study of civilian countermeasures than considering models with a neurologic focus alone.

▶ This article reviews an NIH workshop intended to summarize recent evidence and pertinent questions related to blast injury to the brain. Perhaps the most important observation is that this important problem is poorly understood, in part, because of the difficulty with creation of appropriate experimental models.[1,2]

At this point, the primary transduction pathway for blast injury to the brain remains unclear. While a commonsense approach suggests direct transmission of energy via a transcranial route as marked by tympanic membrane damage, an intriguing series of studies suggest that protection of the chest and abdomen may also be protective of the brain. These experiments suggest that brain injury occurs by propagation of waves of blast energy through the vascular system or the cerebral spinal fluid. Like nonblast traumatic brain injury (TBI), TBI due to blast leads to edema, contusion, diffuse axonal injury, hematoma formation, and hemorrhage. Posttraumatic stress disorder (PTSD) is a common problem in both terrorist and civilian TBI. Ongoing studies of blast TBI suggest a potential biomarker within the family of S100 proteins indicative of PTSD development. New neuroimaging technologies including diffusion tensor imaging detect white and gray matter damage. White matter injury identified with diffusion tensor imaging is frequently undetectable with conventional CT or MRI imaging.

Finally, civilian practitioners facing blast TBI should be aware of the increased morbidity associated with closed-space injury (busses and trains, where reflection of blast waves can magnify injury). Initial CT evaluation in the emergency department is frequently negative in these patients, but later studies demonstrate progression of brain injury. Finally, an underappreciated factor in blast TBI is that occurring secondary to blunt pulmonary trauma in the setting of blast waves. Severe hypoxemia and gas emboli, common phenomena in blast injury to the lung, can be particularly injurious to the sensitized brain.[3]

D. J. Dries, MSE, MD

References

1. Ritenour AE, Blackbourne LH, Kelly JF, et al. Incidence of primary blast injury in US military overseas contingency operations: a retrospective study. *Ann Surg.* 2010;251:1140-1144.

2. Champion HR, Holcomb JB, Young LA. Injuries from explosions: physics, biophysics, pathology, and required research focus. *J Trauma.* 2009;66:1468-1477.
3. DePalma RG, Burris DG, Champion HR, Hodgson MJ. Blast injuries. *N Engl J Med.* 2005;352:1335-1342.

Occult pneumothoraces in patients with penetrating trauma: Does mechanism matter?

Ball CG, Dente CJ, Kirkpatrick AW, et al (Emory Univ, Atlanta, GA; Univ of Calgary, Alberta, Canada)

Can J Surg 53:251-255, 2010

Background.—Supine anteroposterior (AP) chest radiography is an insensitive test for detecting posttraumatic pneumothoraces (PTXs). Computed tomography (CT) often identifies occult pneumothoraces (OPTXs) not diagnosed by chest radiography. All previous literature describes the epidemiology of OPTX in patients with blunt poly-trauma. Our goal was to identify the frequency of OPTXs in patients with penetrating trauma.

Methods.—All patients with penetrating trauma admitted over a 10-year period to Grady Memorial Hospital with a PTX were identified. We reviewed patients' thora-coabdominal CT scans and corresponding chest radiographs.

Results.—Records for 1121 (20%) patients with a PTX (penetrating mechanism) were audited; CT imaging was available for 146 (13%) patients. Of these, 127 (87%) had undergone upright chest radiography. The remainder (19 patients) had a supine AP chest radiograph. Fifteen (79%) of the PTXs detected on supine AP chest radiographs were occult. Only 10 (8%) were occult when an upright chest radiograph was used ($p < 0.001$). Posttraumatic PTXs were occult on chest radiographs in 17% (25/146) of patients. Fourteen (56%) patients with OPTXs underwent tube thoracostomy, compared with 95% (115/121) of patients with overt PTXs ($p < 0.001$).

Conclusion.—Up to 17% of all PTXs in patients injured by penetrating mechanisms will be missed by standard trauma chest radiographs. This increases to nearly 80% with supine AP chest radiographs. Upright chest radiography detects 92% of all PTXs and is available to most patients without spinal trauma. The frequency of tube thora-costomy use in patients with overt PTXs is significantly higher than for OPTXs in blunt and penetrating trauma.

▶ These data come from the Grady Memorial Hospital in Atlanta, where a significant volume of penetrating trauma is seen. Despite the opportunity to perform prospective research, a retrospective design is used. We are told that patients with penetrating mechanism are studied, but penetrating mechanism is not further defined. Clearly, some forms of penetrating trauma carry higher risk of occult or overt pneumothorax than others. It is also important to note that all patients are not imaged equally. Some patients have confirmation by chest computed tomography (CT), while others have only abdominal CT available. Thus, some pneumothoraces could be missed.

I agree completely with the authors that in the setting of penetrating trauma, the supine chest X-ray is ineffective in identifying many presentations of pneumothorax. At the very least, an upright film should be obtained if spine injury is not a concern. The authors indicate a 17% miss rate with standard radiographs. However, these patients do not receive a consistent approach to radiography.

Finally, early work related to the problem of occult pneumothorax indicates that most of these patients will not require chest drain placement, even if they receive positive pressure ventilation. These authors provide no additional data regarding the rationale for their approach to management of the patient with occult pneumothorax after penetrating trauma. Thus, the clinician is left to decide the role of tube thoracostomy in these patients. This study does not add to our knowledge of the natural history of occult pneumothorax in the patient with penetrating trauma.[1]

D. J. Dries, MSE, MD

Reference

1. Brasel KJ, Stafford RE, Weigelt JA, Tenquist JE, Borgstrom DC. Treatment of occult pneumothoraces from blunt trauma. *J Trauma*. 1999;46:987-991.

Predictors for the Selection of Patients for Abdominal CT After Blunt Trauma: A Proposal for a Diagnostic Algorithm
Deunk J, Brink M, Dekker HM, et al (Radboud Univ Nijmegen Med Ctr, The Netherlands)
Ann Surg 251:512-520, 2010

Objective.—To select parameters that can predict which patients should receive abdominal computed tomography (CT) after high-energy blunt trauma.

Summary Background Data.—Abdominal CT accurately detects injuries of the abdomen, pelvis, and lumbar spine, but has important disadvantages. More evidence for an appropriate patient selection for CT is required.

Methods.—A prospective observational study was performed on consecutive adult high-energy blunt trauma patients. All patients received primary and secondary surveys according to the advanced trauma life support, sonography (focused assessment with sonography for trauma [FAST]), conventional radiography (CR) of the chest, pelvis, and spine and routine abdominal CT. Parameters from prehospital information, physical examination, laboratory investigations, FAST, and CR were prospectively recorded for all patients. Independent predictors for the presence of ≥ 1 injuries on abdominal CT were determined using a multivariate logistic regression analysis.

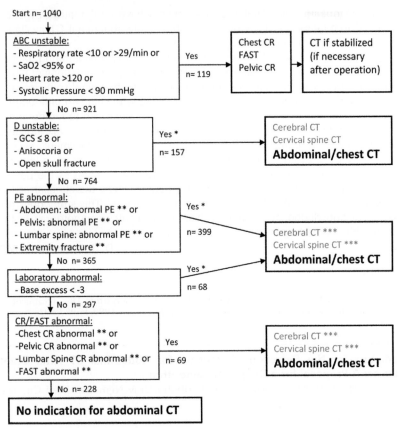

FIGURE 2.—Proposal for a diagnostic algorithm for abdominal evaluation in patients after blunt high-energy trauma. The number (n) of patients that follow the different paths of the algorithm are outlined, if the algorithm were to be used in our population. *Consider chest CR and FAST in case of endotracheal intubation or expected delay before computed tomography performance. **Definitions of abnormalities in PE and CR and extremity fracture, are specified in Table 2. ***Indications for cerebral and cervical spine computed tomography are beyond the scope of the study and this algorithm, but should be considered in these patients. CR indicates conventional radiography; FAST, Focused Sonography for Trauma; PE, physical examination. (Reprinted from Deunk J, Brink M, Dekker HM, et al. Predictors for the selection of patients for abdominal CT after blunt trauma: a proposal for a diagnostic algorithm. *Ann Surg.* 2010;251:512-520.)

Results.—A total of 1040 patients were included, 309 had injuries on abdominal CT. Nine parameters were independent predictors for injuries on CT: abnormal CR of the pelvis (odds ratio [OR], 46.8), lumbar spine (OR, 16.2), and chest (OR, 2.37), abnormal FAST (OR, 26.7), abnormalities in physical examination of the abdomen/pelvis (OR, 2.41) or lumbar spine (OR 2.53), base excess < −3 (OR, 2.39), systolic blood pressure < 90 mm Hg (OR, 3.81), and long bone fractures (OR, 1.61). The prediction model based on these predictors resulted in a R^2 of 0.60, a sensitivity of 97%, and a specificity of 33%. A diagnostic algorithm was subsequently proposed, which could reduce CT usage with 22% as compared with a routine use.

TABLE 2.—Definitions of Potential Predictors in the Present Study

Variable	Definitions*
Abnormal chest CR	Pneumothorax, hemothorax, pulmonary contusion, subcutaneous emphysema, rib fractures, scapular fracture, clavicle fracture, suspected aortic rupture, diaphragm rupture
Abnormal pelvic CR	Pubic bone fracture, acetabulum fracture, iliac wing fracture, sacrum fracture, femoral head fracture, symphysiolysis, sacroiliacal joint luxation, hip luxation
Abnormal lumbar spine CR	Vertebral fracture, transverse processes fracture, abnormal spinal configuration, or distended paraspinal line
FAST-positive	Free fluid on abdominal ultrasound according to the principles of Focused Assessment with Sonography for Trauma (FAST)
Intubation	Endotracheal intubation by prehospital medical services or immediately during initial assessment on the emergency department (ED)
Hypotension	Prehospital systolic blood pressure or first systolic pressure on the ED lower than 90 mm Hg (transient; no shock class 3/4)
Heart rate >120 bpm	Prehospital heart rate or first heart rate on the ED higher than 120 beats per minute
GCS <14	Glasgow Coma Scale (GCS) lower than 14 on initial presentation on the ED or prior to intubation in case of intubation and sedation by prehospital medical services
GCS <11	Glasgow Coma Scale lower than 11 on initial presentation on the ED or prior to intubation in case of intubation and sedation by prehospital medical services
Abnormal physical examination of the abdomen and/or pelvis	Abdominal tenderness, guarding, distention, lacerations, or hematoma of the abdominal wall. Clinical suspicion of a pelvic fracture due to osseous tenderness
Abnormal physical examination of the lumbar spine	Midline lumbar tenderness, lacerations, or abrasions of the back. Neurological deficit with sensory and/or motor loss, suspicious for unstable lumbar spine fractures
Abnormal physical examination of the chest	Decreased breath sounds, tenderness, flail chest, subcutaneous emphysema, lacerations, or hematoma of the chest wall. Breathing frequency >29 or <10/min, pulse-oximetry SaO_2 <95%
Fracture of the extremities	Fractures of the femur, tibia, fibula, humerus, radius, or ulna, confirmed by radiography
Laboratory BE <−3	Base excess (BE) lower than −3 mmoL/L in the initial arterial blood gas
Intoxication	Clinical suspicion of alcohol or dugs intoxication or elevated serum ethanol levels (>0.1 g/L)

CR indicates conventional radiography.
*The presence of any of these findings result in a positive variable.

Conclusions.—Based on parameters from physical examination, laboratory, FAST, and CR, we created a prediction model with a high sensitivity to select patients for abdominal CT after blunt trauma. A diagnostic algorithm was proposed.

▶ There is no question that unnecessary imaging is performed after blunt trauma.[1,2] A review of data provided by these authors indicates that 70% of the study population, even in the setting of high-energy blunt injury, did not have evidence of traumatic injury when CT scans were obtained. Unfortunately, authors differ on the value of physical examination in determination of the need for CT scanning. Some authors argue that minimal physical findings may be present despite life-threatening internal injury.[3]

These authors have constructed a workable clinical algorithm to determine propriety of CT, which is being evaluated in my own trauma center (Table 2 and Fig 2). It is clear, for example, that despite a growing literature supporting its use and advances in ultrasound technology, ultrasound evaluation in the emergency department is frequently followed by CT even if clinical findings suggesting the need for CT are absent.[4]

Clearly, one of the horizons in trauma care is the role of evolving imaging technology in the management of injured patients.[5] The classic question is not what we can do but what we should do. As the public becomes more aware of radiation risk, pressure to reduce unnecessary imaging in the emergency department will grow. This need is particularly important in young patients where the lifetime risk of malignancy goes up with imaging during the first 3 decades.[1] Now we have a well-written study to support thoughtful limitation of CT imaging.

D. J. Dries, MSE, MD

References

1. Brenner DJ, Hall EJ. Computed tomography — an increasing source of radiation exposure. *N Engl J Med.* 2007;357:2277-2284.
2. Martin DR, Semelka RC. Health effects of ionising radiation from diagnostic CT. *Lancet.* 2006;367:1712-1714.
3. Michetti CP, Hanna R, Crandall JR, Fakhry SM. Contemporary analysis of thoracic aortic injury: importance of screening based on crash characteristics. *J Trauma.* 2007;63:18-25.
4. Farahmand N, Sirlin CB, Brown MA, et al. Hypotensive patients with blunt abdominal trauma: performance of screening US. *Radiology.* 2005;235:436-443.
5. Brink M, de Lange F, Oostveen LJ, et al. Arm raising at exposure-controlled multidetector trauma CT of thoracoabdominal region: higher image quality, lower radiation dose. *Radiology.* 2008;249:661-670.

Results of the CONTROL Trial: Efficacy and Safety of Recombinant Activated Factor VII in the Management of Refractory Traumatic Hemorrhage

Hauser CJ, for the CONTROL Study Group (Harvard Med School and Beth Israel Deaconess Med Ctr, Boston, MA; et al)
J Trauma 69:489-500, 2010

Background.—Traumatic coagulopathy contributes to early death by exsanguination and late death in multiple organ failure. Recombinant Factor VIIa (rFVIIa, NovoSeven) is a procoagulant that might limit bleeding and improve trauma outcomes.

Methods.—We performed a phase 3 randomized clinical trial evaluating efficacy and safety of rFVIIa as an adjunct to direct hemostasis in major trauma. We studied 573 patients (481 blunt and 92 penetrating) who bled 4 to 8 red blood cell (RBC) units within 12 hours of injury and were still bleeding despite strict damage control resuscitation and operative management. Patients were assigned to rFVIIa (200 μg/kg initially; 100 μg/kg at 1 hour and 3 hours) or placebo. Intensive care unit management was standardized using evidence-based trauma "bundles" with formal oversight of compliance. Primary outcome was 30-day mortality. Predefined secondary outcomes included blood products used. Safety was assessed through 90 days. Study powering was based on prior randomized controlled trials and large trauma center databases.

Results.—Enrollment was terminated at 573 of 1502 planned patients because of unexpected low mortality prompted by futility analysis (10.8% vs. 27.5% planned/predicted) and difficulties consenting and enrolling sicker patients. Mortality was 11.0% (rFVIIa) versus 10.7% (placebo) ($p = 0.93$, blunt) and 18.2% (rFVIIa) versus 13.2% (placebo) ($p = 0.40$, penetrating). Blunt trauma rFVIIa patients received (mean ± SD) 7.8 ± 10.6 RBC units and 19.0 ± 27.1 total allogeneic units through 48 hours, and placebo patients received 9.1 ± 11.3 RBC units ($p = 0.04$) and 23.5 ± 28.0 total allogeneic units ($p = 0.04$). Thrombotic adverse events were similar across study cohorts.

Conclusions.—rFVIIa reduced blood product use but did not affect mortality compared with placebo. Modern evidence-based trauma lowers mortality, paradoxically making outcomes studies increasingly difficult.

▶ This is the second large multicenter trial using recombinant activated factor VII in traumatic hemorrhage. Similar to the original work by Boffard and others, no difference in mortality is identified but blood product use may be reduced.[1]

The authors make 3 important observations in the discussion of this article. First, recombinant activated factor VII did reduce blood product use, which is consistent with its role as a procoagulative agent. Second, is the drug safe? Other reporters have raised the question of thrombotic events. While a difference in thrombotic complications was not identified in this study, an article in the *New England Journal of Medicine* published at the same time indicates that the risk of thrombotic complications with the use of recombinant activated factor VII increases with age. Note that the CONTROL trial studies a relatively young patient group.[2] Third, the authors argue that improvements in trauma care make it difficult in studies such as this to demonstrate better outcomes. I agree with this observation that small, multicenter, tightly controlled trials are less likely to demonstrate improved outcome in a complex trauma population.

The reader should not give up on clinical trials in trauma, however. The recent Clinical Randomization of an Antifibrinolytic in Significant Hemorrhage 2 (CRASH-2) trial used an Internet-based format, multinational enrollment, and demonstrated that tranexamic acid reduced all-cause mortality in patients with trauma with significant hemorrhage.[3] The reader may consider the methodology in the CRASH-2 studies as a possible pathway to identify better treatment for injured patients.

D. J. Dries, MSE, MD

References

1. Boffard KD, Choong PI, Kluger Y, et al. The treatment of bleeding is to stop the bleeding! Treatment of trauma-related hemorrhage. *Transfusion.* 2009;49: 240S-247S.

2. Levi M, Levy JH, Andersen HF, Truloff D. Safety of recombinant activated factor VII in randomized clinical trials. *N Engl J Med.* 2010;363:1791-1800.
3. CRASH-2 trial collaborators. Effects of tranexamic acid on death, vascular occlusive events, and blood transfusion in trauma patients with significant haemorrhage (CRASH-2): a randomized, placebo-controlled trial. *Lancet.* 2010;376:23-32.

Review of Lodox Statscan in the detection of peripheral skeletal fractures in multiple injury patients

Deyle S, Brehmer T, Evangelopoulos DS, et al (Univ Hosp Bern, Switzerland)
Injury 41:818-822, 2010

Introduction.—As part of the primary survey, polytrauma patients in our emergency department are examined using the new 'Lodox Statscan' (LS) digital low-radiation imaging device. The LS provides full-body anterior and lateral views based on enhanced linear slot-scanning technology, in accordance with the recommended Advanced Trauma Life Support (ATLS) Guidelines. This study's objectives were to establish whether LS appropriately rules out peripheral bone injuries and to examine whether LS imaging provides adequate information for the preoperative planning of such lesions.

Methods.—A total of 245 consecutive polytrauma patients aged 16 years or more undergoing LS imaging were included in this retrospective chart analysis. The results of the LS scans were reviewed and compared to additional plain radiographs or computed tomography scans, whenever further radiological imaging was required to determine consecutive therapy.

Results.—The sensitivity and specificity of the LS scans were 73% and 100%, respectively, for peripheral skeletal injuries. Additional plain radiographs were performed in 50% of cases for (1) superior focussing and more precise resolution of the affected part of the body, (2) additional second or third plane, (3) additional information about fracture type and planning of the surgical approach and (4) for preoperative planning of implant size and positioning on calibrated digitised films, <1% because of the low quality of the LS scan and <1% because the fracture zone had not been fully captured.

Conclusion.—The study demonstrates that despite LS's high sensitivity and specificity in the detection of peripheral skeletal injuries, additional radiological imaging for diagnostic or preoperative reasons was required. Our results imply that LS, although efficient for patient screening in the emergency room, cannot always rule out peripheral skeletal injuries.

▶ The Lodox device provides a full-body anterior and lateral view based on a low-radiation scanning technology. A full-body scan requires as little as 6.5 minutes and uses 10% of the mean conventional radiation dose.[1,2]

This study demonstrates that up to 50% of patients required additional imaging either for operative planning or evaluation of fractures, despite the availability of Lodox evaluation. Most commonly missed injuries are in the hands and the feet. Fortunately, orthopedic injuries to the hands and feet are not life-threatening. Unfortunately, limitations are identified in Lodox scanning of more important and proximal skeletal injuries of the upper and the lower extremities as well.

Some of the early enthusiasm regarding Lodox scanning may not be justifiable. This technology may have a limited role in the unresponsive patient, where physical examination is incomplete, or in the obese patient or the polytrauma patient, where rapid general evaluation is required. At present, I do not believe that the cost of this technology justifies its widespread integration into emergency department practice. Whether resolution can be improved without significant increase in radiation exposure remains to be seen.

D. J. Dries, MSE, MD

References

1. Beningfield S, Potgieter H, Nicol A, et al. Report on a new type of trauma full-body digital X-ray machine. *Emerg Radiol.* 2003;10:23-29.
2. Boffard KD, Goosen J, Plani F, Degiannis E, Potgieter H. The use of low dosage X-ray (Lodox/Statscan) in major trauma: comparison between low dose X-ray and conventional X-ray techniques. *J Trauma.* 2006;60:1175-1183.

Surgical considerations in the management of combined radiation blast injury casualties caused by a radiological dirty bomb
Williams G, O'Malley M (Univ Hosp (Walsgrave Site), Coventry, UK; Warrington Hosp, UK)
Injury 41:943-947, 2010

The capacity for surgical teams to respond appropriately to the consequences caused by the detonation of a radiological dirty bomb will be determined by prior knowledge, familiarity and training for this type unique terrorist event. This paper will focus on the surgical aspects of

Isotope	Radiation type	Radiological half life
Americium (Am-s241)	Alpha	458 years
Caesium (Cs-137)	Beta, Gamma	30 years
Cobalt (Co-60)	Beta, Gamma	5 years
Iridium (Ir-192)	Beta, Gamma	74 days

FIGURE 1.—Isotopes likely to be utilised in the construction a radiological dirty bomb. (Reprinted from Williams G, O'Malley M. Surgical considerations in the management of combined radiation blast injury casualties caused by a radiological dirty bomb. *Injury.* 2010;41:943-947, with permission from Elsevier.)

Category	Body part	Example
Type 1 (blastwave injury)	Gas-filled structures are are the most susceptible (Respiratory, ENT, GIT)	Pulmonary barotrauma Middle ear damage Abdominal haemorrhage / perforation
Type 2 (fragmentation injury from device - primary or debris - secondary)	Any body part	Penetrating ballistic or blunt injury Eye penetration Traumatic wounding
Type 3 (caused by blastwind displacement of the victim)	Any body part	Closed or open brain injury Fracture and traumatic amputation
Type 4 (miscellaneous eg radiation, crush, fire)	GIT, skeletal, bone marrow	Crush injury and compartment syndrome Acute effects of radiation

FIGURE 2.—Types of blast injury.[9] *Editor's Note*: Please refer to original journal article for full references. (Reprinted from Williams G, O'Malley M. Surgical considerations in the management of combined radiation blast injury casualties caused by a radiological dirty bomb. *Injury*. 2010;41:943-947, with permission from Elsevier.)

this scenario with particular emphasis on the management of combined trauma-radiological injury. The paper also describes some of the more serious explosion-contamination incidents from nuclear industrial sources, summarises learning points and parallels taken from these scenarios in relation to subject of a radiological dirty bomb and describes the likely radioactive substances involved (Figs 1, 2, and 5).

▶ This is an excellent overview of clinical considerations where blunt trauma is combined with dispersal of nuclear material. I have included a number of figures from this article because of the relative paucity of literature in this area.

Isotope	Management
Americium (Am-s241)	Chelation with DTPA 1g in 250mls normal saline iv over 2 hours once daily for 5 days)
Caesium (Cs-137)	Ion exchange with Prussian blue 1-3g daily with 200ml water 3 week duration titrated to urinary excretion
Cobalt (Co-60)	Gastric lavage and DTPA 1g in 250mls normal saline iv over 2 hours once daily for 5 days
Iridium (Ir-192)	Unknown

FIGURE 5.—Isotopes of interest, properties and medical treatment.[25] *Editor's Note*: Please refer to original journal article for full references. (Reprinted from Williams G, O'Malley M. Surgical considerations in the management of combined radiation blast injury casualties caused by a radiological dirty bomb. *Injury*. 2010;41:943-947, with permission from Elsevier.)

I will attempt to summarize key points. First, the approach to these patients must begin with the ABCs of blunt trauma. There is no difference between water and chelating agents with regard to success of external decontamination. Hair should probably be shaved, as it is nearly impossible to decontaminate.

Emergency surgical intervention should be complete within 48 hours of an incident before any radiation-induced bone marrow suppression occurs.[1,2] Body bags should be used to transport patients to the operating room, as these do not allow loss of fluid. The operating room should be isolated from the remainder of operating theaters, and the corridors used to reach the operating room should be isolated from other hallways as far as possible. Floors should be protected with disposable coverings and any nonessential operating room equipment removed.

Radiation detectors and simple body irrigation with mild detergents is sufficient for surface decontamination. Wounds should be closed as soon as reasonably possible due to infection related to immune compromise. Wounds that remain contaminated despite debridement and irrigation should be covered with waterproof dressings to limit the spread of contamination.

Wound healing and late extremity loss may occur with progressive effects of isotopes with long half-life. Even small numbers of undebrideable radioactive fragments left in situ could result in the patient accumulating a fatal dose of radiation exposure depending on fragment activity. In these cases, amputation may be considered.

Finally, due to immune consequences of radiation exposure, difficulties with postoperative healing should be anticipated with an increased number of wound complications. Management strategies, however, remain the same.

D. J. Dries, MSE, MD

References

1. Military Medical Operations. http://www.afrri.usuhs.mil/outreach/guidance.htm. Accessed October 31, 2009.
2. Radiation Event Medial Management US Department of Health and Human Services. http://www.remm.nlm.gov. Accessed October 31, 2009.

Variation in Pediatric and Adolescent Firearm Mortality Rates in Rural and Urban US Counties

Nance ML, Carr BG, Kallan MJ, et al (Children's Hosp of Philadelphia, PA; Univ of Pennsylvania, Philadelphia)
Pediatrics 125:1112-1118, 2010

Objective.—We examined whether firearm mortality rates among children varied across US counties along a rural-urban continuum.

Methods.—US vital statistics data were accessed for all pediatric (age: 0–19 years) firearm deaths from 1999 through 2006. Deaths were analyzed according to a modified rural-urban continuum code (based on population size and proximity to metropolitan areas) assigned to each county (3141 counties).

Results.—In the 8-year study period, there were 23 649 pediatric firearm deaths (15 190 homicides, 7082 suicides, and 1377 unintentional deaths). Pediatric nonfirearm mortality rates were significantly higher in the most-rural counties (adjusted rate ratio: 1.36 [95% confidence interval [CI]: 1.13–1.64]), compared with the most-urban counties. The most-rural counties demonstrated virtually identical pediatric firearm mortality rates (adjusted rate ratio: 0.91 [95% CI: 0.63–1.32]), compared with the most-urban counties. The most-rural counties had higher rates of pediatric firearm suicide (adjusted rate ratio: 2.01 [95% CI: 1.43–2.83]) and unintentional firearm death (adjusted rate ratio: 2.19 [95% CI: 1.27–3.77]), compared with the most-urban counties. Pediatric firearm homicides rates were significantly higher in the most-urban counties (adjusted rate ratio: 3.69 [95% CI: 2.00–6.80]), compared with the most-rural counties.

Conclusions.—Children in the most-rural US counties had firearm mortality rates that were statistically indistinguishable from those for children in the most-urban US counties. This finding reflects a greater homicide rate in urban counties counterbalanced by greater suicide and unintentional firearm death rates in rural counties. Nonfirearm mortality rates were significantly greater outside the most-urban US counties.

▶ This detailed analysis uses data from the National Center for Health Statistics National Vital Statistics System from 1999 through 2006. Death certificates were reviewed for each state, and a continuum developed describing mortality site as predominantly rural or urban. Children dying from firearm injuries were concentrated at the older end of the pediatric age range regardless of rural or urban location. Homicide is the most common cause of firearm mortality, but suicide becomes increasingly important as children age. This study challenges the historic bias that mortality in children related to firearm use is concentrated in urban areas.[1]

What social patterns can the intensivist anticipate? (Where should prevention dollars go?) In the cities, control interpersonal violence. In rural areas, teach gun safety and suicide awareness.

D. J. Dries, MSE, MD

Reference

1. Branas CC, Nance ML, Elliott MR, Richmond TS, Schwab CW. Urban-rural shifts in intentional firearm death: different causes, same results. *Am J Public Health.* 2004;94:1750-1755.

11 Neurologic: Traumatic and Non-traumatic

Causes and Outcomes of Acute Neuromuscular Respiratory Failure
Serrano MC, Rabinstein AA (Mayo Clinic, Rochester, MN)
Arch Neurol 67:1089-1094, 2010

Objective.—To identify the spectrum of causes, analyze the usefulness of diagnostic tests, and recognize prognostic factors in patients with acute neuromuscular respiratory failure.

Methods.—We evaluated 85 patients admitted to the intensive care unit (ICU) at Mayo Clinic, Rochester, between 2003 and 2009 with acute neuromuscular respiratory failure, defined as a need for mechanical ventilation owing to primary impairment of the peripheral nervous system. Outcome was assessed at hospital discharge and at last follow-up. Poor outcome was defined as a modified Rankin score greater than 3.

Results.—The median age was 66 years; median follow-up, 5 months. The most frequent diagnoses were myasthenia gravis, Guillain-Barré syndrome, myopathies, and amyotrophic lateral sclerosis (27, 12, 12, and 12 patients, respectively). Forty-seven patients (55%) had no known neuromuscular diagnosis before admission, and 36 of them (77%) had poor short-term outcomes. In 10 patients (12%), the diagnosis remained unknown on discharge; only 1 (10%) had regained independent function. Older age was associated with increased mortality during hospitalization. Longer mechanical ventilation times and ICU stays were associated with poor outcome at discharge but not at the last follow-up. Patients without a known neuromuscular diagnosis before admission had longer duration of mechanical ventilation, longer ICU stays, and worse outcomes at discharge. Electromyography was the most useful diagnostic test in patients without previously known neuromuscular diagnoses. The presence of spontaneous activity on needle insertion predicted poor short-term outcome regardless of final diagnosis. Coexistent cardiopulmonary diseases also predicted poor long-term outcome.

Conclusions.—Among patients with neuromuscular respiratory failure, those without known diagnosis before admission have poorer outcomes.

Patients whose diagnoses remain unclear at discharge have the highest rates of disability.

▶ While neuromuscular causes of acute respiratory failure are a relatively uncommon process in most of our critical care units, it is important for all of us to recognize this group of patients and realize the clinical and prognostic implications of this diagnosis. The data presented by the Mayo group may be a bit different than what you would find at your institution, if yours is not a large national referral center. However, there are a number of important observations we should all take away from this report. Fifty-five percent of the reported patients did not have a prior diagnosis of a neuromuscular disease, and these individuals tended to have longer intensive care unit (ICU) stays, longer duration of mechanical ventilatory support, and a worse outcome at discharge. Most patients with neuromuscular respiratory failure who were discharged from the ICU were severely disabled at the time of discharge. Those individuals who could be supported with noninvasive ventilation as opposed to invasive ventilatory support had the shortest ICU stay. Patients with underlying cardiopulmonary disease had the worst outcome and patients who had diabetes or pneumonia develop as a complication of this treatment had longer ICU stays. Finally, of the 10 patients in whom there was an inability to diagnose the etiology of the neuromuscular disease that resulted in acute respiratory failure, only one was independent at the time of discharge and last follow-up. These data give us a great appreciation for the devastating impact of neuromuscular disease causing acute respiratory failure and will help advise our patients and their families as to the prognosis and impact of this process.

R. A. Balk, MD

Effects of Early Intensive Blood Pressure-Lowering Treatment on the Growth of Hematoma and Perihematomal Edema in Acute Intracerebral Hemorrhage: The Intensive Blood Pressure Reduction in Acute Cerebral Haemorrhage Trial (INTERACT)

Anderson CS, for the INTERACT Investigators (Royal Prince Alfred Hosp and the Univ of Sydney, Australia; et al)
Stroke 41:307-312, 2010

Background and Purpose.—The Intensive Blood Pressure Reduction In Acute Cerebral Haemorrhage Trial (INTERACT) study suggests that early intensive blood pressure (BP) lowering can attenuate hematoma growth at 24 hours after intracerebral hemorrhage. The present analyses aimed to determine the effects of treatment on hematoma and perihematomal edema over 72 hours.

Methods.—INTERACT included 404 patients with CT-confirmed intracerebral hemorrhage, elevated systolic BP (150 to 220 mm Hg), and capacity to start BP-lowering treatment within 6 hours of intracerebral hemorrhage. Patients were randomly assigned to an intensive (target systolic BP 140 mmHg) or standard guideline-based management of BP (target systolic BP 180 mm Hg) using routine intravenous agents. Baseline and repeat CTs (24 and 72 hours) were performed using standardized techniques with digital images analyzed centrally. Outcomes were increases in hematoma and perihematomal edema volumes over 72 hours.

Results.—Overall, 296 patients had all 3 CT scans available for the hematoma and 270 for the edema analyses. Mean systolic BP was 11.7 mm Hg lower in the intensive group than in the guideline group during 1 to 24 hours. Adjusted mean absolute increases in hematoma volumes (mL) at 24 and 72 hours were 2.40 and 0.15 in the guideline group compared with −0.74 and −2.31 in the intensive group, respectively, an overall difference of 2.80 (95% CI, 1.04 to 4.56; $P=0.002$). Adjusted mean absolute increases in edema volumes (mL) at 24 and 72 hours were 6.27 and 10.02 in the guideline group compared with 4.19 and 7.34 in the intensive group, respectively, for an overall difference of 2.38 (95% CI, −0.45 to 5.22; $P=0.10$).

Conclusion.—Early intensive BP-lowering treatment attenuated hematoma growth over 72 hours in intracerebral hemorrhage. There were no appreciable effects on perihematomal edema.

▶ This is a fairly large randomized trial considering the fact that it is rather challenging to conduct such a study in the setting of acute intracerebral hemorrhage (ICH). The topic of blood pressure (BP) management for ICH has been debated for a long time.[1-3] Nonrandomized trials have reported lack of BP control as an independent risk factor for spontaneous hematoma growth, and this is an important study assessing the safety and feasibility of early intensive BP lowering and associated hematoma growth as well as perihematoma edema. The result is in favor of early intensive control, as such therapy was associated with reduced hematoma growth over 72 hours. A few points are worth mentioning. First, the difference in absolute hematoma growth volume between 2 groups was only a couple of milliliters. A 1- to 2-cc difference in hematoma volume may or may not have any significant clinical meaning. What is statistically meaningful may not directly translate into something clinically meaningful. This difference may be secondary to only a small gap in between the mean BP difference between 2 groups. With more dramatic difference in average BP, there could be more profound difference in hematoma growth.

K. Lee, MD

References

1. Brott T, Broderick J, Kothari R, Barsan W, et al. Early hemorrhage growth in patients with intracerebral hemorrhage. *Stroke.* 1997;28:1-5.
2. Kazui S, Minematsu K, Yamamoto H, Sawada T, Yamaguchi T. Predisposing factors to enlargement of spontaneous intracerebral hematoma. *Stroke.* 1997;28: 2370-2375.
3. Fujii Y, Takeuchi S, Sasaki O, Minakawa T, Tanaka R. Multivariate analysis of predictors of hematoma enlargement in spontaneous intracerebral hemorrhage. *Stroke.* 1998;29:1160-1166.

Health-Related Quality of Life in Patients With Multiple Injuries and Traumatic Brain Injury 10+ Years Postinjury

Steel J, Youssef M, Pfeifer R, et al (Univ of Pittsburgh School of Medicine, PA; Univ of Aachen, Germany; et al)
J Trauma 69:523-531, 2010

Background.—The aim of this study was to examine the long-term physical and psychological consequences of multiple blunt forced trauma at ≥10-year follow-up for patients with and without traumatic brain injury (TBI).

Methods.—A total of 620 patients with multiple injuries were assessed with the Medical Outcomes Study-Short Form-12 and a physical reexamination at ≥10-year follow-up. Injury-related characteristics were collected from patients' medical record. Chi-square analysis, Analysis of Variance, and linear and logistic regression were performed to test differences between groups and examine predictors of physical and psychological functioning at ≥10-year follow-up.

Results.—Patients with multiple injuries who sustained a TBI (n = 398) were more likely to be female ($p = 0.001$), younger in age at the time of injury ($p = 0.02$), have higher Injury Severity Scores ($p = 0.001$), shorter ward stays ($p = 0.001$), and a greater number of upper extremity injuries ($p = 0.02$) when compared with those without TBI (n = 222). Patients with TBI reported poorer psychological functioning ($p = 0.02$) and more frequently reported chronic pain ($p = 0.01$). Patients with TBI used medical aids ($p = 0.002$) less frequently at follow-up when compared with patients without TBI. Significant predictors of health-related quality of life at ≥10-year follow-up included age at the time of injury (physical; $p = 0.001$), gender ($p = 0.05$), number of ventilation days ($p = 0.02$), satisfaction with rehabilitation ($p = 0.001$), disability caused by the injury ($p = 0.001$), and use of medical aids (physical $p = 0.02$).

Conclusions.—Prospective studies are needed with a broader range of measures that may be sensitive to the consequences of TBI. Evidence-based interventions to facilitate physical and psychological rehabilitation, designed to target at risk patients, are warranted.

▶ This is an extensive review from the German trauma registry of patients with mild to moderate traumatic brain injury (TBI). There is excellent participation with 80% of potential candidates actually enrolled to provide data to the trial.

There are several important observations. First, the effects of trauma are the most important determinants of long-term outcome. Of potential patients identified with mild to moderate head injury, 37% died of head injury in hospital.[1] On follow-up, 10 years or more after injury, patients with TBI had significantly poorer psychological well-being when compared with patients having multiple orthopedic trauma but no brain injury. Fracture patterns also differed among patient groups. This, I believe, is a simple reflection of the geography of trauma. Patients with head injury were more likely to have upper extremity rather than lower extremity trauma.

Perhaps the most important observation, on closer reading of the article, is the weakness of present tools for evaluating neurologic and quality-of-life outcome in this patient group. This rigorous retrospective work points out the need for good prospective studies.

D. J. Dries, MSE, MD

Reference

1. Ottochian M, Benfield R, Inaba K, Chan LS, Demetriades D. Prospective evaluation of a predictive model of mortality in patients with isolated head injury. *J Trauma.* 2009;67:81-84.

Prediction of Respiratory Insufficiency in Guillain-Barré Syndrome
Walgaard C, Lingsma HF, Ruts L, et al (Erasmus Med Ctr, Rotterdam, the Netherlands; et al)
Ann Neurol 67:781-787, 2010

Objective.—Respiratory insufficiency is a frequent and serious complication of the Guillain-Barré syndrome (GBS). We aimed to develop a simple but accurate model to predict the chance of respiratory insufficiency in the acute stage of the disease based on clinical characteristics available at hospital admission.

Methods.—Mechanical ventilation (MV) in the first week of admission was used as an indicator of acute stage respiratory insufficiency. Prospectively collected data from a derivation cohort of 397 GBS patients were used to identify predictors of MV. A multivariate logistic regression model was validated in a separate cohort of 191 GBS patients. Model performance criteria comprised discrimination (area under receiver operating curve [AUC]) and calibration (graphically). A scoring system for clinical practice was constructed from the regression coefficients of the model in the combined cohorts.

Results.—In the derivation cohort, 22% needed MV in the first week of admission. Days between onset of weakness and admission, Medical Research Council sum score, and presence of facial and/or bulbar weakness were the main predictors of MV. The prognostic model had a good discriminative ability (AUC, 0.84). In the validation cohort, 14% needed MV in the first week of admission, and both calibration and discriminative ability of the model were good (AUC, 0.82). The scoring system ranged from 0 to 7, with corresponding chances of respiratory insufficiency from 1 to 91%.

Interpretation.—This model accurately predicts development of respiratory insufficiency within 1 week in patients with GBS, using clinical characteristics available at admission. After further validation, the model may

TABLE 2.—EGRIS

Measure	Categories	Score
Days between onset of weakness and hospital admission	>7 days	0
	4–7 days	1
	≤3 days	2
Facial and/or bulbar weakness at hospital admission	Absence	0
	Presence	1
MRC sum score at hospital admission	60–51	0
	50–41	1
	40–31	2
	30–21	3
	≤20	4
EGRIS		0–7

EGRIS = Erasmus GBS Respiratory Insufficiency Score; MRC = Medical Research Counsel.

TABLE 3.—Risk Categories for Respiratory Insufficiency According to EGRIS

Category	Derivation Set	Validation Set	Combined Sets
Low risk (EGRIS 0–2)	5/152 (3%)	5/116 (4%)	10/268 (4%; 95% CI, 1–6%)
Intermediate risk (EGRIS 3–4)	42/168 (25%)	13/60 (22%)	55/228 (24%; 95% CI, 19–30%)
High risk (EGRIS 5–7)	36/57 (63%)	9/12 (75%)	45/69 (65%; 95% CI, 54–76%)
Total	83/377 (22%)	27/188 (14%)	110/565 (19%; 95% CI, 16–23%)

Probability of respiratory insufficiency in the first week of hospital admission in the derivation, validation, and combined sets stratified for EGRIS and expressed as number of mechanically ventilated patients/total number of patients (%). EGRIS — Erasmus GBS Respiratory Insufficiency Score; CI = confidence interval for combined sets.

assist in clinical decision making, for example, on patient transfer to an intensive care unit (Tables 2 and 3).

▶ Patients with Guillain-Barré syndrome (GBS) often present a great challenge to the intensivist because most patients will make a complete and full recovery as long as we prevent complications of critical illness and pay attention to details.[1] One of the important complications to recognize and address as early as possible is respiratory failure. This trial identified a large number of patients with GBS and identified findings that were associated with the need for mechanical ventilatory support. Approximately 22% of the patients in the development cohort required mechanical ventilatory support. The 3 factors associated with a need for ventilatory support from the development cohort were then prospectively studied in an evaluation cohort of patients in which 14% required ventilatory support. The 3 factors, Medical Research Council sum score, rate of disease progression, and the presence of facial/bulbar weakness are easy to recognize and would suggest more severe GBS that would be expected to cause a higher risk of respiratory failure.

The ability to determine which GBS patients have a high risk for developing respiratory failure allows the intensivist time to plan for a semielective intubation or even an early tracheostomy. This would decrease the risk associated with emergent intubation. To establish the clinical benefit associated with this clinical tool, we need a prospective evaluation to confirm that the predictive index will continue to predict the GBS patients with a high risk for respiratory failure and need for ventilatory assistance.

R. A. Balk, MD

Reference

1. Dhar R, Stitt L, Hahn AF. The morbidity and outcome of patients with Guillain-Barré syndrome admitted to the intensive care unit. *J Neurol Sci.* 2008;264: 121-128.

The case against confirmatory tests for determining brain death in adults
Wijdicks EFM (Mayo Clinic, Rochester, MN)
Neurology 75:77-83, 2010

The determination of brain death is based on a comprehensive clinical assessment. A confirmatory test—at least, in adult patients in the United States—is not mandatory, but it typically is used as a safeguard or added when findings on clinical examination are unwontedly incomplete. In other countries, confirmatory tests are mandatory; in many, they are optional. These tests can be divided into those that test the brain's electrical function and those that test cerebral blood flow. A false-positive result (i.e., the test result suggests brain death, but clinically the patient does not meet the criteria) is not common but has been described for tests frequently used to determine brain death. A false-negative result (i.e., the test result suggests intact brain function, but clinically the patient meets the criteria) in one test may result in more confirmatory tests and no resolution when the test results diverge. Also, pathologic studies have shown that considerable areas of viable brain tissue may remain in patients who meet the clinical criteria of brain death, a fact that makes these tests less diagnostic. Confirmatory tests are residua from earlier days of refining comatose states. A comprehensive clinical examination, when performed by skilled examiners, should have perfect diagnostic accuracy.

▶ Determining and declaring a patient brain dead requires skill and compassion. Although the exact rules for determining brain death may differ from state to state, the general concept remains the same. Determining brain death typically requires a patient to fail a comprehensive neurologic examination other than reflexive activity. Commonly, the requirement is for the clinicians to perform 2 tests, set a number of hours apart after ensuring certain exclusions are not met. The second examination sometimes includes additional tests like an apnea test. When it is simply not possible to reliably perform this sequence secondary to clinical status, then ancillary tests are usually used. For instance, when a patient has a simultaneous C1-C2 fracture dislocation with cord transaction and a significant traumatic brain event, one would not be able to perform all aspects of the clinical examination, and certainly, one would not be able to perform an apnea test. This author suggests that these ancillary tests are simply not necessary and that the clinical examination is sufficient. In this opinion piece, the author suggests that false positives occur. It is unclear why this should ever be the case, as the ancillary tests should not be performed if the clinical examination does not warrant their use. False negatives are also cited as a concern. The question should not be whether or not false negatives exist, but rather in such scenarios, is it better to declare brain death or to pause? The answer to this question is not a simple yes or no but lies in the perspective used. The safest approach if one desires to be cautious about declaring brain death is to wait an additional period of time and repeat the test. If one is most concerned about the viability of organs for transplant, then a different conclusion may be reached. Because our ethical standards require that we stay focused on the patient in front of us, who has not yet met the criteria for death, it seems prudent to accept a cautious stance, despite the subsequent clinical or financial impact.

T. Dorman, MD

Transfusions and long-term functional outcomes in traumatic brain injury
Warner MA, O'Keeffe T, Bhavsar P, et al (Univ of Texas Southwestern Med Ctr, Dallas; Arizona Health Sciences Ctr, Tucson)
J Neurosurg 113:539-546, 2010

Object.—In this paper, the authors' goal was to examine the relationship between transfusion and long-term functional outcomes in moderately anemic patients (lowest hematocrit [HCT] level 21–30%) with traumatic brain injury (TBI). While evidence suggests that transfusions are associated with poor hospital outcomes, no study has examined transfusions and long-term functional outcomes in this population. The preferred transfusion threshold remains controversial.

Methods.—The authors performed a retrospective review of patients who were admitted with TBI between September 2005 and November 2007, extracting data such as HCT level, status of red blood cell transfusion, admission Glasgow Coma Scale (GCS) score, serum glucose, and length of hospital stay. Outcome measures assessed at 6 months were Glasgow Outcome Scale-Extended score, Functional Status Examination score, and patient death. A multivariate generalized linear model controlling for confounding variables was used to assess the association between transfusion and outcome.

Results.—During the study period, 292 patients were identified, and 139 (47.6%) met the criteria for moderate anemia. Roughly half (54.7%) underwent transfusions. Univariate analyses showed significant correlations between outcome score and patient age, admission GCS score, head Abbreviated Injury Scale score, number of days with an HCT level < 30%, highest glucose level, number of days with a glucose level > 200 mg/dl, length of hospital stay, number of patients receiving a transfusion, and transfusion volume. In multivariate analysis, admission

GCS score, receiving a transfusion, and transfusion volume were the only variables associated with outcome (F = 2.458, p = 0.007; F = 11.694, p = 0.001; and F = 1.991, p = 0.020, respectively). There was no association between transfusion and death.

Conclusions.—Transfusions may contribute to poor long-term functional outcomes in anemic patients with TBI. Transfusion strategies should be aimed at patients with symptomatic anemia or physiological compromise, and transfusion volume should be minimized.

▶ Maintenance of adequate oxygenation of brain tissue following traumatic brain injury (TBI) is a central tenet of the management of such patients and has been demonstrated to be associated with improved outcomes in this patient population. However, transfusion of packed red blood cells (PRBCs) has been equivocal in its utility to achieve this therapeutic goal, and in a significant proportion of patients, it has even been associated with diminished tissue oxygen tension. In this retrospective study, the authors sought to evaluate the relationship between PRBC transfusion and long-term functional outcomes in moderately anemic patients (those with hematocrits between 21% and 30%) suffering from TBI. In the multivariate analysis, the only factors associated with worse functional outcomes were admission Glasgow Coma Score, receipt of PRBC transfusion, and transfusion volume. To assess the impact of transfusion on long-term functional outcome by severity of TBI subgroup analysis was then performed. Among those with mild TBI, receiving a transfusion and transfusion volume were both associated with poor functional outcome; among those with severe TBI, receiving a transfusion was associated with poor functional outcome. There were insufficient patients with moderate TBI to generate statistically meaningful findings. This study suggests that in the head-injured population, similar to many other critically ill and injured patient populations, despite the deleterious effects of anemia and the importance of adequate tissue oxygenation, transfusion of PRBC may not be an effective means of meeting these needs, and the adverse effects of PRBC may in fact often outweigh their frequently limited benefits. Further study is needed to define what population, if any, of TBI patients may benefit from PRBC transfusion and at what hemoglobin/hematocrit or tissue oxygenation threshold.

D. R. Gerber, DO

12 Ethics/Socioeconomic/ Administrative Issues

Miscellaneous

Conflicts in the ICU: perspectives of administrators and clinicians

Danjoux Meth N, Lawless B, Hawryluck L (Critical Care Secretariat, Toronto, Ontario, Canada; St Michael's Hosp, Toronto, Ontario, Canada; Univ Health Network, Toronto, Ontario, Canada)
Intensive Care Med 35:2068-2077, 2009

Purpose.—The purpose of this study is to understand conflicts in the ICU setting as experienced by clinicians and administrators and explore methods currently used to resolve such conflicts when there may be discordance between clinicians and families, caregivers or administration.

Methods.—Qualitative case study methodology using semi-structured interviews was used. The sample included community and academic health science centres in 16 hospitals from across the province of Ontario, Canada. A total of 42 participants including hospital administrators and ICU clinicians were interviewed. Participants were sampled purposively to ensure representation.

Results.—The most common source of conflict in the ICU is a result of disagreement about the goals of treatment. Such conflicts arise between the ICU and referring teams (inter-team), among members of the ICU team (intra-team), and between the ICU team and patients' family/substitute decision-maker (SDM). Inter- and intra-team conflicts often contribute to conflicts between the ICU team and families. Various themes were identified as contributing factors that may influence conflict resolution practices as well as the various consequences and challenges of conflict situations. Limitations of current conflict resolution policies were revealed as well as suggested strategies to improve practice.

Conclusions.—There is considerable variability in dealing with conflicts in the ICU. Greater attention is needed at a systems level to support a culture aimed at prevention and resolution of conflicts to avoid increased sources of anxiety, stress and burnout.

▶ The intensive care unit (ICU) is an emotionally charged environment where patients and their families experience daily stress and doubt. It is the responsibility of the medical team to try to alleviate feelings of uncertainty by presenting information in a confident and cohesive manner. The size of a medical team involved in the daily care of 1 patient can be quite large and includes nurses, clinicians of various subspecialties, and hospital administrators, including bioethicists and social workers. Given the large and complex size of the team, discordance and conflict are bound to arise among the members. Thus, it becomes quite challenging to appear as a consistent and united team to patients about the goals of care. This discordance can only exacerbate a patient's and/or family's anxiety and may lead to distrust or lack of confidence in the competency of a team.

It is important to first recognize how and where conflicts arise to properly prevent and resolve them. This article sampled a large cross-section of typical ICU team members at both academic and community centers in Canada.

The article identified several types of inter- and intrateam conflicts that are centered on the same simple question: is ICU admission warranted? There seems to be a sense that if a patient has a predicted poor outcome, there is comfort in knowing that at least all the available measures to provide the best care were taken and that often includes ICU admission, appropriate or not. While there are differing expectations among teams about the goals of treatment, there should at least be agreement that the ICU is neither palliative nor a necessary avenue to avoid death. The problem of resource allocation and availability also appears to be a major factor in both inter- and intrateam conflicts. This may be especially prominent in Canada, where resources are openly considered limited and finite. In the United States, however, this is not a fully accepted notion among physicians and families. There is a general sense that every patient should and will receive all measures of care regardless of expense and availability.

Conflicts may be alleviated in the ICU by clearly elaborating goals of treatment and consensus on expectations among families and health care teams. Communication is the key to avoiding inter- and intrateam conflicts. Families often have unrealistic expectations not only because they lack or misuse information, but they also have an emotional imperative to preserve a loved one regardless of means or outcome. This only further highlights the importance of medical professionals to provide a cohesive front so as not to cause more confusion and anxiety for patients. The attempt to classify the source of these problems will aid the medical community to more systematically understand and resolve conflicts in the ICU. System-wide adoption of a conflict resolution standard of care, as suggested by the authors, has the potential to minimize damage when conflicts arise. Certainly, in stressful ICUs where life and death issues are being discussed, conflict between patients, families, and physicians or among providers themselves will always occur. Importantly, physicians need to feel supported by hospital administrators, as they attempt to resolve the conflict. This support becomes evident when a hospital-wide policy regarding conflict resolution is clearly stated and standardized. Involvement of patients and their families in the decision-making process provides an opportunity to educate patients and families and give them a sense of autonomy. This education may represent the best defense against family insistence on inappropriate treatment. Early identification of these conflicts and a system-wide, multidisciplinary, standardized response involving staff and patients' families are the keys to rapid resolution of conflict in the ICU setting.

M. Balasta, BA
A. D. Fesnak, BS
V. K. Rajput, MD

Deferred proxy consent in emergency critical care research: Ethically valid and practically feasible
Jansen TC, Kompanje EJO, Bakker J (Erasmus MC Univ Med Ctr Rotterdam, The Netherlands)
Crit Care Med 37:S65-S68, 2009

Important ethical aspects apply to the process of obtaining consent in emergency critical care research: the incapacity of almost all patients for giving informed consent and the emergency and life-threatening nature of the conditions involved, resulting in short therapeutic time frames. We argue that deferred proxy consent is the preferable substitute for informed patient consent in emergency critical care research. However, researchers can face two problems when using this consent procedure. First, can proxies give a valid judgment for consent or refusal in the acute phase of the life-threatening illness of their relative, and second, what should researchers do with already obtained data when study procedures are finished (e.g., because the patient has died) before proxies can be informed and consent be sought? We propose approaching the relatives with information about the trial and asking them for consent only if it is ethically valid to do so. The first psychological distress may prohibit a complete understanding of the information, which is necessary for a true and valid informed proxy consent. In addition, we recommend using the study data if study procedures are finished before proxies can be informed and consent be sought, provided sufficient privacy measures have been applied.

▶ Research in critical care holds many unique challenges, especially obtaining consent to participate in a clinical trial. Deferred consent has been a heavily debated topic, which involves enrolling a patient in a trial and beginning study protocols before getting consent. Details of the study are later discussed with the patient or the family who can grant or deny participation in the study. Informed consent and asking relatives for substitute judgment are both problematic in emergency situations. Authors of this article support deferred proxy consent as an ethical way to conduct critical care research and recommend guidelines for using data from patients who have died before researchers can ask for consent.

Consent by proxy is an ethically questionable practice because relatives do not always accurately represent the patient's philosophy about life and death situations and can be emotionally compromised. Relatives frequently do not decide as a patient would himself, and the surrogate is not always the person whom the patient would choose as a representative. Family members may not be present to give consent and a patient can consequently miss a therapeutic window for an experimental intervention. Moreover, relatives can be in a state of psychological crisis in which they are not competent to understand the facts of a clinical trial and make an informed decision. Asking relatives for consent during times of psychological stress is not recommended because they can be temporarily incompetent when told that their loved one has a poor prognosis.

The authors believe that the inability to give informed consent, when unconscious or cognitively impaired, should not preclude critically ill patients from the benefits of clinical research. Additionally, studies should enroll patients during the best time to test for a treatment effect to guarantee a valid study. The results of the pulmonary artery catheters in management of patients in intensive care (PAC-man) trial illustrate the difficulties of getting informed consent with a critically ill population. Only 2.6% of patients of 500 were able to give informed consent themselves and 81.2% had consent given by a relative.[1] It is beneficent and just to include critically ill patients in trials where deferred consent is used and informed consent is not feasible.

Critically ill populations have high mortality rates, and one of the controversial aspects of deferred consent is whether or not to include data from patients who unfortunately died before consent was obtained. The PAC-man trial showed that of 500 critically ill patients, there was a 60.6% mortality rate.[1] Should a patient die before consent is granted, the authors advocate that it is ethical to include the deceased patient's data in the study without asking for consent. Study procedures and data collection will have already been done. Refusing participation in the study at that point will only introduce selection bias and compromise the validity of the study.

With growing concern that patients would be exploited, the United States tightened regulations on studies that did not require informed consent. In 1992, The Office of Human Research Protections limited the use of deferred consent to studies that posed minimal risk to patients, mainly limiting its use to data collection.[2] However, many researchers disputed the new guideline on behalf of patients who would want experimental treatment in a life-threatening situation but could not participate because they could not give prospective consent. This led to a revision of the guidelines that now state that deferred consent can be used in life-threatening situations, when getting consent is not feasible, and when participation may benefit the patient. Additionally, minimal risk was replaced with appropriate incremental risk, which compares risk of the intervention with the condition of the patient rather than activities of daily life.[2] Deferred consent is rarely used in the United States because of the strict guidelines, which limit its use to data collection and treatment of critical conditions that have no standard effective therapy.

Emergency situations such as head trauma, catastrophic cardiovascular events, and sepsis are just a few conditions that researchers are targeting to improve outcomes and decrease mortality. Unfortunately, getting informed consent is not feasible when patients are unconscious and there is a small therapeutic window. In a limited number of situations, United States guidelines allow the use of deferred consent when it is in the best interest of the patient. Although not ideal, deferred proxy consent is an ethically appropriate alternative to informed consent because when used in correct situations it can produce valid study results and give therapeutic benefit to patients.

K. Keselowsky, BS

V. K. Rajput, MD

References

1. Harvey SE, Elbourne D, Ashcroft J, Jones CM, Rowan K. Informed consent in clinical trials in critical care: experience from the PAC-Man Study. *Intensive Care Med.* 2006;32:2020-2025.
2. Luce JM. Informed consent for clinical research involving patients with chest disease in the United States. *Chest.* 2009;135:1061-1068.

Do hospitals provide lower quality of care to black patients for pneumonia?
Mayr FB, Yende S, D'Angelo G, et al (Univ of Pittsburgh, PA; Washington Univ School of Medicine, St Louis, MO)
Crit Care Med 38:759-765, 2010

Objectives.—Recent studies reported lower quality of care for black vs. white patients with community-acquired pneumonia and suggested that disparities persist at the individual hospital level. We examined racial differences in emergency department and intensive care unit care processes to determine whether differences persist after adjusting for case-mix and variation in care across hospitals.

Design.—Prospective, observational cohort study.

Setting.—Twenty-eight U.S. hospitals.

Patients.—Patients with community-acquired pneumonia: 1738 white and 352 black patients.

Interventions.—None.

Measurements.—We compared care quality based on antibiotic receipt within 4 hrs and adherence to American Thoracic Society antibiotic guidelines, and intensity based on intensive care unit admission and mechanical ventilation use. Using random effects and generalized estimating equations models, we adjusted for case-mix and clustering of racial groups within hospitals and estimated odds ratios for differences in care within and across hospitals.

Main Results.—Black patients were less likely to receive antibiotics within 4 hrs (odds ratio, 0.55; 95% confidence interval, 0.43–0.70; $p < .001$) and less likely to receive guideline-adherent antibiotics (odds ratio, 0.72; 95% confidence interval, 0.57–0.91; $p = .006$). These differences were attenuated after adjusting for casemix (odds ratio, 0.59; 95% confidence interval; 0.46–0.76 and 0.84; 95% confidence interval, 0.66–1.09). Within hospitals, black and white patients received similar care quality (odds ratio, 1; 95% confidence interval, 0.97–1.04 and 1; 95% confidence interval, 0.97–1.03). However, hospitals that served a greater proportion of black patients were less likely to provide timely antibiotics (odds ratio, 0.84; 95% confidence interval, 0.78–0.90). Black patients were more likely to receive mechanical ventilation (odds ratio, 1.57; 95% confidence interval, 1.02–2.42; $p = .042$). Again, within hospitals, black and white subjects were equally likely to receive mechanical ventilation (odds ratio, 1; 95% confidence interval, .94–1.06) and hospitals that served a greater proportion of black patients were more likely to institute mechanical ventilation (odds ratio, 1.13; 95% confidence interval, 1.02–1.25).

Conclusions.—Black patients appear to receive lower quality and higher intensity of care in crude analyses. However, these differences were explained by different case-mix and variation in care across hospitals. Within the same hospital, no racial differences in care were observed.

▶ The United States health care system has been shown to provide a lower quality of care for African Americans when compared with Caucasians.[1] Physicians and health care systems have been aware of this disparity in health care delivery and have sought ways to correct it. Recently, closer monitoring of core health care measures, such as breast cancer screening and testing of low-density lipoprotein cholesterol, in managed health care plans has led to higher-quality health care, which in turn has helped decrease the disparities in care between Caucasians and African Americans.[2] However, despite these changes, disparities are still a reality between both groups.

This prospective observational cohort study evaluated the quality of care for black and white patients with community-acquired pneumonia (CAP) to discern any disparities of care. Patients were recruited from 28 hospitals in Pennsylvania, Connecticut, Michigan, and Tennessee. Quality of care for pneumonia was defined as the delivery of antibiotics within 4 hours and adherence to American Thoracic Society antibiotic guidelines. It was found in the crude analysis that black patients were less likely to receive antibiotics within 4 hours of diagnosis of CAP and so received lower quality of care, as the guidelines for antibiotic administration had not been met. Linking quality of care to receipt of antibiotics within 4 hours is troublesome, as it has been shown that the rush to start antibiotics within 4 hours has led to inappropriate use of antibiotics and inaccurate diagnosis of CAP, both signs of suboptimal care.[3] In addition, while measuring the time of antibiotic administration evaluates the efficiency of care and adherence to a protocol, it may not be the most optimal measure for the effectiveness or quality of care. This underlines the problem that there is no true gold standard for quality of care to be measured and explains why medical society guidelines and recommendations are often used.

Interestingly, it was found in this study that hospitals that served a greater proportion of black patients were less likely to provide timely antibiotics. It has been shown that hospitals with a high proportion of black patients had worse performance scores on pneumonia core measures.[4] Many of these hospitals with large black patient populations are often academic teaching centers. Targeting those select institutions for improvement may lead to an increase in the quality of health care and diminish health care disparities.

When this study examined the care given within hospitals, there was no difference in the quality or the intensity of care (as measured by admission to the intensive care unit and use of mechanical ventilation) between black and white patients. This suggests that it may be the variation in health care across hospitals that cause disparities in health care. More research will be required in this area to fully answer that question.

More effort and resources should be directed at hospitals that are underperforming and providing lower quality of care, especially hospitals that have large proportions of minorities. This may be the most effective solution to decreasing racial disparities in medicine.

S. Patel, MD

V. K. Rajput, MD

References

1. Schneider EC, Zaslavsky AM, Epstein AM. Racial disparities in the quality of care for enrollees in Medicare managed care. *JAMA.* 2002;287:1288-1294.
2. Trivedi AN, Zaslavsky AM, Schneider EC, Ayanian JZ. Trends in the quality of care and racial disparities in Medicare managed care. *N Engl J Med.* 2005;353: 692-700.
3. Kanwar M, Brar N, Khatib R, Fakih MG. Misdiagnosis of community-acquired pneumonia and inappropriate utilization of antibiotics side effects of the 4-h antibiotic administration rule. *Chest.* 2007;131:1865-1869.
4. Jha AK, Orav EJ, Li Z, Epstein AM. Concentration and quality of hospitals that care for elderly black patients. *Arch Intern Med.* 2007;167:1177-1182.

Is Rapid Organ Recovery a Good Idea? An Exploratory Study of the Public's Knowledge and Attitudes
DuBois JM, Waterman AD, Iltis A, et al (Saint Louis Univ, MO; Washington Univ School of Medicine, St Louis, MO)
Am J Transplant 9:2392-2399, 2009

In 2006, the Institute of Medicine (IOM) recommended demonstration projects on uncontrolled donation after cardiac death or rapid organ recovery (ROR). To investigate what the public thinks about key ethical and policy questions associated with ROR, 70 African-American, Caucasian and Latino community members in St. Louis, MO, participated in focus groups and completed surveys, before and after being educated about ROR. Before the focus group, most participants believed mistakenly that they could donate organs following an unexpected cardiac arrest (76%). After the focus group, 84% would want to donate organs after unexpected cardiac arrest; 81% would support organ cooling to enable this. The public generally supported organ cooling without family consent if the individual had joined the donor registry, but were mixed in their opinions about what should be done if they were not on the registry. African-American and Latino participants expressed greater fears than Caucasians that if they consented to organ donation, physicians might do less to save their life; however, support for ROR was not significantly lower in these subgroups. Although this study is exploratory, public support for ROR was present. We recommend that adequate consent processes and safeguards be established to foster trust and support for ROR.

▶ While giving hope to those who had none in previous years, transplant medicine has unfortunately become a victim of its own success; the list of potential recipients has always outpaced the prospective donors, with that lead continuously growing. In an effort to expand the pool of qualified donors, investigations into the practicality of organ recovery after uncontrolled donation after cardiac death (uDCD), also known as rapid organ recovery (ROR), and non-heart beating organ donation were recommended by the Institute of Medicine. This process of temporarily stabilizing organs in situ, following unexpected circulatory collapse (often without family consent because of time constraint), has yet to be adopted in the United States but is widely supported in Europe.

This article surveyed the public's perception of ROR and the possible societal response if this protocol was implemented. Besides revealing a general unfamiliarity with current donation restrictions, the study exposes an overall support for ROR for known consenting donors across racial groups. However, many of these supporters had not consented to being donors themselves. This incongruity could be because of a personal fear concerning donation. Although people realize that donation is beneficial to society, their next words might be "but I could never do that." In the event of a patient of unknown consent status following uDCD, the surveyed public was in favor of pre-emptive organ preservation via catheter insertion until family or proxy could be contacted to express their wishes. European countries have used a presumed consent for nearly 30 years, with a significant increase in the donor pool.[1] The success of this approach may be because of the decidedly more liberal nature of Western European societies and the more homogenous populations involved. Also revealed was a general distrust in the African-American and Latino communities that donor consent would correlate to a less fervent attempt by physicians to save their lives, a distrust that has been well documented in the past.[2] This distrust would only be reinforced with the notion that the teams tasked with saving the patient's life would be the very same ones that initialized the recovery protocol. A test ROR program run in the Washington, DC, area showed that maintaining 2 separate teams was impractical because of manpower and expense constraints.[3] A suspicious public would certainly only grow more hesitant of consenting to organ endowment knowing these circumstances, especially given the long-standing and deep-rooted mistrust between minority groups and the majority over all aspects of society.

Additional education and donation enrollment will not solve the shortage program, but it may buy some time before the ethical quandaries of ROR are ironed out.

V. K. Rajput, MD

References

1. Michielsen P. Presumed consent to organ donation: 10 years' experience in Belgium. *J R Soc Med.* 1996;89:663-666.

2. Siminoff LA, Burant CJ, Ibrahim SA. Racial disparities in preferences and perceptions regarding organ donation. *J Gen Intern Med.* 2006;21:995-1000.

3. Light JA. The Washington, D.C. experience with uncontrolled donation after circulatory determination of death: promises and pitfalls. *J Law Med Ethics.* 2008;36:735-740.

Organ Donation: A Portrait of Family Refusal in Québec
Baran D, Langevin S, Lebeau C (McGill Univ Health Centre/Royal Victoria Hosp, Montréal, Canada; Centre Hospitalier Affilié Universitaire de Québec/ Hôpital de l'Enfant-Jésus, Québec, Canada; Québec-Transplant, Canada)
Transplant Proc 41:3281-3283, 2009

Many studies from around the world have reported different reasons why families refuse organ donation. In Quebec, however, there are no known data on the subject. To enable us to better communicate with families, a research project was conducted from January to December 2007 in hospital centers with personnel who specialize in supporting families. Our objective was to identify the reasons why Quebecers refuse a request for organ donation. The findings demonstrate that knowing the express wishes of the deceased person about organ donation and end-of-life treatment influences the family. When these wishes are not known, the partners of older donors refuse in greater numbers, primarily for familial or circumstantial reasons. Refusal based on religion or ethnicity is rare. Some families approached before neurologic death is diagnosed do not wish to wait until all the criteria for neurologic death are met.

▶ A visit to a hospital-bound loved one is an emotionally charged event for any person; to complicate that encounter with the loved one's shrugging off the mortal coil is to elevate the situation to an entirely new level. The marvels of modern medicine have managed to create an even more affecting toll. For all of the benefit that organ transplantation has offered to the world, a heavy price is often unmentioned; with rare exception, healthy organs can only be procured by the life of another. Temporal constraints require that the attending physician must make a request to the deceased's family for harvest. This time-sensitive yet highly emotional step can result in the refusal by the family. It would be foolish and extremely irresponsible of physicians to not investigate the causes given by families when they say no.

While a set number of refusals are based on the straightforward explanation that it was against the patient's wishes or the family was unsure of the patient's belief in donation, that component accounted for a little more than 40% of refusals. Add in the patient's refusal to be maintained on life support, that percentage reaches only 50%. Of that remaining half, 40% were attributed to factors based on the neurological determination of death, primarily the time delay between the first indication of brain death and the required passage of time to satisfy all criteria. The interesting aspect of this study was the often intangible aspects of donation requests: the who, where, and how. Perhaps unsurprising, the families of those patients who died in the intensive care setting donated more often as opposed to those in the emergency department, secondary to the extra time given to families to cope, which the intensive care unit provided. The use of a physician to make the request, either with or without a resource nurse, had the highest percentage of donation.

While the study was limited to Québec, the motivations for refusal seem to be quite universal. A study from Spain reiterated the same findings that the patient's wish not to donate was the primary cause, and barring known wishes, the family's uncertainty concerning the deceased's desires was the second most common factor.[1] Further exploration of the patient's initial wish against organ donation is required so as to formulate public health campaigns that directly target these beliefs. Explanation was not given in either the Québec or Spain studies for the initial refusal, and it would be curious to see if the mistrust of the medical profession, a complaint often given by minority populations in the United States, is a contributor to the hesitance to donate.[2]

B. J. Smith, BS
V. K. Rajput, MD

References

1. Frutos MA, Ruiz P, Requena MV, Daga D. Family refusal in organ donation: analysis of three patterns. *Transplant Proc.* 2002;34:2513-2514.
2. Siminoff LA, Burant CJ, Ibrahim SA. Racial disparities in preferences and perceptions regarding organ donation. *J Gen Intern Med.* 2006;21:995-1000.

Patients' preferences for enrolment into critical-care trials
Scales DC, Smith OM, Pinto R, et al (Univ of Toronto, Ontario, Canada; Sunnybrook Health Science Centre, Toronto, Ontario, Canada; et al)
Intensive Care Med 35:1703-1712, 2009

Background.—Most critically ill patients are incapable of providing informed consent for research.

Objective.—We sought to determine patients' preferences for different consent frameworks for enrolling incapable patients into critical-care trials.

Design.—Prospective observational and structured interview study.

Setting.—Five university-affiliated hospitals in Ontario.

Patients.—Two-hundred and forty consecutive capable and consenting survivors of critical illness.

Intervention.—Participants considered four frameworks for enrolling incapable patients into clinical trials using a baseline scenario and three permutations for: risk (very low vs. high), treatment type (new vs. currently available), and availability of substitute decision-maker (yes vs. no).

Measurements and Main Results.—For each scenario, patients chose their preferred framework and rated the acceptability of each framework using a seven-point Likert scale. Most (180/240; 76%) patients selected "consent by substitute prior to enrolment" as their preferred framework; this also received the highest baseline acceptability ratings ("acceptable" or "highly acceptable" 207/240; 87%). Modifying risk or treatment type did not substantially change these ratings. A minority of patients rated delayed consent as unacceptable or highly unacceptable in both the baseline scenario (48/240, 20% delayed to substitute; 57/240, 24% delayed to patient) and when a substitute was unavailable (34/240; 15%).

Conclusions.—Most survivors of critical illness found the usual practice of obtaining informed consent from a substitute decision-maker prior to enrolment in a clinical trial to be acceptable. Nearly half of patients considered foregoing informed consent to be unacceptable, whereas a minority considered enrolment followed by delayed consent to be unacceptable even when a substitute was unavailable. These approaches should, therefore, only be considered when deviating from the usual practice of obtaining consent from a substitute decision-maker is truly justified, such as where treatments being tested need to be delivered as soon as possible in order to be effective.

► In critically ill patients, treatment success is usually time dependent. When sufficient equipoise exists between 2 treatment options, or a treatment option and doing nothing, researchers need to be able to ascertain that the experimental treatments meet the ideals of beneficence and nonmaleficence. Given this time-dependent need, the clinical equipoise, and the impaired rational decision-making capacity of patients (due to the severity of their illness and therapies received), clinical trials need an alternative enrollment strategy.

This article establishes normative values for patient wishes based on information given to the families and a surrogate decision maker. The data illustrate the extent to which critically ill patients are comfortable being enrolled in clinical trials by consent from a substitute decision maker before enrollment. These data enable physician-researchers to make a descriptive claim; that is, they are able to make a judgment based on data, rather than expert ethical opinion, as to the appropriate enrollment framework for incapacitated patients.

A more ethically murky area is what to do when a surrogate is not available. In this study, patients preferred enrollment and delayed consent over no consent. A study by Cook et al[1] also concludes that intensivists and researchers prefer a delayed consent process over no consent at all.

It is remarkably selfless that patients trust surrogate decision makers to enroll them in clinical trials mainly aimed to improve therapeutics of future patients. How often do surrogates make the right decision? A recent meta-analysis by Shalowitz et al[2] shows that surrogate decision makers make concordant decisions with the patients' wishes in 68% of cases based on hypothetical case scenarios presented to participants in that study. This suggests that decisions regarding enrollment in clinical trials may need to be explicitly stated just as intubation and resuscitation are now.

J. E. McGinnis, BS
V. K. Rajput, MD

References

1. Cook DJ, Blythe D, Rischbieth A, et al. Enrollment of intensive care unit patients into clinical studies: a trinational survey of researchers' experiences, beliefs, and practices. *Crit Care Med.* 2008;36:2100-2105.
2. Shalowitz DI, Garrett-Mayer E, Wendler D. The accuracy of surrogate decision makers: a systematic review. *Arch Intern Med.* 2006;166:493-497.

Prevalence and Factors of Intensive Care Unit Conflicts: The Conflicus Study

Azoulay É, for the Conflicus Study Investigators and for the Ethics Section of the European Society of Intensive Care Medicine (Univ Paris-7 Paris-Diderot, France; et al)

Am J Respir Crit Care Med 180:853-860, 2009

Rationale.—Many sources of conflict exist in intensive care units (ICUs). Few studies recorded the prevalence, characteristics, and risk factors for conflicts in ICUs.

Objectives.—To record the prevalence, characteristics, and risk factors for conflicts in ICUs.

Methods.—One-day cross-sectional survey of ICU clinicians. Data on perceived conflicts in the week before the survey day were obtained from 7,498 ICU staff members (323 ICUs in 24 countries).

Measurements and Main Results.—Conflicts were perceived by 5,268 (71.6%) respondents. Nurse–physician conflicts were the most common (32.6%), followed by conflicts among nurses (27.3%) and staff-relative conflicts (26.6%). The most common conflict-causing behaviors were personal animosity, mistrust, and communication gaps. During end-of-life care, the main sources of perceived conflict were lack of psychological support, absence of staff meetings, and problems with the decision-making process. Conflicts perceived as severe were reported by 3,974 (53%) respondents. Job strain was significantly associated with perceiving conflicts and with greater severity of perceived conflicts. Multivariate analysis identified 15 factors associated with perceived conflicts, of which 6 were potential targets for future intervention: staff working more than 40 h/wk, more than 15 ICU beds, caring for dying patients or providing pre- and postmortem care within the last week, symptom control not ensured jointly by physicians and nurses, and no routine unit-level meetings.

Conclusions.—Over 70% of ICU workers reported perceived conflicts, which were often considered severe and were significantly associated with job strain. Workload, inadequate communication, and end-of-life care emerged as important potential targets for improvement.

▶ In any setting where there are at least 2 people working in concert, a conflict will be a near inevitability. Place those colleagues in an environment with an inherent stress level greater than most other places, and conflict becomes a question of when and not just if. For all the settings of a hospital, the intensive care unit (ICU) has to be one of the tensest surroundings for an already high-pressure milieu. Ever-observant health care workers have already recognized this concern, previously studying various potential causes and even the effect of dispute on the quality of care; however, the prevalence of conflict and a broad look at potential factors have not been thoroughly scrutinized.

Given the vast cast of actors within an ICU, the origins of conflict are innumerable. The health care worker, be it physician or nursing staff, must deal not only with the physical maladies of the patient but also the complex interactions of the deathly ill with their respective loved ones. The families of the hospitalized must not only work through the emotional mire; they must also sift through the information being presented by the physician staff, especially in terms of end-of-life care. With the intricacy of ICU-based interaction, it should not be surprising that approximately 70% of staff reported perceived conflicts, and families noted conflict rates of up to 80%. One significant form of conflict that was conveyed was the perception of a disregard for nursing input by physicians concerning decision making. Other sources of potential conflict presented by the article have been documented by additional studies as well, including higher staff-to-patient ratios and family perceptions of poor communication between themselves and staff.[1] Interestingly, the role of ethics training for hospital staff increased the perception of conflicts, and this factor was accounted for as a form of selection bias.

A point to be noted in this study was based on the perception of conflict; it is quite possible that it was only a single party who felt there was a conflict present. This argument could be entangled with the higher percentage of dispute reported by those with ethics training; some individuals may be quicker to call something a conflict, while the other party may feel the complete opposite. That possibility notwithstanding, the overarching theme in this study seems to be that a breakdown in communication is the prime cause of ICU-based disputes. Whether it is the nurses being too overloaded with work preventing them from fully interacting with patients and their families or the nursing staff feeling that their input is being ignored by the physicians, the fundamental need to interconnect effectively with all present parties is not being completed.

B. J. Smith, BS

V. K. Rajput, MD

Reference

1. Stricker KH, Kimberger O, Schmidlin K, Zwahlen M, Mohr U, Rothen HU. Family satisfaction in the intensive care unit: what makes the difference? *Intensive Care Med.* 2009;35:2051-2059.

Use of Intensive Care Services during Terminal Hospitalizations in England and the United States

Wunsch H, Linde-Zwirble WT, Harrison DA, et al (Columbia Univ, NY; ZD Associates, Perkasie, PA; Intensive Care Natl Audit & Res Centre, London, UK; et al)
Am J Respir Crit Care Med 180:875-880, 2009

Rationale.—Despite broad concern regarding the provision and cost of health care at the end of life, country-specific patterns of care have rarely been compared.

Objectives.—To assess the use of hospital and intensive care services during terminal hospitalizations in England and the United States, two populations with similar socioeconomic backgrounds and life expectancies.

Methods.—Retrospective cohort study over a 1-year period (2001) using national (England) Hospital Episode Statistics, and regional (seven U.S. states) administrative discharge data as well as English and U.S. census data. We measured hospitalization rates and death rates during hospitalization with and without intensive care.

Measurements and Main Results.—Age-adjusted acute hospitalization rates were 110.5 per 1,000 population in England versus 105.3 in the seven U.S. states, with the same mortality rate (0.9 per 1,000 population) in both countries. Of all deaths, 50.3% occurred in hospital in England and 36.6% in the United States, yet only 5.1% of all deaths in England involved intensive care, versus 17.2% in the United States, representing 10.1% of hospital deaths in England versus 47.1% in the United States. Greater intensive care use in the U.S. was most notable with older age; among decedents 85+ years, intensive care was used for 31.5% of medical deaths and 61.0% of surgical deaths in the United States versus 1.9 and 8.5% of deaths in England.

Conclusions.—Despite similar overall hospitalization rates in England and the United States, there were marked differences in terminal hospitalizations, with far greater use of intensive care services in the United States, especially among medical patients and the elderly population.

▶ The comparison of different health care systems is an incredibly complex task, and one must first reflect upon several basic questions before undertaking that challenge. This study proposed that contrasting hospitalization, intensive care unit (ICU) use, and mortality between England and the United States would provide insight into the provision and cost of end-of-life care. Wunsch et al ask whether the use of intensive care services is high, low, or similar in the United States compared with other countries, assuming that there is indeed a standard or correct rubric upon which to compare. Given the similar life expectancy rates at birth and at 65 years and the overall age distribution, England was a good choice for comparison.

England's health care system, however, differs from the United States' in both structure and basic social premise. England's National Health Service (NHS) is available for all its residents and is funded by government taxes; there are few private options for individuals. The United States has a complex and often disjointed system of private and government insurance that is funded by self, employers, state taxes, and federal taxes. If individuals do not receive health care benefits through an employer nor qualify for government-sponsored aid, then they join the growing uninsured or underinsured population in the United States. Because of its size and mission, the NHS must openly enforce national budgets and rationing of services. This study reveals that while more deaths occurred among patients hospitalized in England, they used the ICU 4 times less than in the United States, and this difference was especially pronounced in the elderly population. In England, the "admission to intensive care is predicated on the balance between resources and the likelihood of benefit." This inherent value judgment is in stark contrast to the United States, where concepts of resource allocation and rationing are generally unacceptable.

This raises the question of whether comparison can lead to an applicable conclusion that affects how we provide care. Perhaps more patients die in England's hospitals because they underuse the ICU, or maybe the United States is simply overusing it. It would be difficult to tease out the truth because of the common belief that everything must be done to preserve life in the United States. A patient may expect aggressive care, and this in turn pressures clinicians to take more aggressive measures than is warranted. Clinicians in England seem to have much more say in end-of-life care than in the United States, and perhaps this translates into patients having less expectations of autonomy. Thus, physicians in England can have more control over resource allocation without the fear of censure, litigation, and emotional disturbance of not fulfilling patient expectations and current standards of practice.

In 2008, the United Kingdom spent 8.7% of its gross domestic product on health care versus over 15% in the United States (see Fig 1 in the original article), a number that is steadily climbing and predicted to be 17% in 2010. This discrepancy likely reflects the tangible and intangible differences of system structure, societal attitudes, patient expectations, and the role of a physician as a decision maker. While it may be difficult to agree on utility, validity, and applicability of comparing health care systems, it is still a valuable exercise. Beyond just gaining knowledge of how other systems function, it importantly allows us greater insight into the strengths and weaknesses of our own.

M. Balasta, BA

V. K. Rajput, MD

Quality of Life/End of Life/Outcome Prediction

End-of-life decisions in an Indian intensive care unit
Mani RK, Mandal AK, Bal S, et al (Fortis Flt Lt Rajan Dhall Hosp, Vasant Kunj, New Delhi, India)
Intensive Care Med 35:1713-1719, 2009

Background.—There is a paucity of data on end-of-life decisions (EOLD) for patients in Indian intensive care units (ICUs).

Objective.—To document the end-of-life and full-support (FS) decisions among patients dying in an ICU, to compare the respective patient characteristics and to describe the process of decision-making.

Design.—Retrospective, observational.

Patients.—Consecutive patients admitted to a 12-bed closed medical-surgical ICU.

Exclusions.—Patients with EOLD discharged home or transferred to another hospital.

Measurements and Results.—Demographic profile, APACHE IV at 24 h, ICU outcome, type of limitation, disease category, pre-admission functional status, reasons for EOLD, interventions and therapies within 3 days of death, time to EOLD, time to death after EOLD and ICU length of stay. Out of 88 deaths among 830 admissions, 49% were preceded by EOLD. Of these 58% had withholding of treatment, 35% had do-not-resuscitate orders (DNR) and 7% had a withdrawal decision. Mean age and APACHE IV scores were similar between EOLD and FS groups. Functional dependence before hospitalization favored EOLD. Patients receiving EOLD as opposed to FS had longer stays. Fifty-three percent of limitations were decided during the first week of ICU stay well before the time of death. Escalation of therapy within 3 days of death was less frequent in the EOLD group.

Conclusions.—Despite societal and legal barriers, half the patients dying in the ICU received a decision to limit therapy mostly as withholding or DNR orders. These decisions evolved early in the course of stay and resulted in significant reduction of therapeutic burdens.

▶ The decision to apply limits to the administration of medical or surgical interventions offered to patients in the intensive care unit (ICU) setting is complex. Seldom is the scope of the narrow doctor-patient dyad as widened as in this setting. Often included in decision making are not only the patient's family but also hospice directors, chaplains, and hospital ethics representatives, to name but a few. Communication between these interested parties is vital. Of particular importance is a clear understanding on the part of patients and their families as to what medical science can and cannot offer and thorough familiarity on the part of physicians as to their legal and ethical rights and responsibilities. The failure to communicate this crucial information can result in decisions by patients and their families to continue indefinitely futile and costly intervention, while physicians may retreat in frustration from any attempt to change this course out of fear of legal consequences. Challenges to effective communication arise at least in part from the social, cultural, religious, and legal context in which these decisions are made. The authors of this study sought to show that limitations to therapy can be discussed and agreed upon in an ethical manner in a significant number of cases of ICU admissions in an Indian hospital despite these challenges.

The unique Indian context of this study is one in which a public culture of fighting till the end is complemented by perceived risks of initiating or sustaining discussions of end-of-life decisions (EOLDs) on the part of physicians. One particularly undesirable outcome of this situation is that instances of patients who leave against medical advice (LAMA) is common, as the private-sector dominance of health care delivery promotes the decision to continue care without limits until the financial burden mounts to a level that patients and their families cannot bear. Care is then simply and abruptly withdrawn, which in this context is classified as LAMA. Furthermore, this approach of delivering full care until funds run out is tacitly welcome to physicians, who thereby circumvent perceived legal liability, according to the authors. As it is not uncommon for physicians in India to hold a financial stake in medical treatment over and above the consultations they provide, there exists a strong incentive to prolong futile care.

Roughly half of the families of patients in this study engaged in EOLD, with the remainder receiving full support, defined as provision of all measures needed to support hemodynamics, metabolism, and ventilation. Most patients and families who made EOLD decided to withhold life support, with advanced chronic disease and unresponsiveness to treatment being cited as the most typical reasons. From an economic point of view, these patients had fewer interventions performed and therefore generated a significantly reduced cost burden to their loved ones. What this means is that EOLD allows patients and their families to make well-informed and rational decisions about their care, while preventing or reducing paralyzing financial hardship. Perhaps more importantly, it offers a feeling of control over the conditions that ultimately allow for a good death.

This study suggests that implementing a strategy of early and gradual dialog, conducted in a formal way over days to weeks, can result in reaching consensus successfully among physicians, patients, and families. Family conferencing, which was regular and repeated, was effectively substituted for incidental bedside discussions of prognosis and treatment plan. It remains to be studied as to what degree more widespread physicians' understanding of their financial or legal rights in such matters may contribute to the success of these discussions. Specifically, physicians should be made to understand their right under the law to advise patients and their families about the possibility of withholding care, and their moral responsibility to do exactly that. In addition, further characterization of families' religious commitments and their application to EOLD, which was not possible in this study, would be of benefit in learning how to address their concerns.

T. C. Foster, PhD

V. K. Rajput, MD

Ethnic differences in do-not-resuscitate orders after intracerebral hemorrhage
Zahuranec DB, Brown DL, Lisabeth LD, et al (Univ of Michigan Med School, Ann Arbor; et al)
Crit Care Med 37:2807-2811, 2009

Objective.—To explore ethnic differences in do-not-resuscitate orders after intracerebral hemorrhage.

Design.—Population-based surveillance.

Setting.—Corpus Christi, Texas.

Patients.—All cases of intracerebral hemorrhage in the community of Corpus Christi, TX were ascertained as part of the Brain Attack Surveillance in Corpus Christi (BASIC) project.

Interventions.—None.

Measurements and Main Results.—Medical records were reviewed for do-not-resuscitate orders. Unadjusted and multivariable logistic regression were used to test for associations between ethnicity and do-not-resuscitate orders, both overall ("any do-not-resuscitate") and within 24 hrs of presentation ("early do-not-resuscitate"), adjusted for age, gender, Glasgow Coma Scale, intracerebral hemorrhage volume, intraventricular hemorrhage, infratentorial hemorrhage, modified Charlson Index, and admission from a nursing home. A total of 270 cases of intracerebral hemorrhage from 2000–2003 were analyzed. Mexican-Americans were younger and had a higher Glasgow Coma Scale than non-Hispanic whites. Mexican-Americans were half as likely as non-Hispanic whites to have early do-not-resuscitate orders in unadjusted analysis (odds ratio 0.45, 95% confidence interval 0.27, 0.75), although this association was not significant when adjusted for age (odds ratio 0.61, 95% confidence interval 0.35, 1.06) and in the fully adjusted model (odds ratio 0.75, 95% confidence interval 0.39, 1.46). Mexican-Americans were less likely than non-Hispanic whites to have do-not-resuscitate orders written at any time point (odds ratio 0.37, 95% confidence interval 0.23, 0.61). Adjustment for age alone attenuated this relationship although it retained significance (odds ratio 0.49, 95% confidence interval 0.29, 0.82). In the fully adjusted model, Mexican-Americans were less likely than non-Hispanic whites to use do-not-resuscitate orders at any time point, although the 95% confidence interval included one (odds ratio 0.52, 95% confidence interval 0.27, 1.00).

Conclusions.—Mexican-Americans were less likely than non-Hispanic whites to have do-not-resuscitate orders after intracerebral hemorrhage although the association was attenuated after adjustment for age and other confounders. The persistent trend toward less frequent use of do-not-resuscitate orders in Mexican-Americans suggests that further study is warranted.

▶ Ethnic differences in do-not-resuscitate (DNR) orders are known to exist, with most studies focusing on African-Americans and historically little data on Hispanics. With the United States Census Bureau projecting Hispanic-Americans to account for nearly one-quarter of the American population by 2050,[1] physicians will need to become more cognizant of Hispanic-American preferences for end-of-life care. Recent studies have focused on this issue and have shown that people of Hispanic ethnicity are against potentially life-shortening palliative drugs[2] and are one-third as likely as Caucasians to have DNR orders.[3] It is important to know these facts about Hispanic-Americans, as they are known to suffer the devastating event of an intracerebral hemorrhage (ICH) more frequently than non-Hispanic-Americans,[4] and their beliefs can dictate whether DNR orders, along with other palliative care measures, will be instituted.

This retrospective, population-based, surveillance study examined the issue of ethnic differences in end-of-life care by evaluating the differences in DNR orders among different ethnicities after an ICH. The study population involved 7 nonacademic medical centers in the community of Corpus Christi, Texas. It was found that Mexican-Americans were less likely than non-Hispanic whites to have DNR orders after an ICH. When adjusted for age, this association, while less strong, remained statistically significant. However, when adjusted with additional confounders, such as gender, admission from a nursing home, Glasgow Coma Scale, hemorrhage volume, and location of hemorrhage, the association became nonsignificant. This seems to indicate that ethnicity may not be the sole factor, but just one among many, that affects the decision to have DNR orders after a devastating medical event. Previous studies have tried to examine what influences DNR orders and found that patients with DNR orders were significantly older, had abnormal mental status, and were diagnosed with a malignancy, while being less likely to have had myocardial infarction, stroke, or chronic obstructive pulmonary disease when compared with patients in whom resuscitation was attempted.[5]

Limitations to this study included a small sample size and not having data on other potential confounders such as religion, education, and socioeconomic status. The participants were recruited from a single region in Texas, which may introduce a bias based on local sampling of Hispanic-Americans and hinder the ability for the study results to be generalized to other regions in the United States. Furthermore, the retrospective nature of the study prevented the acquisition of data from physicians and patient families on the attitudes toward DNR orders and reasons for not implementing them.

Prognosis in ICH is always complex, and families often need time to adjust to the tragedy that they are facing. By attempting to understand the contributing factors that go into making the decision on DNR orders, more appropriate information can be given to those who are required to make this decision. In turn, understanding the Hispanic-American culture and their beliefs on death and dying will aid physicians in their ability to provide culturally sensitive end-of-life care.

T. Cartwright, MD

S. N. Patel, MD

References

1. Day JC. *Population Projections of the United States by Age, Sex, Race, and Hispanic Origin: 1995 to 2050*. U.S. Bureau of the Census, Current Population Reports, p. 25–1130. Washington, DC: U.S. Government Printing Office; 1996. Table 1: Percent Distribution of the Population by Race and Hispanic Origin: 1990-2050. Pg 13.
2. Barnato AE, Anthony DL, Skinner J, Gallagher PM, Fisher ES. Racial and ethnic differences in preferences for end-of-life treatment. *J Gen Intern Med*. 2009;24: 695-701.
3. Degenholtz HB, Arnold RA, Meisel A, Lave JR. Persistence of racial disparities in advance care plan documents among nursing home residents. *J Am Geriatr Soc*. 2002;50:378-381.

4. Bruno A, Qualls C. Risk factors for intracerebral and subarachnoid hemorrhage among Hispanics and non-Hispanic whites in a New Mexico community. *Neuroepidemiology.* 2000;19:227-232.

5. Bedell SE, Pelle D, Maher PL, Cleary PD. Do-not-resuscitate orders for critically ill patients in the hospital. How are they used and what is their impact? *JAMA.* 1986; 256:233-237.

Expanding the paradigm of the physician's role in surrogate decision-making: An empirically derived framework

White DB, Malvar G, Karr J, et al (Univ of Pittsburgh Med Ctr, PA; Univ of California, San Francisco; et al)
Crit Care Med 38:743-750, 2010

Background.—Little is known about what role physicians take in the decision-making process about life support in intensive care units.

Objective.—To determine how responsibility is balanced between physicians and surrogates for life support decisions and to empirically develop a framework to describe different models of physician involvement.

Design.—Multi-centered study of audio-taped clinician–family conferences with a derivation and validation cohort.

Setting.—Intensive care units of four hospitals in Seattle, Washington, in 2000 to 2002 and two hospitals in San Francisco, California, in 2006 to 2008.

Participants.—Four hundred fourteen clinicians and 495 surrogates who were involved in 162 life support decisions.

Results.—In the derivation cohort (n = 63 decisions), no clinician inquired about surrogates' preferred role in decision-making. Physicians took one of four distinct roles: 1) informative role (7 of 63) in which the physician provided information about the patient's medical condition, prognosis, and treatment options but did not elicit information about the patient's values, engage in deliberations, or provide a recommendation about whether to continue life support; 2) facilitative role (23 of 63), in which the physician refrained from providing a recommendation but actively guided the surrogate through a process of clarifying the patients' values and applying those values to the decision; 3) collaborative role (32 of 63), in which the physician shared in deliberations with the family and provided a recommendation; and 4) directive role (1 of 63), in which the physician assumed all responsibility for, and informed the family of, the decision. In 10 out of 20 conferences in which surrogates requested a recommendation, the physician refused to provide one. The validation cohort revealed a similar frequency of use of the four roles, and frequent refusal by physicians to provide treatment recommendations.

Conclusions.—There is considerable variability in the roles physicians take in decision-making about life support with surrogates but little negotiation of desired roles. We present an empirically derived framework that provides a more comprehensive view of physicians' possible roles.

▶ While physicians are commonly perceived as lifesavers, the harsh reality of the world is that they will fall short of that goal. This truth especially holds true in the world of critical care medicine, where the intensely ill often succumb to their afflictions. This unfortunate familiarity with death has forced intensive care unit physicians to become the bearers of bad news on a regular basis; but given that their patients regularly are in such poor health that they cannot speak for themselves, the physicians have become additionally tasked with playing a role in the surrogate decision-making process. Precisely what that role entails, however, has never been clarified or even categorized. To further complicate this situation, such decisions are only loosely associated with medical facts and instead rely heavily on personal values. This study sought to determine exactly how physicians fulfill their portion of the surrogate decision process and perhaps create a model that can serve as a further tool in the training of future health care professionals.

As with any process that involves individual persons, physicians were found to have a variety of approaches to surrogate decision making, yet interestingly, none asked the surrogates how they wanted to proceed in the discussions. Physicians would self-select into 1 of 4 general categories: the directive, the collaborative, the facilitative, and the informative. While being polar opposites, the authoritative directive and the passive informative methods use little to no surrogate input, with the former having the physician simply dictating how things will proceed, and the latter simply having the physician stating the medical facts, leaving any decisions to the proxy. Frankly, the directive approach is an archaic nod to the age of paternalistic medicine and tends to be at odds with the Patient Self-Determination Act,[1] while the informative may be perceived as cold and sterile, a just-the-facts approach. The collaborative and facilitative methods are quite similar, save for the recommendations given in the collaborative route that are absent in the facilitative approach. Regardless of the differences between the latter 2, physicians interact with the surrogate to come to a hopefully amenable resolution. An important note to recall is that even within this study, physicians were witnessed to use at least two of the roles in daily practice, and it was not uncommon to use 2 in the same conversation dependent upon how the surrogates responded.

While being far from a definitive answer on how to approach and how to train physicians to approach the highly emotional surrogate decision-making discussion, this study gives a framework on which to build a more thorough system. Now, by no means should the recommendations of authors be taken as a checklist of how to approach such a value and ethically laden meeting, nor does it give ethical judgment on the 4 identified approaches. This study also overlooks the questionable accuracy of the decisions made by surrogates.[2] While not the end-all and be-all solution to surrogate decision making, the authors did help define a physician's role in the decision-making process. From this basis, physicians can be cognizant of their own personal approach and refine it accordingly; a solid foundation to any attempt to revise a system that was never formally installed.

B. J. Smith, BS

V. K. Rajput, MD

References

1. Patient Self-Determination Act of 1990. http://www.fha.org/acrobat/Patient%20 Self%20Determination%20Act%201990.pdf. Accessed November 29, 2010.
2. Shalowitz DI, Garrett-Mayer E, Wendler D. The accuracy of surrogate decision makers: a systemic review. *Arch Intern Med.* 2006;166:493-497.

Family satisfaction in the intensive care unit: what makes the difference?
Stricker KH, Kimberger O, Schmidlin K, et al (Bern Univ Hosp [Inselspital] and Univ of Bern, Switzerland; Med Univ of Vienna, Austria; Inst for Social and Preventive Medicine, Finkenhubelweg, Bern, Switzerland)
Intensive Care Med 35:2051-2059, 2009

Purpose.—To assess family satisfaction in the ICU and to identify parameters for improvement.

Methods.—Multicenter study in Swiss ICUs. Families were given a questionnaire covering overall satisfaction, satisfaction with care and satisfaction with information/decision-making. Demographic, medical and institutional data were gathered from patients, visitors and ICUs.

Results.—A total of 996 questionnaires from family members were analyzed. Individual questions were assessed, and summary measures (range 0–100) were calculated, with higher scores indicating greater satisfaction. Summary score was 78 ± 14 (mean ± SD) for overall satisfaction, 79 ± 14 for care and 77 ± 15 for information/decision-making. In multivariable multilevel linear regression analyses, higher severity of illness was associated with higher satisfaction, while a higher patient:nurse ratio and written admission/discharge criteria were associated with lower overall satisfaction. Using performance-importance plots, items with high impact on overall satisfaction but low satisfaction were identified. They included: emotional support, providing understandable, complete, consistent information and coordination of care.

Conclusions.—Overall, proxies were satisfied with care and with information/decision-making. Still, several factors, such as emotional support, coordination of care and communication, are associated with poor satisfaction, suggesting the need for improvement.

▶ The nature of the intensive care unit (ICU) creates a unique environment in medicine where the health care personnel often must perform their duties in front of not only the patient but also his/her loved ones. Given the recent movement to a focus on quality of life and quality of the dying process, hospitals have become aware of the importance of family satisfaction in the process of care. This is not unlike the business model of customer satisfaction. This emphasis on satisfaction is only magnified within the ICU, perhaps because of the critical nature of illness in the ICU and the increasing presence of family during the daily routine. This study served to measure determinants of family satisfaction and identify where changes can be made to improve satisfaction.

As with any complex equation, family satisfaction was found to be multifactorial, with the patient-to-nurse ratio, the presence of written admission/discharge criteria, and severity of acute illness being important factors. The severity of acute illness will obviously not change; however, the patient-to-nurse ratio and written criteria are parameters that could be altered to increase satisfaction. The latter can be done but should be in a general fashion only. The former is dictated by resources, and although it is natural for a family to want more nursing presence, the family wishes do not match the system capabilities. Perhaps counterintuitively, the severity of illness also fell into this realm, as more severe illnesses open the door to increased provider-family communication. While this study did reveal new aspects to family satisfaction, the overarching theme is that the increased communication between hospital personnel and the loved ones of the patients leads to greater perceptions of care quality. This knowledge is by no means new, with the influence of communication on satisfaction being documented as far back as 1968.[1]

With the mounting evidence that patient-provider communication is linked to health outcomes,[2] the further promotion of communication between patient and provider should certainly be encouraged. Patient satisfaction can be used as a crude tool to assess the effectiveness of that communication. Even with all the new technology present, especially in the ICU, successful medicine still starts from the face-to-face interaction between patient (or surrogate) and provider.

B. J. Smith, BS

V. K. Rajput, MD

References

1. Korsch BM, Gozzi EK, Francis V. Gaps in doctor-patient communication: 1. Doctor-patient interaction and patient satisfaction. *Pediatrics*. 1968;42:855-871.
2. Street RL Jr, Makoul G, Arora NK, Epstein RM. How does communication heal? Pathways linking clinician-patient communication to health outcomes. *Patient Educ Couns*. 2009;74:295-301.

Identification of Variables That Influence Brain-Dead Donors' Family Groups Regarding Refusal

Sotillo E, Montoya E, Martínez V, et al (Natl Transplantation Organization of Venezuela [NTOV], Caracas; et al)
Transplant Proc 41:3466-3470, 2009

Objective.—To identify the variables that influenced brain-dead donor family groups to refuse donation.

Methods.—The Tissue and Organ Procurement System in Venezuela designed a tool to register some phases of a family interview performed by transplant coordinators. This tool analyzed three phases. The first phase of the interview allowed the coordinator to evaluate the communication quality with the family group during a brain-death notification. The second phase assessed how families understood this notification, and the third phase identified the family grief sequence. Among the 186 interviews during 2007 to procure tissues and organs for transplantation, 37.63% ($n = 70$) concluded as family refusals. A retrospective study sought to analyze these results.

Results.—The average time between notification of brain death and the first approach to the family was 8.78 hours. Setting a place for interviews was done in 91.10% of cases. Previous knowledge about donation was seen in only 53.33% of cases. The main phase of family grief identified was denial (80%). The five reasons for family denial were: absolute denial, family disagreement, uncertainty about the destination of the donated organs and tissues, fear about deformation of the donor's body, and lack of acceptance of brain death.

Conclusions.—Brain-death notification produced a deep sadness among family groups. There was a lack of knowledge regarding donation of tissues and organs. It was impossible to quantify the time needed by families to understand and accept brain death and to identify the grief sequence in order to avoid family refusals.

▶ The economics of organ and tissue transplantation present a formidable challenge. Demand for transplants continues to outpace availability from deceased donors. Among the obstacles to increasing supply of donations is the refusal on the part of potential donors' family groups. The authors of this study represent groups interested in the identification of potential donors and procurement of viable organ and tissue donations. The study identified aspects of the interview process that may subvert attempts to obtain consent for donation from families. Complex psychological factors seem to play a major role in this subversion. For example, the sudden and unexpected nature of the insult contributes to families' unpreparedness or unwillingness to consider donation. This is understandable, as families who find themselves in a state of shock and disbelief often need time to understand the details surrounding the unexpected and tragic event, then somehow attempt to obtain reconciliation with this knowledge through grief. For those who grieve a sudden loss, the idea that they would be asked for the organs of their recently lost loved ones can be interpreted as an insult.

It may not be surprising, then, that one-third of family groups reported mistrust with respect to the way their relatives were treated by their health care providers, and they cited institutional resentment as a reason for their refusal to consent to donation. Half of the families were characterized as refusing because of a lack of knowledge of the meaning of brain death. These results suggest that improvements in trust and communication with health care providers may positively influence families' willingness to consent.

The sudden and unexpected circumstances surrounding many of the patients' injuries were a heavy influence on their unwillingness to accept the brain death. Finally, it is worth noting that nearly one-third of the families did not offer a reason for their refusal, which may again betray a lack of trust toward those performing the study. Several key parameters measured, like well-structured families and an interview environment that was adequate, lacked satisfactory elucidation. Increasing the precision of how these variables are defined in future studies may offer ideas for interventions and improvements in organ donation. These improvements would do well to focus on instilling and increasing affected families' understanding and feelings of trust in the process of donation. The confidence in deciding to donate is all too often threatened, as this study suggests, by the actions and attitudes of health care providers antecedent to the interview. If this suggestion is correct, then any lasting improvement to family consent rates must confront that issue as part of a comprehensive strategy. In particular, physicians cannot shirk their responsibility to inform the families of brain-dead patients in a timely, patient, and empathetic manner.

T. C. Foster, PhD

V. K. Rajput, MD

In their own words: Patients and families define high-quality palliative care in the intensive care unit

Nelson JE, Puntillo KA, Pronovost PJ, et al (Mount Sinai School of Medicine, NY; Univ of California, San Francisco; Johns Hopkins Univ School of Medicine, Baltimore, MD; et al)
Crit Care Med 38:808-818, 2010

Objective.—Although the majority of hospital deaths occur in the intensive care unit and virtually all critically ill patients and their families have palliative needs, we know little about how patients and families, the most important "stakeholders," define high-quality intensive care unit palliative care. We conducted this study to obtain their views on important domains of this care.

Design.—Qualitative study using focus groups facilitated by a single physician.

Setting.—A 20-bed general intensive care unit in a 382-bed community hospital in Oklahoma; 24-bed medical–surgical intensive care unit in a 377-bed tertiary, university hospital in urban California; and eight-bed medical intensive care unit in a 311-bed Veterans' Affairs hospital in a northeastern city.

Patients.—Randomly-selected patients with intensive care unit length of stay ≥5 days in 2007 to 2008 who survived the intensive care unit, families of survivors, and families of patients who died in the intensive care unit.

Interventions.—None.

Measurements and Main Results.—Focus group facilitator used open-ended questions and scripted probes from a written guide. Three investigators independently coded meeting transcripts, achieving consensus on themes. From 48 subjects (15 patients, 33 family members) in nine focus groups across three sites, a shared definition of high-quality intensive care unit palliative care emerged: timely, clear, and compassionate communication by clinicians; clinical decision-making focused on patients' preferences, goals, and values; patient care maintaining comfort, dignity, and personhood; and family care with open access and proximity to patients, interdisciplinary support in the intensive care unit, and bereavement care for families of patients who died. Participants also endorsed specific processes to operationalize the care they considered important.

Conclusions.—Efforts to improve intensive care unit palliative care quality should focus on domains and processes that are most valued by critically ill patients and their families, among whom we found broad agreement in a diverse sample. Measures of quality and effective interventions exist to improve care in domains that are important to intensive care unit patients and families.

▶ Most hospital deaths occur in the intensive care unit (ICU) in the United States.[1] Therefore, it has become important to provide the highest-quality palliative care to patients and their families in this setting. Before an institution can put into place guidelines to provide such care, an accurate definition of high-quality palliative care must be established. Defining high-quality palliative care in the intensive care setting, however, can be challenging. Professional-derived definitions do exist,[2,3] but patients and their families may differ in their thoughts and perceptions on what defines high-quality palliative care. Obtaining patients' and families' perspectives on high-quality palliative care is useful and critical in guiding future palliative care practices in the ICU.

This study makes use of facilitated group interviews with former ICU patients and family members of former patients. The facilitator began the interview with open-ended questions, asking patients to define high-quality care. Importantly, the facilitator did not initiate the use of the term palliative care, but rather the patient/family group chose to discuss the issue independently. After a period of open-ended questions, the facilitator then asked probe questions to assure that all necessary information was obtained. The data gathered from these interviews were compiled, coded, and reviewed by 3 independent investigators. The results revealed that patients and their families stressed the importance of 4 areas of ICU palliative care: (1) communication, (2) patient-focused decision making, (3) maintaining the patient's comfort, dignity, personhood, and privacy, and (4) care for the family.

The patients and their families felt that it is important for physicians to have an honest, open, consistent, and continuous discussion with both patients and families throughout the ICU stay. In this way, the families felt that the patients' dignity and personhood could be respected without compromising high quality of care. This study provides clinicians with a unified theory of the fundamental issues that patients and their families find crucial to high-quality palliative care in the ICU setting. Often, in high-stress ICU settings, complex family dynamics and complicated life-threatening illnesses make it difficult to discern what patients and families need and how to deliver this care. Through analysis of the responses from the group of ICU patients and families, we begin to see that common fundamental themes characterize patient and family desires. Patients and families want an open and honest communication, on a level that they can understand. Families want their loved ones to be the drivers of decisions and be respected as persons. Lastly, this study suggests that both patients and family members feel that families are important members in the entire process. In short, the group expressed the desire to feel involved and respected.

A. D. Fesnak, BS

V. K. Rajput, MD

References

1. Angus DC, Barnato AE, Linde-Zwirble WT, et al. Use of intensive care at the end of life in the United States: An epidemiologic study. *Crit Care Med.* 2004;32: 638-643.
2. National Consensus Project for Quality Palliative Care. Clinical Practice Guidelines for Quality Palliative Care. http://www.nationalconsensusproject.org. Accessed June 30, 2009.
3. Clarke EB, Curtis JR, Luce JM, et al. Quality indicators for end-of-life care in the intensive care unit. *Crit Care Med.* 2003;31:2255-2262.

Surviving critical illness: Acute respiratory distress syndrome as experienced by patients and their caregivers
Cox CE, Docherty SL, Brandon DH, et al (Duke Univ, Durham, NC; Duke Univ School of Nursing, Durham, NC; et al)
Crit Care Med 37:2702-2708, 2009

Objective.—To characterize the effects of critical illness in the daily lives and functioning of acute respiratory distress syndrome survivors. Survivors of acute respiratory distress syndrome, a systemic critical illness, often report poor quality of life based on responses to standardized questionnaires. However, the experiences of acute respiratory distress syndrome survivors have not been reported.

Design.—We conducted semistructured interviews with 23 acute respiratory distress syndrome survivors and 24 caregivers 3 to 9 mos after intensive care unit admission, stopping enrollment after thematic saturation was reached. Transcripts were analyzed, using Colaizzi's qualitative methodology, to identify significant ways in which survivors' critical illness experience impacted their lives.

Setting.—Medical and surgical intensive care units of an academic medical center and a community hospital.

Patients.—We recruited consecutively 31 acute respiratory distress syndrome survivors and their informal caregivers. Eight patients died before completing interviews.

Interventions.—None.

Measurements and Main Results.—Participants related five key elements of experience as survivors of acute respiratory distress syndrome: 1) pervasive memories of critical care; 2) day-to-day impact of new disability; 3) critical illness defining the sense of self; 4) relationship strain and change; and 5) ability to cope with disability. Survivors described remarkable disability that persisted for months. Caregivers' interviews revealed substantial strain from caregiving responsibilities as well as frequent symptom minimization by patients.

Conclusions.—The diverse and unique experiences of acute respiratory distress syndrome survivors reflect the global impact of severe critical illness. We have identified symptom domains important to acute respiratory distress syndrome patients who are not well represented in existing health outcomes measures. These insights may aid the development of targeted interventions to enhance recovery and return of function after acute respiratory distress syndrome.

▶ In many metrics of research, the patient's voice is missing. This study obtains the first-person perspective from critical care survivors and caregivers as to what life is like after acute respiratory distress syndrome (ARDS). The survivors commonly experience many posttraumatic stress disorder–like symptoms, such as vivid and terrifying memories of intubations, ventilators, and the inability to speak.

Once discharged, the patients report that their day-to-day life is yoked to their new physical and functional disabilities. The interviews are enlightening because of the immediacy in the patients' words. They feel profoundly weak and previous tasks seem insurmountable. Another study linked pulmonary function with quality of life posthospitalization.[1] Taken together, these studies suggest a close link between body function and future quality of life.

What can be done with this qualitative knowledge? It has been shown that social support is correlated with better quality of life after ARDS.[2] This highlights the need to ensure adequate support from family and staff during and after the intensive care unit stay. This study also points out that the impact of the disabilities extends to the family and caregivers. Therefore, information about what to expect and adequate support should be provided to both patients and their caregivers.

This research complements research done with quantitative questionnaires assessing patient well-being. While it may lack some of the generalizability of quantitative studies, the patients' own words can be more accurate and poignant than choosing a value between 1 and 10.

J. E. McGinnis, BS
V. K. Rajput, MD

References

1. Heyland DK, Groll D, Caeser M. Survivors of acute respiratory distress syndrome: relationship between pulmonary dysfunction and long-term health-related quality of life. *Crit Care Med.* 2005;33:1549-1556.
2. Deja M, Denke C, Weber-Carstens S, et al. Social support during intensive care unit stay might improve mental impairment and consequently health-related quality of life in survivors of severe acute respiratory distress syndrome. *Crit Care.* 2006;10:R147.

The role of doctors' religious faith and ethnicity in taking ethically controversial decisions during end-of-life care

Seale C (Queen Mary Univ of London, UK)
J Med Ethics 36:677-682, 2010

Background and Aims.—The prevalence of religious faith among doctors and its relationship with decision-making in end-of-life care is not well documented. The impact of ethnic differences on this is also poorly understood. This study compares ethnicity and religious faith in the medical and general UK populations, and reports on their associations with ethically controversial decisions taken when providing care to dying patients.

Method.—A postal survey of 3733 UK medical practitioners, of whom 2923 reported on the care of their last patient who died.

Findings.—Specialists in care of the elderly were somewhat more likely to be Hindu or Muslim than other doctors; palliative care specialists were somewhat more likely to be Christian, religious and 'white' than others. Ethnicity was largely unrelated to rates of reporting ethically controversial decisions. Independently of speciality, doctors who described themselves as nonreligious were more likely than others to report having given continuous deep sedation until death, having taken decisions they expected or partly intended to end life, and to have discussed these decisions with patients judged to have the capacity to participate in discussions. Speciality was independently related to wide variations in the reporting of decisions taken with some intent to end life, with doctors in 'other hospital' specialities being almost 10 times as likely to report this when compared with palliative medicine specialists, regardless of religious faith.

Conclusions.—Greater acknowledgement of the relationship of doctors' values with clinical decision-making is advocated.

▶ End-of-life care presents various legal, moral, and ethical challenges to physicians of all faiths and ethnicities. Differing cultural backgrounds often produce different perspectives on end-of-life care. These attitudes have been previously explored.[1] However, how these perspectives affect the decisions made by medical professionals is still poorly understood. The data gathered from this self-reported postal survey have shed some light on how faith and ethnicity affect medical practitioners' participation in end-of-life care.

The data obtained depict 2 populations of respondents. On the one hand, palliative care physicians and those who report strong religious faith are less likely to provide sedation until death, make decisions with an intent to hasten death, or discuss these decisions with patients. On the other hand, physicians who report no religious affiliation, those physicians who report being very or extremely nonreligious, or physicians in fields other than palliative care are more likely to provide continuous sedation until death, make decisions with some degree of intent to hasten death, discuss these decisions with patients and families, and support the legalization of assisted dying. Interestingly, while strength of religious faith and specialty are independently associated with these decisions, ethnicity is less correlative.

Physicians' attitudes toward end-of-life care are particularly meaningful when they impact actual decisions that those physicians make. These decisions themselves can even be inconsequential, so long as they are in line with the patient's desires. For instance, if a patient and a physician agree that continuous sedation should not be administered under any circumstances, then no conflict exists, and the illusion of patient autonomy is maintained. If however, the patient's feelings are at odds with his/her physician's, it is important to determine why these disconnections exist and if there is any action to be taken to rectify the situation. Certainly, ethnicity and faith inform most of a physician's perspective on health care in general. When the medical population's ethnic and faith demographics do not match with the patient population's ethnicity and faith, special care needs to be taken by the practitioner to respect and understand the patient's background. Regarding the controversial issue of end-of-life care, it is important for physicians to ensure that they do not impose their cultural values on the patient, while simultaneously acting ethically and upholding the Hippocratic oath.

A. D. Fesnak, BS

V. K. Rajput, MD

Reference

1. Pugh EJ, Song R, Whittaker V, Blenkinsopp J. A profile of the belief system and attitudes to end-of-life decisions of senior clinicians working in a National Health Service Hospital in the United Kingdom. *Palliat Med.* 2009;23:158-164.

Three-Year Outcomes for Medicare Beneficiaries Who Survive Intensive Care
Wunsch H, Guerra C, Barnato AE, et al (Columbia Univ, NY; Univ of Pittsburgh, PA; et al)
JAMA 303:849-856, 2010

Context.—Although hospital mortality has decreased over time in the United States for patients who receive intensive care, little is known about subsequent outcomes for those discharged alive.

Objective.—To assess 3-year outcomes for Medicare beneficiaries who survive intensive care.

Design, Setting, and Patients.—A matched, retrospective cohort study was conducted using a 5% sample of Medicare beneficiaries older than 65 years. A random half of all patients were selected who received intensive care and survived to hospital discharge in 2003 with 3-year follow-up through 2006. From the other half of the sample, 2 matched control groups were generated: hospitalized patients who survived to discharge (hospital controls) and the general population (general controls), individually matched on age, sex, race, and whether they had surgery (for hospital controls).

Main Outcome Measure.—Three-year mortality after hospital discharge.

Results.—There were 35 308 intensive care unit (ICU) patients who survived to hospital discharge. The ICU survivors had a higher 3-year mortality (39.5%; n = 13 950) than hospital controls (34.5%; n = 12 173) (adjusted hazard ratio [AHR], 1.07 [95% confidence interval {CI}, 1.04-1.10]; *P* < .001) and general controls (14.9%; n = 5266) (AHR, 2.39 [95% CI, 2.31-2.48]; *P* < .001). The ICU survivors who did not receive mechanical ventilation had minimal increased risk compared with hospital controls (3-year mortality, 38.3% [n = 12 716] vs 34.6% [n = 11 470], respectively; AHR, 1.04 [95% CI, 1.02-1.07]). Those receiving mechanical ventilation had substantially increased mortality (57.6% [1234 ICU survivors] vs 32.8%[703 hospital controls]; AHR, 1.56 [95%CI, 1.40-1.73]), with risk concentrated in the 6 months after the quarter of hospital discharge (6-month mortality, 30.1% (n = 645) for those receiving mechanical ventilation vs 9.6%(n = 206) for hospital controls; AHR, 2.26 [95% CI, 1.90-2.69]). Discharge to a skilled care facility for ICU survivors (33.0%; n = 11 634) and hospital controls (26.4%; n = 9328) also was associated with high 6-month mortality (24.1% for ICU survivors and hospital controls discharged to a skilled care facility vs 7.5% for ICU survivors and hospital controls discharged home; AHR, 2.62 [95% CI, 2.50-2.74]; *P* < .001 for ICU survivors and hospital controls combined).

Conclusions.—There is a large US population of elderly individuals who survived the ICU stay to hospital discharge but who have a high mortality over the subsequent years in excess of that seen in comparable controls. The risk is concentrated early after hospital discharge among those who require mechanical ventilation.

▶ Life expectancy as well as intensive care unit (ICU) survivors have been steadily increasing. These 2 factors have placed an increase in the number of patients occupying ICU beds and/or receiving ICU-level care outside of the traditional ICU. Institutions attempting to accommodate the increase in the critically ill have been expanding their ICUs to include more beds and create intermediate care units to help throughput. But are we placing our emphasis on survival to discharge or improving short-term survival with concern for future quality of life or resource use?

Wunsch and colleagues studied a 5% sample of Medicare beneficiaries. The study examined the 3-year outcomes and health care resource use of ICU survivors older than 65 years, identifying subgroups and periods in which patients were at the highest risk of death. The findings suggest that those patients older than 65 years who survived the ICU stay, received mechanical ventilation, and were discharged to a skilled care facility may be at higher risk of mortality compared with hospital and general controls. Do we need to consider a previous ICU admission in a patient older than 65 years as a potential risk factor for mortality, with an even higher risk if they were transferred to a skilled care facility and/or received mechanical ventilation?

The results of this study raise a few distressing social issues as the growing aged lack the social support to be discharged home, which may decrease one of the mortality risks. Addressing end-of-life care questions prior to a critical illness may also prove to be what the patient would have preferred.

As caregivers and consumers, we may need to rethink how the measure of quality of life does not necessarily equal survival to long-term 24-hour nursing care with an increased risk of rehospitalization. Returning to a time when families cared for their sick elders can offer comfort to the patients in addition to decreasing resource utilization and perhaps another hospital admission.

C. A. Schorr, RN, MSN

13 Pharmacology/ Sedation-Analgesia

A protocol of no sedation for critically ill patients receiving mechanical ventilation: a randomised trial
Strøm T, Martinussen T, Toft P (Odense Univ Hosp, Denmark; Univ of Southern, Denmark)
Lancet 375:475-480, 2010

Background.—Standard treatment of critically ill patients undergoing mechanical ventilation is continuous sedation. Daily interruption of sedation has a beneficial effect, and in the general intesive care unit of Odense University Hospital, Denmark, standard practice is a protocol of no sedation. We aimed to establish whether duration of mechanical ventilation could be reduced with a protocol of no sedation versus daily interruption of sedation.

Methods.—Of 428 patients assessed for eligibility, we enrolled 140 critically ill adult patients who were undergoing mechanical ventilation and were expected to need ventilation for more than 24 h. Patients were randomly assigned in a 1:1 ratio (unblinded) to receive: no sedation (n=70 patients); or sedation (20 mg/mL propofol for 48 h, 1 mg/mL midazolam thereafter) with daily interruption until awake (n=70, control group). Both groups were treated with bolus doses of morphine ($2 \cdot 5$ or 5 mg). The primary outcome was the number of days without mechanical ventilation in a 28-day period, and we also recorded the length of stay in the intensive care unit (from admission to 28 days) and in hospital (from admission to 90 days). Analysis was by intention to treat. This study is registered with ClinicalTrials.gov, number NCT00466492.

Findings.—27 patients died or were successfully extubated within 48 h, and, as per our study design, were excluded from the study and statistical analysis. Patients receiving no sedation had significantly more days without ventilation (n=55; mean $13 \cdot 8$ days, SD $11 \cdot 0$) than did those receiving interrupted sedation (n=58; mean $9 \cdot 6$ days, SD $10 \cdot 0$; mean difference $4 \cdot 2$ days, 95% CI $0 \cdot 3$–$8 \cdot 1$; p=$0 \cdot 0191$). No sedation was also associated with a shorter stay in the intensive care unit (HR $1 \cdot 86$, 95% CI $1 \cdot 05$–$3 \cdot 23$; p=$0 \cdot 0316$), and, for the first 30 days studied, in hospital ($3 \cdot 57$, $1 \cdot 52$–$9 \cdot 09$; p=$0 \cdot 0039$), than was interrupted sedation. No difference was recorded in the occurrences of accidental extubations, the need for CT or MRI brain scans, or ventilator-associated pneumonia.

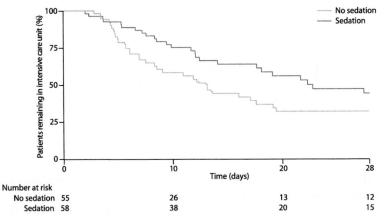

FIGURE 2.—Kaplan-Meier plot of length of stay in the intensive care unit and number at risk from admission to 28 days. (Reprinted from Strøm T, Martinussen T, Toft P. A protocol of no sedation for critically ill patients receiving mechanical ventilation: a randomised trial. *Lancet.* 2010;375:475-480, with permission from Elsevier.)

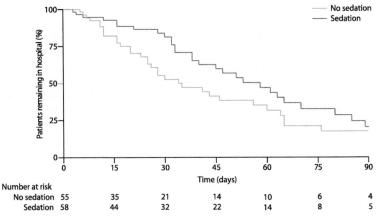

FIGURE 3.—Kaplan-Meier plot of length of stay in hospital and number at risk from admission to 90 days. (Reprinted from Strøm T, Martinussen T, Toft P. A protocol of no sedation for critically ill patients receiving mechanical ventilation: a randomised trial. *Lancet.* 2010;375:475-480, with permission from Elsevier.)

Agitated delirium was more frequent in the intervention group than in the control group (n=11, 20% *vs* n=4, 7%; p=0·0400).

Interpretation.—No sedation of critically ill patients receiving mechanical ventilation is associated with an increase in days without ventilation. A multicentre study is needed to establish whether this effect can be reproduced in other facilities.

▶ Sedation use in critically ill patients had been growing until studies began to show a benefit of a daily sedation holiday in appropriate patients. This study takes that concept one step further and evaluates no sedation as an alternative.

TABLE 2.—Outcome Data

	No Sedation (n=55)	Sedation (n=58)	p value
Days without mechanical ventilation (from intubation to day 28)	13·8 (11·0); 18·0 (0–24·1)	9·6 (10·0); 6·9 (0–20·5)	0·0191*†
Length of stay (days)			
Intensive care unit	13·1 (5·7–··)‡	22·8 (11·7–··)‡	0·0316*§
Hospital	34 (17–65)	58 (33–85)	0·0039*§¶
Mortality			
Intensive care unit	12 (22%)	22 (38%)	0·06
Hospital	20 (36%)	27 (47%)	0·27
Drug doses (mg/kg)‖			
Propofol (per h of infusion)**	0 (0–0·515)	0·773 (0·154–1·648)	0·0001
Midazolam (per h of infusion)	0 (0–0)	0·0034 (0–0·0240)	<0·0001
Morphine (per h of mechanical ventilation)	0·0048 (0·0014–0·0111)	0·0045 (0·0020–0·0064)	0·39
Haloperidol (per day of mechanical ventilation)	0 (0–0·0145)	0 (0–0)	0·0140
Tracheostomy	16 (29%)	17 (29%)	0·98
Ventilator-associated pneumonia	6 (11%)	7 (12%)	0·85

Data are mean (SD), median (IQR), or number (%). ··=data not available because of censoring at day 28.
*Corrected for baseline variables: age, sex, weight, acute physiology and chronic health evaluation (APACHE II), simplified acute physiology score (SAPS II), and sequential organ-failure assessment (SOFA) at day 1.
†Calculated from multiple linear regression.
‡More than 25% of patients remained in the intensive care unit for more than 28 days (figure 2).
§Calculated from Cox regression analysis.
¶Calculated for the first 30 days to agree with the proportional hazards assumption.
‖Drug dose (mg) as a proportion of bodyweight (kg).
**Maximum dose during 48 h of treatment.

As can be seen in Table 2, this approach was associated with fewer days of mechanical ventilation and a shorter length of stay (LOS) but did not translate into a reduction in mortality. Figures 2 and 3 not only show the shortened LOS but also show that the differences in LOS started after about 5 days for intensive care unit (ICU) LOS and after about 10 days for hospital LOS. This is as one might expect, as the cumulative effect of a sedative approach is more likely to impact LOS. Importantly, this study only evaluated patients out to 24 days, and a longer evaluation is important as a full assessment on recovery is also warranted. These gains were attained at the cost of a higher rate of delirium and a need for increased resources to manage unsedated patients. Given these negative findings and the fact that posttraumatic stress disorder for the patients and their families was not assessed, most would agree that a wholesale adoption of this approach is not warranted at this time. In addition, there was an almost 20% failure rate of this approach. This study does, however, provide additional strong evidence that minimizing sedation can be done and will likely be beneficial.

T. Dorman, MD

Use of intravenous infusion sedation among mechanically ventilated patients in the United States

Wunsch H, Kahn JM, Kramer AA, et al (Columbia Univ, NY; Univ of Pennsylvania School of Medicine, Philadelphia; Cerner Corporation, Vienna, VA; et al)
Crit Care Med 37:3031-3039, 2009

Objective.—Many studies compare the efficacy of different forms of intravenous infusion sedation for critically ill patients, but little is known about the actual use of these medications. We sought to describe current use of intravenous infusion sedation in mechanically ventilated patients in U.S. intensive care units.

Design.—Retrospective cohort study of intravenous infusion sedation among mechanically ventilated patients. Intravenous sedatives examined included benzodiazepines (midazolam and lorazepam), propofol, and dexmedetomidine. Use was defined as having received an intravenous infusion for any time period during the stay in intensive care.

Setting.—One hundred seventy-four intensive care units contributing data to Project IMPACT from 2001 through 2007.

Patients.—All patients who received mechanical ventilation.

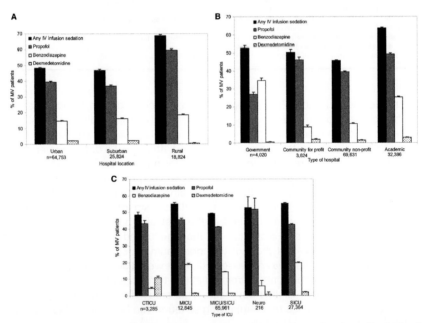

FIGURE 3.—Hospital and intensive care unit (*ICU*) level characteristics of mechanically ventilated (*MV*) patients who received intravenous (*IV*) infusion sedation. *A*, Use of IV infusion sedation by hospital location. *B*, Use of IV infusion sedation by type of hospital. *C*, Use of IV infusion sedation by type of ICU. *CTICU*, cardiothoracic ICU; *MICU*, medical ICU; *SICU*, surgical ICU; *Neuro*, neurological. (Courtesy of Wunsch H, Kahn JM, Kramer AA, et al. Use of intravenous infusion sedation among mechanically ventilated patients in the United States. *Crit Care Med.* 2009;37:3031-3039.)

TABLE 3.—Factors Associated with Receiving Intravenous (IV) Infusion Sedation in Mechanically Ventilated Patients[a]

Variable	OR	(95% CI)	p
Patient characteristics			
Gender (female)	0.80	(0.77–0.81)	<.001
Age	0.91[b]	(0.90–0.92)	<.001
Admission type			<.001
Elective	1.00	—	—
Emergent	1.10	(1.05–1.16)	<.001
Medical	1.14	(1.03–1.20)	.005
Cardiopulmonary resuscitation in 24 hrs before admission	0.76	(0.70–0.81)	<.001
MPM_0–III mortality probability[b]	0.89[c]	(0.88–0.90)	<.001
Log of total length of MV	1.63	(1.62–1.65)	<.001
Location before ICU admission			.07
Hospital ward	1.00	—	—
Emergency department	0.99	(0.94–1.05)	.78
Operating room	0.95	(0.87–1.03)	.17
Other	0.94	(0.89–1.00)	.04
Chronic comorbidity	0.82	(0.79–0.84)	<.001
Mechanical ventilation on admission	0.85	(0.82–0.89)	<.001
Diagnostic category			<.001
Respiratory	1.00	—	—
Cardiovascular	0.95	(0.90–0.99)	<.03
Gastrointestinal	0.85	(0.80–0.90)	<.001
Neurologic	0.76	(0.72–0.80)	<.001
Renal/metabolic	0.78	(0.69–0.87)	<.001
Other	0.77	(0.74–0.81)	<.001
Admission year			<.001
2001	1.00	—	—
2002	1.21	(1.13–1.29)	<.001
2003	1.42	(1.34–1.52)	<.001
2004	1.71	(1.61–1.83)	<.001
2005	2.01	(1.89–2.14)	<.001
2006	2.50	(2.34–2.66)	<.001
2007	2.78	(2.57–3.00)	<.001
Hospital and ICU characteristics			
Hospital location			
Rural	1.00	—	—
Suburban	0.36	(0.34–0.38)	<.001
Urban	0.24	(0.22–0.25)	<.001
Hospital region			
New England	1.00	—	—
Central	0.80	(0.76–0.85)	<.001
Mid-Atlantic	1.30	(1.21–1.38)	<.001
Mountain	1.05	(0.96–1.15)	.30
South Atlantic	0.76	(0.72–0.81)	<.001
West	2.01	(1.84–2.20)	<.001
Hospital licensed beds			<.001
≤300	1.00	—	—
301–450	1.06	(0.99–1.12)	.08
451–800	0.67	(0.63–0.70)	<.001
>800	1.16	(1.08–1.24)	<.001
Hospital type			<.001
Government	1.00	—	—
Academic	1.66	(1.52–1.82)	<.001
Community	1.09	(1.00–1.19)	.05
ICU type			<.001
Surgical	1.00	—	—
Cardiothoracic	2.11	(1.64–2.71)	<.001
Medical	1.09	(1.03–1.16)	.004

(Continued)

TABLE 3. (*continued*)

Variable	OR	(95% CI)	*p*
Mixed medical/surgical	0.72	(0.69–0.75)	<.001
Neurologic	1.81	(1.34–2.45)	<.001
Intensivist physician staffing			<.001
Mandatory CC coverage	1.00	—	—
Discretionary CC coverage	0.75	(0.72–0.78)	<.001
No CC coverage	0.60	(0.49–0.74)	<.001

OR, odds ratio; CI, confidence interval; MPM, Mortality Probability Model; MV, mechanical ventilation; ICU, intensive care unit; CC, intensivist.

[a]Race was included in the model, despite the fact that it was not associated with receiving IV infusion sedation in univariable analysis;

[b]the odds ratio for each 5-yr increase in age. The observed number of patients receiving any sedation was 47,738 while 47,506 patients were predicted to be sedated (ratio = 1.005, $p > .10$). Calibration as measured by the Hosmer–Lemeshow statistic was 12.8 ($p = .12$) and by the Brier statistic was 0.19. Both measures suggest that the model calibrated well. The area under the receiver operating characteristic curve was 0.78, indicating moderately good discrimination;

[c]the odds ratio for each 10% increase in MPM0-III probability.

Interventions.—None.

Measurements and Main Results.—Of 109,671 mechanically ventilated patients, 56,443 (51.5%, 95% confidence interval 51.2–51.8) received one or more intravenous infusion sedatives. Sedative use increased over time, from 39.7% (38.7–40.6) of patients in 2001 to 66.7% (65.7–67.7) in 2007 ($p < .001$). Most patients who received intravenous infusion sedation received propofol (82.2%, 81.9–82.5) vs. benzodiazepines (31.1%, 30.7–31.5) or dexmedetomidine (4.0%, 3.8–4.2). Of the patients, 66.2% (65.8–66.6) received only propofol, and 16.2% (15.9–16.5) only benzodiazepines. Among patients mechanically ventilated >96 hrs, propofol infusions were more common. Intravenous infusion narcotics (fentanyl, morphine, or hydromorphone) were used more frequently among patients who received benzodiazepines (70.1%, 69.1–71.0) compared with propofol (23.9%, 23.5–24.3), $p < .001$.

Conclusions.—The percentage of mechanically ventilated patients receiving intravenous infusion sedation has increased over time. Sedation with an infusion of propofol was much more common than with benzodiazepines or dexmedetomidine, even for patients mechanically ventilated beyond 96 hrs.

▶ Understanding the trend in use of sedation is important, as the world of critical care has become more aware of the benefits of minimizing such medication. Table 3 demonstrates that there was a trend toward greater use over time and not lower use. These authors also found a greater use of porpofol for time frames even greater than the generally recommended maximum of 48 hours. These findings taken individually and together are concerning. Severity of illness data across these time frames might be elucidating. At the top of Fig 3 one can see the prolonged use of propofol as well as see that there are differences in type of ICU. This raises the question as to the inclusion of anesthesiologists as intensivists in these units as one might hypothesize that this type of intensivist may have a different approach to the use of these medications that they use daily in the operating room. Fig 3 also shows an increased use in rural settings, a finding that needs further investigation and one that is worrisome.

T. Dorman, MD

Aminoglycoside clearance is a good estimate of creatinine clearance in intensive care unit patients
Jones TE, Peter JV, Field J (The Queen Elizabeth Hosp, Woodville South, Australia)
Anaesth Intensive Care 37:944-952, 2009

The aim of this study was to determine whether creatinine clearance can be estimated as well by clearance of gentamicin/tobramycin as by routine, non-invasive estimates in the intensive care unit.

The volume of distribution and clearance values for gentamicin/tobramycin were obtained using first order kinetics and an estimate of creatinine clearance derived. Seven estimates of renal function (Cockroft-Gault, MDRD4 and MDRD6 equations, two- and 24-hour urine estimates, two equations utilising Cystatin C concentrations) were compared to the gentamicin/tobramycin clearance estimate in 100 intensive care unit patients.

The gentamicin clearance estimate was at least as reliable as other estimates. The two-hour was less reliable than the 24-hour urine estimate. The Cockroft-Gault appeared to out-perform the MDRD equation estimates. The MDRD4 was not as reliable as the MDRD6 estimate. Cystatin C estimates appeared not as reliable as the gentamicin estimate of renal function.

The gentamicin/tobramycin estimate is at least as good as other estimates and it is available sooner than most others. It should be used in all patients who are prescribed gentamicin. The two-hour urine and MDRD4 estimates should not be used in the intensive care unit.

▶ This study adds to the body of literature that demonstrates aminoglycoside clearance is highly correlated with creatinine clearance in critically ill patients (Fig 1). This is clinically useful information if one uses kinetic dosing models for aminoglycosides, as it permits one to adjust other medications that are renally eliminated earlier so that changes in creatinine may be noted. Unfortunately, the study is not a randomized trial, and thus confounders may be present and unaccounted for. It is quite surprising given the body of literature on the significant increase in the volume of distribution seen during critical illness and injury that these authors were surprised to find elevations in this variable that were consistent with previous reports. The article does not fully explain the methodology used for the 2- and 24-hour urine collections, and thus

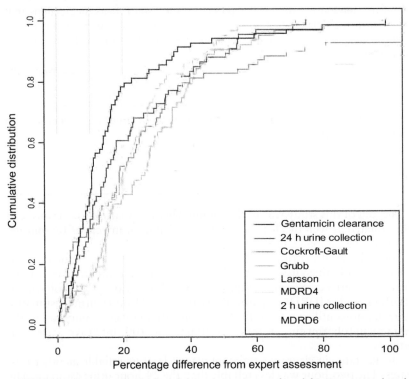

FIGURE 1.—Cumulative distribution of the various estimates of renal function compared to the 'expert assessment' value of renal function. Important clinical set points of 10%, 20% and 50% are shown on the vertical lines. Colour version available on the website. (Reprinted from Jones TE, Peter JV, Field J. Aminoglycoside clearance is a good estimate of creatinine clearance in intensive care unit patients. *Anaesth Intensive Care.* 2009;37:944-952, with permission of the Australian Society of Anaesthetists.)

some of the variability noted in these parameters may be related to the methods of collection.

T. Dorman, MD

Efficacy and safety of quetiapine in critically ill patients with delirium: A prospective, multicenter, randomized, double-blind, placebo-controlled pilot study

Devlin JW, Roberts RJ, Fong JJ, et al (Northeastern Univ School of Pharmacy, Boston, MA; Massachusetts College of Pharmacy, Worcestor; et al)
Crit Care Med 38:419-427, 2010

Objective.—To compare the efficacy and safety of scheduled quetiapine to placebo for the treatment of delirium in critically ill patients requiring as-needed haloperidol.

Design.—Prospective, randomized, double-blind, placebo-controlled study.

Setting.—Three academic medical centers.

Patients.—Thirty-six adult intensive care unit patients with delirium (Intensive Care Delirium Screening Checklist score ≥4), tolerating enteral nutrition, and without a complicating neurologic condition.

Interventions.—Patients were randomized to receive quetiapine 50 mg every 12 hrs or placebo. Quetiapine was increased every 24 hrs (50 to 100 to 150 to 200 mg every 12 hrs) if more than one dose of haloperidol was given in the previous 24 hrs. Study drug was continued until the intensive care unit team discontinued it because of delirium resolution, therapy ≥10 days, or intensive care unit discharge.

Measurements and Main Results.—Baseline characteristics were similar between the quetiapine (n = 18) and placebo (n = 18) groups. Quetiapine was associated with a shorter time to first resolution of delirium [1.0 (interquartile range [IQR], 0.5–3.0) vs. 4.5 days (IQR, 2.0–7.0; $p = .001$)], a reduced duration of delirium [36 (IQR, 12–87) vs. 120 hrs (IQR, 60–195; $p = .006$)], and less agitation (Sedation-Agitation Scale score ≥5) [6 (IQR, 0–38) vs. 36 hrs (IQR, 11–66; $p = .02$)]. Whereas mortality (11% quetiapine vs. 17%) and intensive care unit length of stay (16 quetiapine vs. 16 days) were similar, subjects treated with quetiapine were more likely to be discharged home or to rehabilitation (89% quetiapine vs. 56%; $p = .06$). Subjects treated with quetiapine required fewer days of as-needed haloperidol [3 [(IQR, 2–4)] vs. 4 days (IQR, 3–8; $p = .05$)]. Whereas the incidence of QTc prolongation and extrapyramidal symptoms was similar between groups, more somnolence was observed with quetiapine (22% vs. 11%; $p = .66$).

Conclusions.—Quetiapine added to as-needed haloperidol results in faster delirium resolution, less agitation, and a greater rate of transfer to home or rehabilitation. Future studies should evaluate the effect of quetiapine on mortality, resource utilization, post-intensive care unit cognition, and dependency after discharge in a broader group of patients (Fig 2, Table 6).

▶ Delirium is an important consideration in critically ill patients, and there is a growing body of data that demonstrates its association with worse outcomes. This study looks at the preemptive administration of quetiapine to see whether the incidence of delirium can be reduced. Fig 2 shows the efficacy seen in reducing the proportion of patients who were diagnosed with delirium during the study. However, this was accomplished with trends toward much higher rates of sedation. The scale used was not the most commonly used scale, CAM-ICU, and so the impact of a different scale on both the efficacy and safety of such an approach is unclear. This study is also quite small, but given the possible benefits from lower rates of delirium, a large trial is justifiable. Quetiapine is commonly used in rehabilitation facilities for sleep. Thus, it is an attractive agent for critically ill patients who need adequate restorative sleep. If such utilization was associated with lower rates of delirium at an acceptable safety

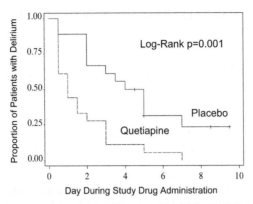

FIGURE 2.—Proportion of patients with first resolution of delirium over time between quetiapine (n = 18) and placebo (n = 18) groups. Both groups of patients were treated using the same as-needed intravenous haloperidol protocol. (Courtesy of Devlin JW, Roberts RJ, Fong JJ, et al. Efficacy and safety of quetiapine in critically ill patients with delirium: a prospective, multicenter, randomized, double-blind, placebo-controlled pilot study. *Crit Care Med*. 2010;38:419-427.)

TABLE 6.—Safety Outcomes During Study Drug Administration[a]

	Quetiapine (n = 18)	Placebo (n = 18)	p
Adverse events[b]	54	69	.29
Study drug-related adverse events[c]	6	2	.39
Subjects who experienced a study drug-related adverse event, %[d]	28	11	.4
Episodes of somnolence	5	2	.56
Subjects experiencing somnolence, %[d]	22	11	.66
Episodes of hypotension	1	0	.79
Subjects experiencing hypotension, %[d]	6	0	1.0
Episodes of EPS	0	0	1.0
Serious study drug-related adverse events[e]	0	0	1.0
Episodes of QTc interval >60 msec above baseline	20	34	.7
Subjects experiencing QTc interval >60 msec above baseline, %[f]	39	44	1.0
Episodes of QTc interval prolongation[g]	30	41	.32
Subjects experiencing QTc prolongation, %[f,g]	50	72	.31
Episodes of QTc interval >500 msec	8	8	1.0
Subjects experiencing QTc interval >500 msec, %[d,f]	22	28	1.0

[a] p values calculated using a Yates-corrected chi-square test when percentages are presented, unless noted otherwise.
[b] all adverse events experienced by subjects during period of study drug administration.
[c] all adverse events possibly or probably related to the study drug.
[d] p value calculated using Fisher's exact test.
[e] all adverse events possibly or probably related to the study drug deemed to be serious and reportable as per FDA MED-WATCH criteria.
[f] subjects experiencing ≥1 episode of QTc prolongation are included only once regardless of the number of episodes of QTc prolongation experienced.
[g] QTc interval prolongation was defined as >450 msec for males and >470 msec for females.

profile, then this would be a welcome addition to our management of these patients. Given its sedative effects, one must wonder whether future studies should restrict its use to bedtime.

T. Dorman, MD

Article Index

Chapter 1: Airways/Lungs

Chapter 2: Cardiovascular

Chapter 3: Hemodynamics and Monitoring

Chapter 4: Burns

Chapter 5: Infectious Disease

Chapter 6: Postoperative Management

Chapter 7: Sepsis/Septic Shock

Chapter 8: Metabolism/Gastrointestinal/Nutrition/Hematology-Oncology

Chapter 9: Renal

Chapter 10: Trauma and Overdose

Chapter 11: Neurologic: Traumatic and Non-traumatic

Chapter 12: Ethics/Socioeconomic/Administrative Issues

Chapter 13: Pharmacology/Sedation-Analgesia

Author Index

Printed and bound by CPI Group (UK) Ltd, Croydon, CR0 4YY

08/05/2025

01864677-0008